The Molecular Aspects of Autoimmunity

Academic Press Rapid Manuscript Reproduction

The Molecular Aspects of Autoimmunity

Edited by

Nadir R. Farid

Division of Endocrinology and Metabolism
Faculty of Medicine
Memorial University of Newfoundland
St. John's, Newfoundland, Canada

Constantin A. Bona

Department of Microbiology
Mount Sinai School of Medicine
New York, New York

ACADEMIC PRESS, INC.

Harcourt Brace Jovanovich, Publishers

San Diego New York Berkeley Boston
London Sydney Tokyo Toronto

This book is printed on acid-free paper. ♾

Academic Press, Inc.
San Diego, California 92101

United Kingdom Edition published by
Academic Press Limited
24–28 Oval Road, London NW1 7DX

Library of Congress Cataloging-in-Publication Data

The Molecular aspects of autoimmunity / edited by Nadir R. Farid, Constantin A. Bona.
p. cm.
Contains a selection of papers presented at the first of a series of biannual meetings on molecular aspects of autoimmunity held in L'Esterel, Quebec, Canada from Oct. 30 through Nov. 2, 1988.
ISBN 0-12-249040-1 (alk. paper)
1. Autoimmunity--Molecular aspects--Congresses. 2. Autoantibodies--Congresses. 3. Autoimmune diseases--Pathogenesis--Congresses. I. Farid, Nadir R. II. Bona, Constantin A.
[DNLM: 1. Autoantibodies--immunology--congresses. 2. Autoimmune Diseases--immunology--congresses. 3. Immunity, Cellular--congresses. WD 305 M718 1988]
QR188.3.M65 1990
616.97'8--dc20
DNLM/DLC
for Library of Congress 89-18223
CIP

Printed in the United States of America
90 91 92 93 9 8 7 6 5 4 3 2 1

CONTENTS

Contributors *vii*
Preface *xi*

The Expression of LY-1 and Immunoglobulin Variable Gene Families in Hybridomas Producing Autoantibodies of Various Specificities 1
Raoul Mayer, Habib Zagouani, Azad Kaushik, Kuppuswamy Kasturi, Vincenzo Fidanza, and Constantin Bona

Structural Characteristics of Human IgM Autoantibodies 29
Fernando R. Goñi, Pojen P. Chen, and Blas Frangione

Molecular Genetics of Human Autoantibodies 41
Pojen P. Chen

Molecular Characterization of Human Anti-DNA Antibodies 59
Katherine A. Siminovitch

From Idiotypic Expression of Lupus Anti-DNA Antibodies to Diversification of Ig Variable Region Genes 73
Moncef Zouali

Murine Autoantibodies Specific for Bromelinized Red Blood Cells Use Restricted Set of Genetic Elements and Their Heavy Chains Define a Novel VH Family 91
Jean-Claude Jaton and Luc Reininger

Molecular Analysis of Murine Lupus-Associated Humoral Anti-Self Response 107
Reinhard Kofler, Frank J. Dixon, and Argyrios N. Theofilopoulos

Establishment of V-Gene Repertoires in Normal Mice 125
Dan Holmberg and Antonia Freitas

Characterization of a Regulatory Idiotope by Antibody Engineering 129
Maurizio Sollazzo, Daniele Castiglia, Rosario Billetta, and Maurizio Zanetti

Epibodies in the Immune Response to the Acetylcholine Receptor 139
Donard S. Dwyer and Joachim Bartels

Interspecies Idiotypes on Anti-Sm Antibodies 155
Howard Dang, Masami Takei, and Norman Talal

Specificities and Idiotypy of Anti-Histone H1 Autoantibodies 161
Marc Monestier and Thomas M. Fasy

Experimental Models of T Cell Tolerance 175
Lorise C. Gahring and William O. Weigle

Genomic and Expressed T Cell Antigen Receptor Repertoire in Autoimmune Murine Models 189
Argyrios N. Theofilopoulos and Paul A. Singer

Structure of the Human Interleukin 2 Receptor and the Biochemical Basis for Its Regulation 219
Dean W. Ballard, Marion R. Fung, Ernst Böhnlein, and Warner C. Greene

Viruses as a Triggering Factor of Autoimmune Type I Diabetes 231
Ji-Won Yoon, Sung-Hee Ihm, and Robert G. McArthur

Mapping Susceptibility to Rheumatoid Arthritis into a Conformationally Equivalent Region of MHC Class II Molecules Encoded by Different Alleles 241
Robert Winchester

In Vitro Model Systems for the Study of Thyroid Autoimmunity: Regulation of Rat MHC Class II Antigens 265
T. F. Davies, W. Hirose, and D. S. Nuefeld

The Molecular Basis of MHC Association with Disease 277
Nadir R. Farid

Basic Role for Anti-Idiotype Autoantibodies in the Prevention of Experimental Autoimmune Thyroiditis 289
C. Bédin, C. Roubaty, B. Texier, H. Tang, M. A. Franco, and J. Charreire

Index 299

CONTRIBUTORS

Numbers in parentheses indicate the pages on which the authors' contributions begin.

C. Bédin (289), INSERM U. 283, Hôpital Cochin, 75674 Paris Cedex 14, France

Dean W. Ballard (219), Howard Hughes Medical Institute, Departments of Medicine and Microbiology/Immunology, Duke University Medical Center, Durham, North Carolina 27710

Joachim Bartels (139), Neuropsychiatry Research Program, University of Alabama at Birmingham, Birmingham, Alabama 35294

Rosario Billetta (129), Department of Medicine, University of California, San Diego, San Diego, California 92103

Ernst Böhnlein (219), Howard Hughes Medical Institute, Departments of Medicine and Microbiology/Immunology, Duke University Medical Center, Durham, North Carolina 27710

Constantin Bona (1), Department of Microbiology, Mount Sinai School of Medicine, New York, New York 10029

Daniele Castiglia (129), Department of Medicine, University of California, San Diego, San Diego, California 92103

J. Charreire (289), INSERM U. 283, Hôpital Cochin, 75674 Paris Cedex 14, France

Pojen P. Chen (29, 41), Department of Molecular and Experimental Medicine, Scripps Clinic and Research Foundation, La Jolla, California 92037

Howard Dang (155), Clinical Immunology Section, Audie L. Murphy Memorial Veterans Hospital, and the Department of Medicine, The University of Texas Health Sciences Center, San Antonio, Texas 78284-7874

T. F. Davies (265), Division of Endocrinology, Department of Medicine, Mount Sinai School of Medicine, New York, New York 10029

Frank J. Dixon (107), Department of Immunology, Research Institute of Scripps Clinic, La Jolla, California 92037

Donard S. Dwyer (139), Neuropsychiatry Research Program, University of Alabama at Birmingham, Birmingham, Alabama 35294

Nadir R. Farid (277), Thyroid Research Laboratory, Health Sciences Centre, Memorial University of Newfoundland, St. John's, Newfoundland, A1B 3V6, Canada

Thomas M. Fasy (161), Department of Pathology, Mount Sinai School of Medicine of the City University of New York, New York, New York 10029

Vincenzo Fidanza (1), Department of Microbiology, Mount Sinai School of Medicine, New York, New York 10029

M. A. Franco (289), INSERM U. 283, Hôpital Cochin, 75674 Paris Cedex 14, France

Blas Frangione (29), Department of Pathology, New York University Medical Center, New York, New York 10016

Antonia Freitas (125), Unité d'Immunobiologie, Départment d'Immunologie, Institut Pasteur, Paris Cedex 15, France

Marion R. Fung (219), Howard Hughes Medical Institute, Departments of Medicine and Microbiology/Immunology, Duke University Medical Center, Durham, North Carolina 27710

Lorise C. Gahring (175), Department of Immunology, Research Institute of Scripps Clinic, La Jolla, California 92037

Fernando R. Goñi[1] (29), Department of Pathology, New York University Medical Center, New York, New York 10016

Warner C. Greene (219), Howard Hughes Medical Institute, Departments of Medicine and Microbiology/Immunology, Duke University Medical Center, Durham, North Carolina 27710

W. Hirose (265), Division of Endocrinology, Department of Medicine, Mount Sinai School of Medicine, New York, New York 10029

Dan Holmberg (125), Unit of Applied Cell and Molecular Biology, University of Umeå, Umeå, Sweden

Sung-Hee Ihm (231), Division of Virology, Department of Microbiology and Infectious Diseases, and Laboratory of Viral and Immunopathogenesis of Diabetes, Julia McFarlane Diabetes Research Centre, The University of Calgary, Calgary, Alberta, Canada T2N 4N1

Jean-Claude Jaton (91), Department of Medical Biochemistry, Medical Center of the University of Geneva, CH-1211 Geneva 4, Switzerland

Kuppuswamy Kasturi (1), Department of Microbiology, Mount Sinai School of Medicine, New York, New York 10029

Azad Kaushik (1), Department of Microbiology, Mount Sinai School of Medicine, New York, New York 10029

Reinhard Kofler (107), Institute for General and Experimental Pathology, University of Innsbruck, Medical School, Innsbruck, Austria, and Department of Immunology, Research Institute of Scripps Clinic, La Jolla, California 92037

Raoul Mayer (1), Department of Microbiology, Mount Sinai School of Medicine, New York, New York 10029

[1]Present address: The L. F. Kimball Research Institute of The New York Blood Center, New York, New York 10021.

Robert G. McArthur (231), Department of Pediatrics, Julia McFarlane Diabetes Research Centre, The University of Calgary, Calgary, Alberta, Canada T2N 4N1

Marc Monestier (161), Institute of Molecular Immunology, Center for Molecular Medicine and Immunology, University of Medicine and Dentistry of New Jersey, Newark, New Jersey 07103

D. S. Nuefeld (265), Division of Endocrinology, Department of Medicine, Mount Sinai School of Medicine, New York, New York 10029

Luc Reininger (91), Department of Pathology, Medical Center of the University of Geneva, CH-1211 Geneva 4, Switzerland

C. Roubaty (289), INSERM U. 283, Hôpital Cochin, 75674 Paris Cedex 14, France

Katherine A. Siminovitch (59), Department of Medicine, Toronto Western Hospital, Univeristy of Toronto, Toronto, Ontario, Canada

Paul A. Singer (189), Department of Immunology, Research Institute of Scripps Clinic, La Jolla, California 92037

Maurizio Sollazzo (129), Department of Medicine, University of California, San Diego, San Diego, California 92103

Masami Takei[2] (155), Clinical Immunology Section, Audie L. Murphy Memorial Veterans Hospital, and the Department of Medicine, The University of Texas Health Sciences Center, San Antonio, Texas 78284-7874

Norman Talal (155), Clinical Immunology Section, Audie L. Murphy Memorial Veterans Hospital, and the Department of Medicine, The University of Texas Health Sciences Center, San Antonio, Texas 78284-7874

H. Tang (289), INSERM U. 283, Hôpital Cochin, 75674 Paris Cedex 14, France

B. Texier (289), INSERM U. 283, Hôpital Cochin, 75674 Paris Cedex 14, France

Argyrios N. Theofilopoulos (107, 189), Department of Immunology, Research Institute of Scripps Clinic, La Jolla, California 92037

William O. Weigle (175), Department of Immunology, Research Institute of Scripps Clinic, La Jolla, California 92037

Robert Winchester (241), Hospital for Joint Diseases and Division of Rheumatology, Department of Medicine, New York University Medical Center, New York, New York 10016

Ji-Won Yoon (231), Division of Virology, Department of Microbiology and Infectious Diseases, and Laboratory of Viral and Immunopathogenesis of Diabetes, Julia McFarlane Diabetes Research Centre, The University of Calgary, Calgary, Alberta, Canada T2N 4N1

Habib Zagouani (1), Department of Microbiology, Mount Sinai School of Medicine, New York, New York 10029

[2]Present address: Nihon University, First Department of Medicine, Tokyo, Japan.

Maurizio Zanetti (129), Department of Medicine, University of California, San Diego, San Diego, California 92103

Moncef Zouali[3] (73), Department of Biochemistry, Tufts University, Medical School, Boston, Massachusetts 02111

[3]Present address: Immunogénétique Cellulaire, Institut Pasteur, 28 rue du Docteur Roux, 75724 Paris Cedex 15, France.

PREFACE

This book contains a selection of the papers presented at the first of a series of biannual meetings on molecular aspects of autoimmunity held in L'Esterel, Quebec, Canada from October 30 through November 2, 1988. The topics covered include the usage of immunoglobulin V genes in autoantibodies, the structural basis for autoantibody cross-reactivities, regulation of the immune response, T Cell usage in autoimmune animals, and MHC Class II associations with disease.

The organizers of this first meeting and the participants thank the following sponsors for their support: Medical Research Council of Canada; Faculty of Medicine, Memorial University of Newfoundland; Nordisk Canada Ltd.; Connaught-Nova Canada Ltd.; IAF Biochem International Inc.; Ames Educational Institute; Otisville Biopharm Inc.

NADIR R. FARID
CONSTANTIN A. BONA

THE EXPRESSION OF LY-1 AND IMMUNOGLOBULIN VARIABLE GENE FAMILIES IN HYBRIDOMAS PRODUCING AUTOANTIBODIES OF VARIOUS SPECIFICITIES

Raoul Mayer, Habib Zaghouani, Azad Kaushik, Kuppuswamy Kasturi, Vincenzo Fidanza and Constantin Bona[1]

Department of Microbiology, Mount Sinai School of Medicine, New York, New York

I. INTRODUCTION

Since theoretically the potential immune repertoire covers the entire antigenic dictionary, it therefore must be made up of lymphocytic clones able to recognize all foreign as well as self antigens. For a long time however, it was considered that autoreactive clones can be detected only in pathological conditions leading to the occurrence of autoimmune phenomena. Since the breaking of self tolerance was believed to occur only in pathological conditions, it was postulated that under normal physiological conditions the self-reactive clones are deleted early in the development of the immune system (1). As a corollary, autoimmunity was considered to be related to the activation of "forbidden" autoreactive clones, or alternatively to the somatic mutation of clones initially programed to recognize foreign antigens (2).

[1] This work was supported by grant no. 2092 from The Council For Tobacco Research Inc., U.S.A. and grant no. AITC1PO1AI24671 from the National Institute of Allergy and Infectious Diseases. Raoul Mayer is a trainee of the United States Public Health Service, Medical Scientist Training Grant GM07280 from the National Institute of General Medical Sciences.

With the advent of hybridoma technology and of more sensitive immunochemical techniques numerous studies have demonstrated that self reactive B and T cell clones are part of the normal immune repertoire (3,4,5) and that immunoglobulins interacting with self antigens are detectable in the serum of normal animals or healthy human subjects (6,7). These findings raised new questions rather than improve our understanding of autoimmune phenomena.

Since autoreactive clones are part of the normal immune repertoire (8,9) and self-reactive antibodies are almost invariably found in healthy subjects, it was envisioned that at least some autoantibodies have a physiological role. If indeed certain autoantibodies have a physiological role, such as clearance of metabolites or aged cells, a major question remaining unanswered deals with the origin of pathogenic autoantibodies.

Several possibilities may be envisioned concerning the occurrence of pathogenic autoantibodies:

a) that they are produced by a distinct subset of clones which differs from the subset of clones producing physiological autoantibodies.

b) that pathogenic autoantibodies are encoded by immunoglobulin (Ig) variable (V) genes derived from a discrete subset of germline genes which are found only in the animals prone to autoimmune diseases. These V genes would rearrange at some developmental stage of the immune system when they would be transcribed at a high level. They could be associated in linkage disequilibrium with other genes such as those controlling the immune response located at the MHC locus. This implies that polymorphic germ line gene differences between normal and autoimmune strains should be detectable and that pathogenic autoantibodies should be encoded by V genes derived from germ line genes found only in animals or individuals prone to autoimmune diseases.

c) that pathogenic autoantibodies are produced by clones specific for non-self antigens or those producing physiological autoantibodies which mutate subsequent to the expansion caused by foreign antigens or polyclonal activation. This concept implies that the structure of V genes encoding pathogenic autoantibodies should be similar to the structure of V genes encoding antibodies specific for foreign antigens and that somatic mutation occurring in anti-non-self antibodies would confer self binding properties. Only one example, provided by a study reported by Diamond and Scharff (10) supports this concept.

d) that clones producing pathogenic autoantibodies are "forbidden" but subsequently become activated as a consequence of disregulation or massive release of self antigens into circulation. This release of autoantigens can be related to a primary injury or molecular mimicry between foreign and self antigens; immune disregulation on the other hand can be due to anti-idiotypic antibodies specific for regulatory idiotopes shared by non-self and self reactive clones, or by the escape from the regulatory control exerted by suppressor T cells.

Therefore, it appears that a major challenge for immunopathologists remains the elucidation of cellular and molecular mechanisms which determine the expression of the self repertoire and the activation of harmful clones which produce autoantibodies.

Recently, important progress was made in the understanding of the mechanisms responsible for the diversification of V germ line genes.
Subsequent to rearrangement of DNA segments, the diversity of immunoglobulin receptors is further increased by random pairing of V_H and V_L gene products, somatic mutation and gene conversion.

The major questions related to the production of autoantibodies are as follows:
a) are they produced by clones which are phenotypically different from those producing anti-non-self antibodies?
b) do they use a restricted set of V gene families?
c) do the V genes encoding autoantibodies use unmutated germline genes or are they highly mutated?

We are addressing these questions by studying the expression of the Ly-1 gene, the usage of V gene families and the structure of V genes of hybridomas producing autoantibodies with various specificities obtained from various murine strains.

II. EXPRESSION OF THE LY-1 GENE IN HYBRIDOMAS PRODUCING AUTOANTIBODIES

Ly-1 (CD5) is a pan T lymphocyte differentiation antigen with a molecular weight of 67 Kd. In 1978 the presence of Leu-1, the human equivalent of Ly-1, was first reported on B cells in a human leukemia study (11). This expression was confined to immunoglobulin $(Ig)^+$ cells from B cell chronic lymphocytic leukemia (B-CLL) patients and small lymphocytic lymphoma (SLL) patients (12-16). Ig^+ cells from acute leukemias, Burkitt's lymphomas and other B cell proliferative disorders were all Leu-1 negative (12-16). In the same year, Lanier et al reported a high incidence of murine B cell lymphomas in a new strain of mouse called B10-H-2^a H-4^b (2^a4^b) which were induced by hyperimmunization with sheep red blood cells (SRBC) (17). Several malignant B lymphoma lines (CH lines) were obtained from these mice. At about the same time, Slavin and Strober also reported a case of murine B cell leukemia (BCL1) which developed spontaneously in an old BALB/c mouse and was characterized by prominent splenomegaly and a very high lymphocyte count (>200,000/µl) (18). BCL1 has been subsequently used as a model of human B-CLL based on phenotypic and morphologic markers. The CH and BCL1 lines were shown to express variable levels of the Ly-1 cytodifferentiation antigen (19,20).

In the case of mouse and human B cell malignancies expressing CD5 on their surface, their large numbers in the spleen and other lymphoid organs made them easily detectable by staining. Since the CD5 B cells are rare in normal animals and human subjects their detection proved to be difficult. With improved immunofluorescence techniques, particularly the development of FACS, the Ly-1 B population in mice was better characterized. The Ly-1 expressing B cells were detected in the spleen and peripheral blood at a very low frequency (1-2%) in most adult mouse strains tested. A higher proportion (10-40%) of Ly-1^+ B cells was found among peritoneal B cells (21). Ly-1 B cells are however undetectable in the bone marrow, lymph nodes and Peyer's patches. When young mice (1 week old) were studied a higher proportion (>30%) of Ly-1 B cells was found among splenic and peritoneal IgM^+ cells (21,22). This high proportion of IgM^+ Ly-1 B cells is however maintained throughout adulthood only in the peritoneum (21). While most B cells die after a short time when cultured in vitro, Ly-1 B cells demonstrate prolonged survival and spontaneous IgM secretion (23).

Bone marrow reconstitution experiments showed a dichotomy in the differentiation of Ly-1^+ and Ly-1^- B cells which probably originates at the stem cell level. Liver cells from fetal mice (the liver is the site of hematopoiesis in early stages of fetal development) reconstituted both sets, while bone marrow cells originating from adult animals were able to reconstitute only the Ly-1^- B cell population (24). As a corollary to these results, it was shown that IgM^+ B cells from adult peritoneum or Ig^+ B cells from newborn mice were able to reconstitute almost exclusively the Ly-1^+ population (23). In view of these findings, most researchers today regard the Ly-1 B cells as a distinct subset of B cells which appears early in ontogeny and is maintained independently of the bone marrow. These characteristics as well as the ability to spontaneously secrete Igs when cultured in vitro clearly distinguish the Ly-1$^+$ B cell subset from the conventional, Ly-1$^-$ B cell subset.

The Ly-1 B cell subset was studied in a variety of inbred mouse strains, including several immunodefective strains. One of the common features shared by these mice is the spontaneous autoantibody production. At one end of the spectrum, SJL and CBA/N mice show a lower level of expression (21,25,26). The proportion of Ly-1 B cells is distinctly higher in NZB mice (22,27). Interestingly, an oligoclonal proliferation of the Ly-1 B subset was observed in NZB mice (28). Phenotypic analysis on NZB peritoneal B cells revealed hyperdiploidy which is believed to represent a pre-malignant stage (28). This appears to be due to a selective expansion of the Ly-1 B cells as a functionally distinct subset. A large fraction of the IgM spontaneously secreted by NZB mice are autoantibodies with specificities restricted to Fc gamma, ssDNA and thymocytes (29). It therefore appears that Ly-1 B cells in NZB mice are responsible for the spontaneous autoantibody production of of the IgM isotype. The viable motheaten (<u>me</u>^{v}) autoimmune strain carries a mutation mapping to chromosome 6 (30,31). These mice die at a young age, and display severe immunodeficiency and autoimmunity (31). Even though the overall number of B cells is decreased nearly all of them are Ly-1$^+$ (32). The high level of spontaneous autoantibody production observed in <u>me</u>^{v} mice must also be due to the Ly-1 B cells since this subset is predominant in <u>me</u>^{v} mice. Sidman et al showed that in this strain the increased Ig secretion is promoted by a B-cell derived maturation factor uniquely elevated in <u>me</u>^{v} mice (33). Interestingly enough, when normal mouse strains were examined a close correlation between the Ly-1 B expression and autoantibody secretion was observed. Following in vivo LPS stimulation, a large fraction of Ly-1$^+$ sorted B cells were shown to be specific for bromelein treated mouse red blood cells (BrMRBC) (34). These cells are consistently enriched in the peritoneal cavity of normal adult mice (35,36). The same correlation between Ly-1 expression and BrMRBC specificity was observed among the CH mouse lymphoma lines; almost all CH murine B lymphoma lines show erythrocyte specificities and Ly-1 expression (37-39). Further, detailed analysis identified the phosphotydil choline determinant on RBC membranes as the epitope recognized by antibodies produced by CH mouse lymphomas which bound bromelein treated erythrocytes (39).

The cDNA cloning of the mouse Ly-1 gene was recently reported (40). We used this probe to study the expression of the Ly-1 gene in a panel of hybridomas producing autoantibodies obtained from various mouse strains. We selected in our study hybridomas obtained from NZB and $\underline{me}^{v}$ mice since these autoimmune strains are characterized by spontaneous autoantibody production and increased proportions of Ly-1 B cells (22,27-32). As controls we used hybridomas producing autoantibodies obtained from BALB/c and DBA/1J mice. Both of these strains showed normal levels of Ly-1 B cells. If we assume that all spleen lymphocytes have approximatively the same chance of being immortalized via the fusion event ($1:10^{-3}$ - $1:10^{-4}$) we would theoretically expect a larger fraction of NZB and $\underline{me}^{v}$ hybridomas to be Ly-1 positive by Northern analysis. If autoantibodies producing hybridomas obtained from murine strains not prone to autoimmune disease are also derived from the Ly-1 B subset, then we would expect similar proportions in both panels.

RNA extracted from murine thymus, two CH mouse lymphoma lines (CH12 and CH31) and one Ly-1 genomic amplified transfectant (S1A5-6) were initially studied since these cells stain intensly with monoclonal anti - Ly-1 reagents. The study of the expression of the Ly-1 gene in T cells shows that the Ly-1 cDNA probe hybridized strongly with thymic RNA (Fig 1).

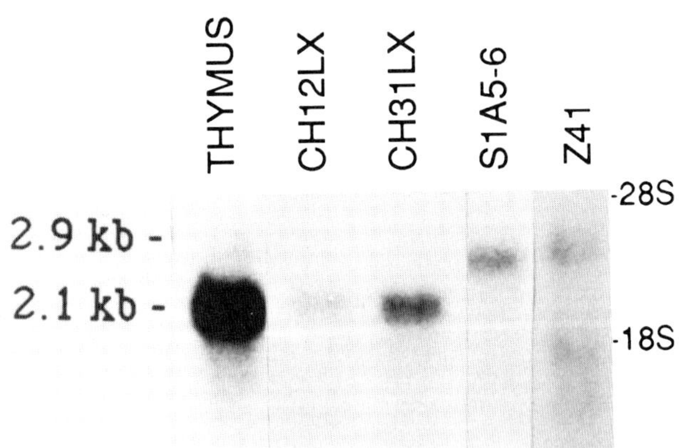

Fig. 1. Northern blot hybridization of RNA obtained from thymus, two lymphoma lines (CH12, CH31), S1A5-6 Ly-1 genomic transfectant and Z41 hybridoma (NZB origin).

Two bands of 2.1 Kb and 2.9 Kb were observed, differing markedly in intensity, suggesting that the less intense 2.9 Kb band probably represents the nuclear precursor of the mature 2.1 Kb mature transcript. Only the 2.1 Kb transcript was detected in RNA extracted from the CH12LX and CH31LX lymphomas, cells which also stain intensly with Ly-1 specific monoclonal antibodies in immunofluorescence studies. The RNA extracted from the Ly-1 amplified genomic transfectant S1A5-6 also hybridizes strongly with the Ly-1 cDNA probe; however, only a 2.7 Kb transcript is detected as previously described (40).

Prior to our study there was a striking discrepancy between data demonstrating the contribution of the Ly-1 B cell subset to the production of murine autoantibodies and the lack of detection of the Ly-1 cytodifferentiation antigen on hybridomas producing autoantibodies. Studies employing hybridomas on the other hand have the definite advantage of allowing the detailed characterization of antibody specificities. Therefore it was important to use a more sensitive approach such as Northern analysis in order to resolve this apparent discrepancy. Our study of 131 hybridomas producing autoantibodies with various specificities, shows that Ly-1 transcripts were detected in 32 out of 72 hybridomas obtained from NZB mice, 6 out of 22 hybridomas obtained from MRL/lpr mice, 7 out of 8 hybridomas obtained from viable $\underline{me}^{v}$ mice, 1 out of 6 C_3H/HeJ hybridomas, 2 out of 7 BALB/c hybridomas and 1 out of 8 CBA/N x BALB/c hybridomas (Table I). These hybridomas show 2.9 Kb and 1.6 Kb transcripts. No Ly-1 transcripts were seen in 7 hybridomas obtained from DBA/1J mice immunized with type II collagen. It is important to mention that most Ly-1 positive hybridomas, as demonstrated by Northern analysis originate from NZB and $\underline{me}^{v}$ mice and produce autoantibodies specific for dsDNA, MRBC, thymocytes, intrinsic factor, thyroglobulin or exhibiting RF activity.

TABLE I. Ly-1 Gene Expression In Hybridomas Producing Autoantibodies

	Total Hyb.	MRL/ lpr	DBA/1	$\underline{me}^{v}$	NZB	C_3H	BALB/c	CBA/N
$Ly\text{-}1^{+}$	49	6	0	7	32	1	2	1
$Ly\text{-}1^{-}$	82	16	8	1	40	5	5	7

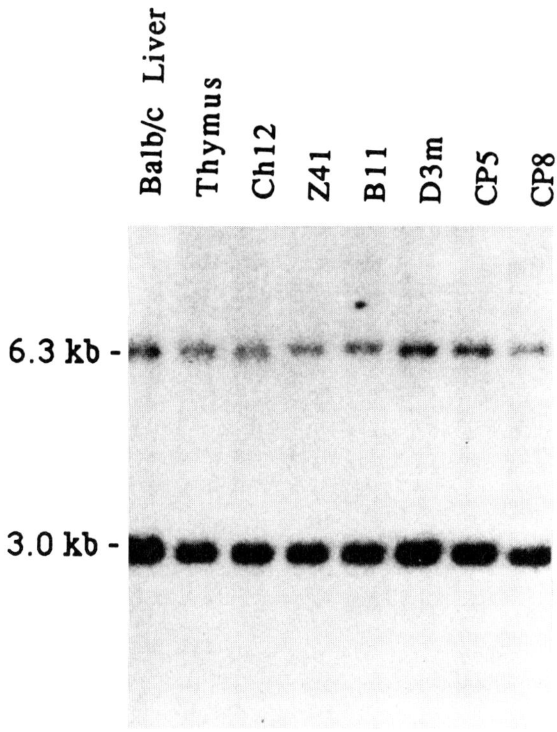

Fig. 2. Southern blot analysis of HindIII digested genomic DNA prepared from liver, thymus, one lymphoma line (CH12), and representative hybridomas.

Representative Ly-1 negative hybridomas were probed with the C_K probe as control, demonstrating in all cases the expected transcript of 1.1 Kb therefore proving the active transcription of functional genes.

Southern blot analysis using Hind III digests of representative Ly-1 positive as well as negative hybridomas demonstrates a hybridization pattern identical in all cases to the liver and thymic DNA (Fig. 2). Consequently, the lack of transcription of the Ly-1 gene in the negative hybridomas cannot be related to the preferential loss of chromosome 19, the locus to which the Ly-1 gene is mapped.

It is important to note that the 2.9 Kb transcript seen in the positive hybridomas corresponds to the precursor thymic transcript. The intensity of the 2.9 and 1.6 Kb bands detected in the positive hybridomas is however significantly weaker, requiring very long exposures, which suggests a much lower level of transcription of the Ly-1 gene in hybridomas as compare to thymocytes and CH lymphoma cells. It is important to emphasize that Ly-1 transcripts were detected mostly in hybridomas obtained from autoimmune strains, namely NZB, $\underline{me}^{v}$ and MRL/lpr. In $\underline{me}^{v}$ mice nearly all B cells express the Ly-1 antigen (32) and the majority of hybridomas obtained from these mice produce autoantibodies (41). These results are consistent with data showing that the Ly-1 subset is involved in the spontaneous production of RFs and autoantibodies specific for DNA, thymocytes and BrMRBC (22,41-43).

Our molecular studies of the Ly-1 gene expression in hybridomas also enabled us to get at least an estimate of the contribution of the Ly-1^{+} and Ly-1^{-} B cell subsets to the production of certain autoantibodies. We have previously determined the specificities of 112 of the 131 hybridomas which were used in our study. Our most significant findings are that 11 out of 19 hybridomas producing anti-DNA autoantibodies, 3 out of 7 hybridomas producing RF, 2 out of 2 hybridomas producing antibodies against Br-MRBC and 12 out of 47 hybridomas producing multispecific autoantibodies originate from the Ly-1^{+} B cell subset. All 7 hybridomas producing CII specific autoantibodies on the other hand originate from the Ly-1^{-} B cell subset. These results are in agreement with prior findings demonstrating a significant contribution of the Ly-1 B cell subset for the production of autoantibodies specific for DNA and RF. No data is available on the Ly-1 B cell V gene structure and usage. Presently we are conducting studies aimed at determining the V gene structure and usage in hybridomas originating from the Ly-1 B cell subset.

III. V GENE UTILIZATION BY MURINE B LYMPHOCYTES

Antibody diversity results from four processes: the combinatorial association of 3 V_H gene segments and 2 V_L segments, the random association of V_H and V_L proteins during the synthesis of the antibody molecule, the somatic mutation of rearranged V_H and V_L genes, and the creation of novel amino acid condons at the junction of V gene segments by addition and deletion of nucleotides prior to joining of DNA segments. During the generation of the immune repertoire intrinsic factors can restrict the potential diversity by preferentially utilizing some V genes for certain subsets of B lymphocytes, by restricting the combinatorial association of various DNA segments and by imposing constraints on V_H:V_L pairing. Consequently, the study of V gene expression at various stages of development of the B cell lineage can provide important information on the molecular mechanisms which contribute to the generation of the repertoire for foreign and self antigens.

The murine V_H genes estimated between 100-200 and V_K genes estimated between 100-300 have been classified in 11 and 30 V gene families, respectively. In the case of V_H gene families, there is generally at least 80% DNA homology between members of a given family which is reflected in the low degree of cross hybridization observed in Southern blotting analysis. This low degree of cross hybridization has permitted an estimation of the genomic complexity of V_H gene families and the classification of various murine strains in haplotypes (44,45). The V_K families were initially classified in subgroups based on the N-terminal sequences of various myeloma proteins (46) and later based on DNA homology. In contrast to V_H genes, there is a significant degree of homology between some V_K families.(e.g. V_K9 shows 80% homology with V_K10, V_K28 shows 87% homology with V_K8 and 82% homology with V_K22, etc.).

Studies of the genomic complexity of V_K families which were carried out by various groups provided discordant information due to the degree of DNA homology of various V_K probes used and in some instances due to such trivial factors such as utilization of low stringency conditions in Southern blots or the utilization of probes from rearranged V_K genes containing J_K and C_K coding sequences. Thus whereas Kasturi et al. (47) and d'Hoostelaere et al. (48) using a probe containing only V_K24 coding sequence under high stringency conditions found only two bands in various murine strains in Southern blotting analysis, Kofler et al. using rearranged M167 (V_K24 J_K5) gene as V_K24 probe and low stringency conditions reported five hybridization bands. Therefore, the high genomic V_K family complexity reported by Kofler et al (49) probably represents an overestimation related to the peculiar conditions used by the authors for the RFLP analysis. The utilization of probes containing only V_K coding sequence and high stringency conditions in Southern blots are key elements for a correct estimation of genomic complexity of V gene families as well as their utilization by B cell clones.

The utilization and mode of expression of V genes by B lymphocytes clones during the ontogeny of the immune system is not well understood. Most of the data available presently describes the frequencies of different V genes used during neonatal and adult stages. Little is known, however, about the mode of expression of various genes during B cell development. The percent frequencies of V_H and V_K genes expressed among mitogen stimulated B lymphocyte clones from neonatal and adult mice are outlined in Table 2. The neonatal B cells were observed to preferentially utilize the most D-proximal V_H genes, as was earlier noted in pre-B cells (54) and fetal B cells (55). Such a programmed pattern of V_H gene expression during fetal and neonatal stages has been suggested to be physiologically relevant (56). In the adult mouse, V_H gene usage appears to be random (52,57-61) as their expression parallels the relative genomic complexity. Certain strain-related differences in V_H gene usage noted by several authors might be due to the methods of detection employed or variations in the numbers of functional V_H gene segments in different mouse strains. Nevertheless, the consensus data suggests a non-random V_H gene usage by neonatal B lymphocyte clones that gradually randomizes during adulthood.

The contribution of V_K genes to the generation of immune diversity is comparable to the contribution of V_H genes, since about 95% of murine immunoglobulin molecules bear kappa light chains. We investigated the V_K gene expression in lipopolysaccharide (LPS) stimulated C57BL/6 B splenocyte clones from neonatal (18,462 clones) and adult (28,106 clones) animals. The analysis of neonatal B cell clones showed a biased expression of V_K1 and V_K9, gene families located in the center of the locus (53). In fact, V_K1, V_K9, and V_K8 constituted about 77% of the V_K gene repertoire in neonates. The most J-proximal family, V_K21, was not expressed in a census of 4,490 B lymphocyte clones analyzed from neonatal mice. Unlike V_H genes, V_K gene expression did not conform to the genomic complexity (53) in adult C57BL/6 mice (Table 2). Most of the studies mentioned above utilized B cell clones or hybridomas obtained after in vivo or in vitro polyclonal activation by LPS. The use of LPS does not seem to influence V_H gene expression in murine B splenocytes (60). Such information

TABLE II. V Gene Usage By B Cell Hybridomas or B Splenocytes From Neonatal and Adult Mice*

Percent V_H Gene Usage By BALB/c Mice							
Gene Order[a] : 5′	---J558--- (60)[b]	J606---- (10)	36-60--- (5)	S107--- (4)	X24---- (2)	Q52---- (15)	7183---3′ (12)
Neonate[c]	18	4	7	4	0	26	22
Adult[d]	34	7.6	10	5.9	4.7	19.6	12.1

Percent V_K Gene Usage By C57BL/6 Mice[f]										
Gene Order[e]: 5′	-VK2--- (5)	VK22--- (7)	VK24--- (2)	(VK1, (3)	VK9)--- (11)	(VK4, (8)	VK8, (12)	VK10, (5)	VK19)--- (10)	VK21-3′ (10)
Neonate	4.7	<0.1	0	40.1	23.0	5.4	13.8	0.3	1.2	0
Adult	1.7	4.3	0.3	25.8	5.1	3.3	9.0	1.4	6.1	2.6

* All these studies do not exclude a bias, if any introduced as a result of LPS stimulation.

a Gene order as mapped by Brodeur et al. (50).

b Genomic complexity based on RFLP pattern of genomic DNA.

c Holmberg (51).

d Jeong et al. (52).

e Gene order as shown by D'Hoostelaere et al. (48).

f Kaushik et al. (53).

is not available on V_K gene usage by B cells. Thus, an exclusion of possible bias introduced by LPS would require an analysis of B cell clones stimulated by several other mitogens or growth factors.

IV. EXPRESSION OF V GENE FAMILIES IN AUTOANTIBODIES

It is well documented that while antibodies specific for haptens and polysaccharide are encoded by genes derived from a restricted number of V gene families and in some occasions of restricted V_H:V_K pairing, the antibodies specific for protein antigens use genes derived from various families. Since the majority of autoantigens are of protein or glycoprotein origin it is important to study the usage of various V genes families by autoantibodies.

During the past 5 years we have studied the usage of V gene families in a large panel of hybridomas producing autoantibodies with various specificities. These hybridomas originate from LPS stimulated lymphocytes from normal strains such as BALB/c, CBA/J, C57BL/6, strains able to develop autoimmune diseases subsequent to immunization with autoantigens such as DBA/1 (collagen induced arthritis) and SJL (encephalitis), or strains prone to autoimmune diseases such as NZB, motheaten and MRL/lpr. The data presented in Table 3 summarizes the V_H gene usage among 180 hybridomas producing autoantibodies. The results clearly indicate that V_H 7183, the most D proximal family, is the most frequently used, followed by Q52. The high frequency usage of J558 reflects the gene complexity of this gene family rather then a positionally related expression.

Similarly, the V_K gene usage analysis of 164 hybridomas secreting autoantibodies, presented in Table 4, shows that V_K1, V_K4, V_K8 and V_K10 genes are used more frequently. Although V_K21 is the most J proximal gene family, it is seldom used in neonates as well as in normal or autoimmune disease prone adult animals. It is also notable that V_K1 is the most frequently used V_K gene family in both neonates and adult animals, for both the normal and autoimmune repertoire. It is also striking that there is a bias in the usage of V_K4 and V_K10 gene families by autoantibodies. These two gene families are represented only at low frequencies in neonatal as well as in normal adult antibody repertoire.

TABLE III. Frequency of V_H families among monoclonal autoantibodies with various specificities*

Specificity of mAbs	V_H FAMILIES 36-60	X24	36-09	J606	VGAM	V_H11	J558	S107	QPC52	7183	NI	Total Studied
DNA	2		1				11	2	1	8	1	26
H_2b							1					1
Sm		1					3	1		6		11
NA								1				1
TG							5	1	1	5		12
MBP							2					2
IF							1					1
Collagen II	2	2	1				6		1	2		14
RF	1	1		1			9		2	5		19
Ach R										2		2
TSH R										1		1
Br-MRBC						9	1		2			12
Coombs							1				4	5
Thymocytes			1	3	2		2					8
Skin								1		2		3
GBM								2				2
Microfibrils									1	1		2
Actin							1			2		3
Multispecific			2	6		1	15	2	11	18		55
Frequency of V_H families	2.7	2.2	2.7	5.5	1.1	5.5	31.9	5.5	10.4	28.5	2.6	|180|
Gene complexity	5	2	20	10	5	2	100	4	15	12		

* Abbreviations : H_2b - histone 2b; Sm - Smith antigen ; NA - nuclear antigen; TG - thyroglobulin; MBP - myelin basic protein; IF - intrinsic factor; RF - rheumatoid factor; Ach R - acetyl choline receptor; TSH R - TSH receptor; Br-MRBC - bromelein treated mouse red blood cells; GBM - glomerular basement membrane; NI - not identified.

TABLE IV. Frequency of V_K families among monoclonal autoantibodies with various specificities*

Specificity of mAbs	V_K FAMILIES 1	2	4	8	9	10	19	21	22	23	24	28	NI	Total Studied
DNA	2		3	1	2	3	1		4			1	7	24
H_2b	1													1
Sm	2		1	3			1						1	8
NA													1	1
TG	1		3	1		3	2						1	11
MBP							1						1	2
IF						1								1
Collagen II	1				1	4			2				5	13
RF	3		4	1	1	1		1					6	17
Ach R	1												1	2
TSH R													1	1
Br-MRBC	1			1	9									11
Coombs	2		1							1			1	5
Thymocytes					2	1								3
Skin	1												2	3
GBM							2							2
Microfibrils	1												1	2
Actin	2		1											3
Multispecific	23		5	1	3	6	2	2	2	2	1		7	54
Frequency of V_K families	25.0	0.	10.9	4.8	10.9	11.5	5.5	1.8	4.9	1.8	0.6	0.6	21.3	|164|
Gene complexity	2-5	ND	6-9	7-8	3-4	2	9	4-8	1	5-6	1-2	ND		

* Abbreviations : H_2b - histone 2b; Sm - Smith antigen ; NA - nuclear antigen; TG - thyroglobulin; MBP - myelin basic protein; IF - intrinsic factor; RF - rheumatoid factor; Ach R - acetyl choline receptor; TSH R - TSH receptor; Br-MRBC - bromelein treated mouse red blood cells; GBM - glomerular basement membrane; NI - not identified.

Tables 5 and 6 present the data of V_H and V_K gene usage by normal and autoimmune disease prone mouse strains. The number of autoantibodies included in this study is variable for each strain. It is clear, however, that the utilization of V gene families is consistant with the data presented earlier. These results taken together indicate that the utilization of V genes by clones producing autoantibodies resembles the V gene expression seen in neonatal clones since the same V gene families are used more frequently. The V_H J558 and 3′ V_H gene families and the V_K families 1, 4, 8 and 10 are used more frequently by hybridomas producing autoantibodies. When comparing hybridomas producing autoantibodies originating from normal animals or strains prone to autoimmune disease, no significant difference in V gene usage was observed. Consequently, the bias in V gene usage appears to be related to the antigenic specificity rather than the strain of origin.

V. STRUCTURAL CHARACTERISTICS OF V GENES ENCODING AUTOANTIBODIES

The study of the structure of V genes can provide important information on the origin of autoantibodies. There are two major concepts attempting to explain the origin of autoantibodies: One states that antibodies for foreign and self antigens are encoded by V genes derived from the same pool of germline genes. During the proliferation of clones induced by foreign antigens, some progeny mutates and acquires self reactivity. In the last few years it was shown that cells producing antibodies specific for bacterial antigens can bind to self antigens subsequent to a somatic mutation which occurred in the V region (10). According to this concept, the somatic mutation is responsible for the appearance of "forbidden" clones endowed with self reactive properties.

The second concept considers autoantibodies to be encoded by a certain subset of germline genes and, that these genes are the origin for the V genes encoding autoantibodies. These clones when stimulated by foreign antigens will further mutate and therefore will acquire higher affinity for foreign antigens but lose autoreactivity. This concept is supported by data which showed that A/J hybridomas selected for the expression of V_H 36-65 germline gene and CRI of anti-arsonate antibodies exhibited reactivity for self antigens (DNA and

TABLE V. Frequency of V_H families among 168 monoclonal antibodies obtained from various strains

	MOUSE STRAINS*											
V_H family	C57 BL/6	nu/nu C57	me^v	SJL	DBA/1	CBA/ J	C_3H/ HeJ	MRL/ lpr	BALB/c spl.	BALB/c per.	NZB spl.	NZB per.
36-60					2						3	
X24			1		1			1				
36-09	1	1	1								1	
J606		2	4					2		2		
VGAM			2									
VH11						2				4	1	3
J558	1		5	1	6	4	3	10	4		13	
S107		1	3					2			2	
QPC52					1	1	1	7	2	1	5	
7183	2		5		3	1	3	8	15	1	17	
NI	1										5	
Total mAb studied	5	4	21	1	13	8	7	30	21	8	47	3

* Abbreviations : spl. - spleen; per. - peritoneal; NI - not identified.

TABLE VI. Frequency of V_K families among 164 monoclonal antibodies obtained from various strains

	MOUSE STRAINS*											
V_K family	C57 BL/6	nu/nu C57	me^v	SJL	DBA/1	CBA/ J	C_3H/ HeJ	MRL/ lpr	BALB/c spl.	BALB/c per.	NZB spl.	NZB per.
1			4		1	1		7	6	3	20	
2												
4	1	1	2		2			6	3		3	
8						1		5		1	1	
9					1	2		3		4	3	3
10	2	2	4		4		1	1	4	2	2	
19		1	2	1		2	1	1	1			
21										1	2	
22	1				1		2	1			2	
23											2	
24								1				
28											1	
NI	1		4		2		3	7	6		11	
Total mAbs. studied	5	4	16	1	11	7	7	32	20	11	47	3

* Abbreviations : spl. - spleen; per. - peritoneal; NI - not identified.

cytoplasmic antigens) and arsonate. The V_H genes expressed in these hybridomas generally were unmutated genes. In contrast, hybridomas selected from secondarily immunized mice were generally devoid of self-reactivity, exhibited a higher affinity for arsonate and generally had mutated V_H genes (62). Another observation supporting the germline gene origin of autoantibodies is that germ-free, chemically fed mice produce immunoglobulins, most of which exhibit reactivity to self antigens (63,64). The wide idiotype cross reactivity observed among autoantibodies present in individuals of outbread species (65) as well as among autoantibodies produced by various inbred animal strains (66) constitutes additional indication of the germline gene origin of autoantibodies.

In a recent study, we carried out nucleotide sequence analysis of either mono or polyspecific autoantibodies derived from both normal and autoimmune disease prone animals. Table 7 summarize the origin, isotype, and specificity of the autoantibodies analyzed. As can be seen, the antibody GP138-10 obtained from MRL/lpr mouse, a strain prone to lupus and arthritis-like disease, immunized with the GT (glutamic acid tyrosine) polymer displayed reactivity to both foreign (GT) and self (DNA, Sm, and Fc IgG_2a) antigens (67). The antibody H45-5 obtained from MRL/lpr treated with the HP20 anti-idiotype antibody carrying the internal image of GT also displayed the same pattern of reactivity (67). Both antibodies are encoded by V_H genes derived from the V_H J558 family (Table 8) and V_K genes derived from the V_K1 and V_K4 gene families respectively (Table 9). The V_H region of GP138-10 and H45-4 show >90% homology with two J558 germ line genes, H13-1 and H18 respectively. The majority of mutations were observed in CDR1 and CDR2. While the D segments of these antibodies vary in length, the J segments are unmutated. With respect to V_K genes, one can see that the GP138-10 V_K gene has 99.7% homology with the V_K germ line gene K5.1 and the single base pair change in CDR3 is a silent mutation. The V_K gene used by H45-5 exhibits several replacement mutations in the Fr1 and CDR3 compared to the V_K4 germ line gene Hy-Gal1. The J_K segments associated with these V_K genes are unmutated.

Two other antibodies M56 obtained from LPS stimulated 1 month old MRL/lpr splenocytes and Y19-10 obtained from Balb/c splenocytes immunized with Y. enterolitica were found to belong to the V_H J558 family. Both antibodies are monospecific (see Table 7) and have V_K genes derived from the V_K8 and V_K4 families respectively. As can be seen in Table 9, the V_K8 gene of M56 has 93% homology to the consensus V_K8 sequence. The silent and replacement

TABLE VII. Origin and specificity of autoantibodies subsequently analyzed by nucleotide sequencing

Autoantibody*	Origin	Isotype	Specificity
GP138-10	MRL/lpr immunized with GT antigen	IgM	GT, DNA, Sm, Fc IgG_{2a}
H45-5	MRL/lpr immunized with HP20	IgM	GT, DNA, Sm, Fc IgG_{2a}
S14-2	Normal me^{v} splenocytes	IgG_1	thymocytes
UN34-11	LPS stimulated me^{v} splenocytes	IgM	thymocytes
UN42-5	LPS stimulated me^{v} splenocytes	IgM	thymocytes
M56	LPS stimulated MRL/lpr splenocytes	IgM	Sm
Z26	LPS stimulated NZB splenocytes	IgM	Sm
Y19-10	BALB/c immunized with Y. enterolitica	IgG_{2b}	rheumatoid factor

* All hybridomas were obtained from splenocytes fused with the nonsecreeting myeloma cell line SP2/0. GT - polymer of glutamic acid and tyrosine, Sm - Smith antigen, and HP20 - a monoclonal anti-idiotypic antibody carrying the internal image of GT.

mutations are homogeneously distributed with the exception of the CDR2 which has 100% homology to the CDR2 of the consensus sequence. When compared to J558 V_H germline genes, both antibodies show a higher number of base pair changes in CDRs than in FRs. Most nucleotide changes led to amino acid replacements, especially in the case of Y19-10 where the CDR1 has only 20% amino acid homology with the corresponding germ line gene. Like M56, the antibody Z26 is also specific for Sm. It was obtained from LPS stimulated NZB splenocytes and derived its V_K from the V_K8 family and its V_H from the V_H7183 family. The Z26 V_H has 93% homology to the germ line gene 37.1. Nucleotide changes were found in the CDRs, and most of them led to amino acid replacement. The Z26 J_H has only 93% homology to the J_H1 germ line segment (Table 8). The Z26 V_H may represent a mutated gene. The Z26 V_K gene, like the M56 V_K gene, has 93% homology to a consensus V_K8 gene. One can note that the CDR2 of both V_K Z26 and V_K M56 are unmutated compared to the consensus sequence (Table 9). Since both antibodies are specific for the Sm antigen and expresse the idiotype found on anti-levan antibodies (77), one may speculate that the CDR2 is important for one or both of these functions.

The V genes of three other autoantibodies specific for thymoctyes and RBC obtained from me^v mice were also sequenced in our laboratory. As can be seen in Table 9 the three antibodies UN42-5, UN34-11, and S14-2 use light chain genes derived from the V_K9 family. The V_K genes of UN42-5 and UN34-11 have 99.7% homology to the germ line CP5 V_K9 gene, with a single nucleotide change in the CDR3. Since this change affects the last nucleotide of the variable region, one can assume that this occurred during the joining process. One can note that both antibodies have unmutated J_K1 segments. The antibody S14-2 derived its V_K gene from another germ line gene of the V_K9 family, namely MOPC41. Only one nucleotide change was found at position 123. This change is silent, leading to an amino acid sequence 100% homologous to the germ line gene. These findings suggests that all three antibodies use unmutated germ line genes deriving from two different members of the V_K9 family. While the antibodies UN42-5 and S14-2 derived their V_H genes from the J606 family, the antibody UN34-11 derived its V_H gene from the S107 family. As can be seen in Table 8, the UN34-11 V_H has 100% homology to the S107 germ line gene VB6.5, and has an unmutated J segment. The antibodies UN42-5 and S14-2 have 92% and 91% homology respectively to a J606 germ line gene, $V_H22.1$. However when compared to each other one can see 99% homology in both the nucleotide and the amino acid

TABLE VIII. Comparison of the nucleotide and amino acid sequences of autoantibody heavy chain variable regions with their corresponding germline genes

Antibody	V	FR1	CDR1	FR2	CDR2	FR3	CDR3 D	CDR3 J_H
				% Nucleotide homology* / % Amino acid homology				
GP138-10:J558	87 / 87	83 / 85	67 / 50	98 / 100	82 / 76	94 / 96	SP2. 3-4	100 / 100
H45-5:J558	91 / 84	96 / 93	75 / 75	93 / 80	88 / 76	92 / 76	FL16.1	100 / 100
UN42-5:J606	92 / 90	98 / 97	73 / 60	100 / 100	76 / 55	93 / 95	Q52	100 / 100
S14-2:J606	91 / 88	98 / 97	67 / 40	100 / 100	76 / 55	91 / 93	SP2. 6 or 7	100 / 100
UN34-11:S107	100 / 100	NS	100 / 100	100 / 100	100 / 100	100 / 100	SP2. 2 or 3-4	100 / 100
Z26:7183	93 / 83	94 / 83	80 / 60	93 / 86	90 / 76	94 / 88	DFL 16.1	95 / 93
M56:J558	88 / 83	83 / 76	73 / 80	95 / 93	89 / 76	92 / 88	SP2.5, 7 or 8	95 / 93
Y19-10:J558	88 / 76	96 / 93	67 / 20	83 / 71	82 / 53	90 / 81	SP2. 6 or 7	100 / 100
UN42-5/S14-2	99.3 / 99	100 / 100	100 / 100	100 / 100	100 / 100	98.3 / 98.3	Q52 / SP2. 6 or 7	100 / 100

* The percentage of nucleotide or amino acid homology of a given region was calculated as follows : the number of nucleotide or amino acid changes within a given region as compared to the corresponding germline gene over the total number of nucleotides or amino acids within the same region. In each case the comparison was made with the closest germline gene. The germline genes used for comparison are: The J558, H13-1 (68) for GP138-10; the J558, H18 (68) for H45-5;the J606, V_H22.1 (69) for S14-2 and UN42-5; the S107, VB6.5 (70) for UN34-11; the 7183, 37-1 (69) for Z26; the J558, V_H23 (71) for M56; and the J558, 33 (72) for Y19-10. The antibodies UN42-5 and S14-2 were also compared to each other(bottom line). The name of each antibody is followed by its corresponding V_H family. V -, variable region, FR - framwork, CDR - complementarity determining region, NS - not sequenced.

TABLE IX. Comparison of the nucleotide and aminoacid sequences of autoantibodies light chain V regions with their corresponding germline genes or consensus sequences

% Nucleotide homology* / % Amino acid homology

Antibody	V	FR1	CDR1	FR2	CDR2	FR3	CDR3	J_K
GP138-10:K1	99.7 / 100	100 / 100	100 / 100	100 / 100	100 / 100	100 / 100	95 / 100	100 / 100
H45-5[a]:K4	80	56	91	73	71	97	44	100
UN42-5:K9	99.7 / 100	100 / 100	100 / 100	100 / 100	100 / 100	100 / 100	95 / 100	100 / 100
UN34-11:K9	99.7 / 100	100 / 100	100 / 100	100 / 100	100 / 100	100 / 100	95 / 100	100 / 100
S14-2:K9	99.7 / 100	100 / 100	100 / 100	97 / 100	100 / 100	100 / 100	100 / 100	100 / 100
Z26:K8	93 / 89	93 / 78	90 / 94	84 / 80	100 / 100	98 / 97	81 / 86	97 / 92
M56:K8	93 / 89	94 / 83	88 / 88	87 / 87	100 / 100	99 / 94	81 / 86	97 / 92

* The percentage of homology was calculated as described in Table VIII. The V_K genes used for comparison are: the V_K1, K5.1 (73) for GP138-10; the V_K4, HyGal (74) for H45-5; the V_K9, CP5 (75) for UN34-11 and UN42-5; the V_K9,MOPC41 (76) for S14-2, and a consensus V_K8 sequence for Z26 and M56. This consensus sequence was obtained from the V_K8 of PY102 (77), Am13 and Am14 (78), and Z26 and M56 sequences.

[a] Comparison was made with amino acid sequence only. No nucleotide sequence is available.

sequences. Only a TAC codon at position 72 is changed to ATC in UN42-5 leading to a replacement of a tyrosine with an isoleucine. Even though these antibodies were obtained from two different mice (S14-2 from 3 weeks old me^v and UN42-5 from 8 week old me^v mice) and are of different isotype, they use the same V_H genes. Our studies of the structure of V_H and V_K genes of hybridomas obtained from animals prone to autoimmune diseases such as me^v, MRL/lpr and NZB, which are specific for different autoantigens such as Sm, thymocytes-RBC, or multispecific antibodies, show that some of them - such as those obtained from me^v - use unmutated germline genes or germline genes with limited somatic mutation. MRL and NZB derived antibodies and the RF antibody obtained from BALB/c mice showed more extensive somatic mutation when compared with the available V_HJ558 germ line gene sequences. However, this does not preclude the posibility that the rearranged V_H gene expressed in these hybridomas have a higher homology with germ line genes not yet identified. The most striking conclusion which can be drawn from our studies is that despite extensive V_H and V_K gene polymorphism observed in inbred mice, unmutated germ line gene nucleotide sequences can be found in rearranged V_H or V_K genes expressed in autoantibodies obtained by various strains.

REFERENCES

1. Burnet, F. M. (1959). Cambridge University Press, London.
2. Burnet, M., & Holmes, M.C. (1965). Nature. (London). 207, 368.
3. Welch, M.J., Fong, S., Vaugham, J.H., & Carson, D.A. (1983). Clin. Exp. Immunol. 51, 299.
4. Dighiero, G., Lymberi, P., Guilbert, B. Ternynck, T., & Avrameas, S. (1986). Ann. N.Y. Acad. Sci. 475, 135.
5. Glimcher, L.H., & Shevach, E.M. (1982). J. Exp. Med. 156, 660.
6. Guilbert, B., Dighiero, G., & Avrameas, S. (1982). J. Immunol. 128, 2774.
7. Lymberi, P., Dighiero, G., Ternynck, T., & Avrameas, S. (1985). Eur. J. Immunol. 15,702.
8. Bellon, B., Manheimer-Lory, A., Monestier, M., Moran, T., Dimitriu-Bona, A., Alt, F., & Bona, C. (1987). J. Clin. Invest. 79, 1044.

9. Logtenberg, T., Kroon, A., Gmeling-Meyling, F.H.J., & Ballieux, R.E. (1987). Eur. J. Immunol. 17, 855.
10. Diamond, B., & Scharff, M.D., (1984). Proc. Nat. Acad. Sci. U.S.A. 81, 5841.
11. Boumsell, L., Bernard, A., & Dausset, J. (1978). Eur. J. Immunol. 8, 900.
12. Boumsell, L., Coppin, H., Dausset, J., & Bernard, A. (1980). J. Exp. Med. 152, 229.
13. Wang, C.Y., Good, R.A., & Evans, R.L. (1980). J. Exp. Med. 151, 1539.
14. Royston, I. Majda, J.A., & Griffiths, J.C.(1980). J. Immunol. 125, 25.
15. Kamoun, M., Kadin, M.F., & Hansen, J.A.(1981) J. Immunol. 127,987.
16. Knowles, D.M., Halper, J.P., & Wang, C.Y. (1983). Cancer. 52, 1369.
17. Lanier, L.L., Lynes, M.A., Haughton, G., & Wettstein, P. (1978). Nature. 271, 554.
18. Slavin, S., & Strober, S.(1978). Nature. 272, 624.
19. Lanier, L.L, Warner, N.L., & Herzenberg, L.A. (1981). J. Exp. Med. 153, 998.
20. Lanier, L.L., Arnold, L.W., & Haughton, G. (1982). Immunogenetics. 16, 367.
21. Hayakawa, K., Hardy, R.R., & Herzenberg, L.A. (1986). Eur. J. Immunol. 16, 450.
22. Hayakawa, K., Hardy, R.R., Parks, D.R., & Herzenberg, L.A. (1983). J. Exp. Med. 157, 202.
23. Braun, J. (1983). J.Immunol. 130, 2113.
24. Hayakawa, K., Hardy, R.R., Herzenberg, L.A., & Herzenberg, L.A. (1985). J. Exp. Med. 161, 1554.
25. Hayakawa, K., Hardy, R.R., & Herzenberg, L.A. (1984). In Progress in Immunology V., eds., Yamamura, Y., and Tada, T. 661.
26. Hayakawa, K., Ishii, R., Kishimoto, T, Herzenberg, L.A., & Hardy, R.R. (1987). In New Horizons in Animal Models for Autoimmune Disease, ed. Kyogaku, M., and Wigzell, H. Tokyo : Academic Press.
27. Manohar, V., Brown, E., & Chused, T.M. (1982). J. Immunol. 129, 532.
28. Raveche, E.S., Alabaster, O., & Steinberg, A.D. (1981). J. Immunol. 126, 154.
29. Manny, N., Datta, S.K., & Schwartz, R. (1979). J. Immunol. 122, 1220.
30. Green, M.C., & Shultz, L.D. (1975). Genetics and Pathology. J. Hered. 66, 250.
31. Shultz, L.D., Coman, D.R., & Sidman, C.L. (1984). Am. J. Pathology. 116, 179.
32. Sidman, C.L., Shultz, L.D., Hardy, R.R., Hayakawa,K., & Herzenberg, L.A. (1986). Science. 232, 1423.

33. Sidman, C.L., Shultz, L.D., & Evans, R. (1985). J. Immunol. 135, 870.
34. Hayakawa, K., Hardy, R.R., & Herzenberg, L.A.(1984). Proc. Natl. Acad. Sci. U.S.A. 81, 2494.
35. Pages, J., & Bussard, A. (1975). Nature. 257, 316.
36. Steele, E.J., & Cunningham, A.J. (1978). Nature. 274, 483.
37. Haughton, G., Arnold, L.W., & Mercolino, T.J. (1986). Immunol. Rev. 93, 35.
38. Pennell, C.A., Arnold, L.W., & Haughton, G. (1985). Proc. Natl. Acad. Sci. U.S.A. 82, 3799.
39. Mercolino, T.J., Arnold, L.W., & Haughton, G. (1986). J. Exp. Med. 163, 155.
40. Huanng, H.-J.S., Jones, N.H., Strominger, J.L., & Herzenberg, L.A. (1987). Proc. Natl. Acad. Sci. U.S.A. 84, 204.
41. Painter, C., Monestier, M., Chew, Sidman., C., & Bona, C. (1988). J. Exp. Med. 167, 1137.
42. Casali, P., Burastero, S.E., Nakamura, M., Inghirami, G., & Notkins, A.L. (1987). Science. 236, 77.
43. Hardy, R.R., Hayakawa,K., & Kishimoto, T. (1987). Science. 236, 81.
44. Brodeur, P.H., & Riblet, R. (1984). Eur. J. Immunol. 14, 922.
45. Dildrope, R. (1984). Immunology Today. 5, 85.
46. Potter, M., Newell, J., B., Rudikoff, S., & Heber, E., (1982). Mol. Immunol. 19, 1619.
47. Kasturi, K., Monestier, M., Mayer, R., & Bona, C. (1988). Mol. Immunol, 25, 213.
48. D'Hoostelaere, L.A., Huppi, K., Mock, B., Malett, C., & Potter, M. (1988). J. Immunol. 141, 652.
49. Kofler, R., Duchosal, M.A., & Dixon, J. (1989). Immunogenetics. 29, 65.
50. Brodeur, D.M., Osam, G.E., Mackle, J. & Lalor, T.M.(1988). J. Exp. Med. 168, 2261.
51. Holmberg, S. (1987). Eur. J. Immunol. 17, 399.
52. Jeong, H.D., Komisar, J.L., Kraig, E. & Teale, J.M. (1988). J. Immunol. 140, 2436.
53. Kaushik, A., Schulze, D.H., Bona, C.A., & Kelsoe, G., (1989). J. Exp. Med. (In press).
54. Yancopoulos, G.D., Desiderio, D.V., Paskind, M., Kearney, J.F., Baltimore, D., & Alt, F.W. (1984). Nature. 311, 757.
55. Perlmutter, R. M., Kearney, J. F., Chang, S. P., & Hood, L. E. (1985). Science, 127, 1597.
56. Jeong, H.D., & Teale, J.M. (1988). J. Exp. Med. 168, 589.
57. Manser, T. Huang, S-Y., & Gefter, M. (1984). Science. 226, 1213.

58. Dildrope, R., Krawinklel, V., Winter, E., & Rajewsky, K., (1985). Eur. J. Immunol. 15, 1154.
59. Schulz, D.H., & Kelsoe, G. (1987). J. Exp. Med. 16, 163.
60. Yancopoulos, G.D., Malynn, B.A., & Alt. F.A. (1988). J. Exp. Med. 168, 417.
61. Dighiero, G., Lim, A., Lembezet, M., Kaushik, A., Andrade, L. & Freitas, A. (1988). Eur. J. Immunol. 18, 1979.
62. Naparstek, Y., Andre-Schartz, J., Manser, T., Wysoki, L.J., Breitman, L., Sttollar, B.D., Gefter, M., & Schwartz, R.S. (1986). J. Exp. Med. 164, 614.
63. Hooijkaas, H., Benner, R., Pleaants, J.R., & Wostman. B.S. (1984). Eur. J. Immunol. 14, 1127.
64. Pereira, P., Forni, l., Larson, L., Cooper, M.D., Heusser,C., & Coutinho, A. (1986). Eur. J. Immunol. 16, 685.
65. Isenberg, D. A. A., Shoenfeld, Y., Madaio, M.P., Rauch, J., Reichlin, M., Stollar, B.D., & Schwartz, R.S. (1984). Lancet. ii, 417.
66. Monestier, M., Bonin, B., Migliorini, P., Dang, H., Datta, S., Kupper, R., Rose, N., Maurer, P., Talal, N., & Bona, C. (1987). J. Exp. Med. 166, 1109.
67. Bailey, N.C., Fidanza, V., Mayer, R., Mazza, G., Fougereau, M., & Bona, C. Submitted.
68. Schiff, C., Milili, M., & Fougereau, M. (1985). Embo J. 4, 1225.
69. Hartman, A.B., & Rudikoff, S. (1984). Embo J. 3, 3023.
70. Pennel, C.A., Arnold, L.W., Haughton, G., & Clarke, S.H. (1988). J. Immunol. 141, 2788.
71. Bothwell, A.L.M., Paskind, M., Reth, K., Imanishi-kari, T., Rajewsky, K., & Baltimore, D. (1981). Cell. 24, 625.
72. Manheimer-leory, A.J., Monestier, M., Bellon, B., Alt, F., & Bona, C. (1986). Proc. Natl. Acad. Sci. U.S.A. 83, 8293.
73. Corbet, S., Milili, M., Fougereau, M., & Schiff, C. (1987). J. Immunol. 138, 932.
74. Pawlita, M., Potter, M., & Rudikoff, S. (1982). J. Immunol. 129, 615.
75. Reininger, L., Ollier, P., Poncet, P., Kaushik, A., & Jaton, J.C. (1987). J.Immunol. 138, 316.
76. Seidman, J.G., Max. E.E., & Leder, P. (1979). Nature. 280, 370.
77. Zaghouani, H., Bonilla, F.A., Meek, K., & Bona, C.A. (1989). Proc. Natl. Acad. Sci. U.S.A. (In press).
78. Schlomchik, M.J., Marshak-Rothstein, A., Wolfowicz, C.B., Rothstein, T.L., & Weigert, M.J. (1987). Nature. 328, 805.

STRUCTURAL CHARACTERISTICS OF HUMAN IgM AUTOANTIBODIES

Fernando R. Goñi[1]
Department of Pathology
New York University Medical Center
New York, New York 10016

Pojen P. Chen
Scripps Clinic and Research Foundation
La Jolla, California 92037

Blas Frangione[2]
Department of Pathology
New York University Medical Center
New York, New York 10016

I. INTRODUCTION

The initial characterization, by Kunkel, Capra, and coworkers, of human monoclonal IgM rheumatoid factors (RF) demonstrated that, serologically, they could be divided into distinct cross-reactive idiotypic (CRI) groups: Wa, Po and Bla. They are preferentially associated to kappa light (L) chains which share remarkably similar variable (V_k) regions (1-4). Later, we found that autoantibodies with anti-low density lipoprotein activity (LDL), anti-intermediate filaments (IF), and anti-I antigen cold agglutinins (CA) also show the same pattern of restriction in their L chain and the expression of the V_{kIIIb} sub-subgroup (5-8). In contrast to the preferential association of the kIIIb sub-

[1]*Present address: The L.F. Kimball Research Institute of the New York Blood Center New York, New York 10021.*
[2] *Supported by N.I.H. Grant #AR 01431 and AR 02594.*

subgroup with IgM autoantibodies, only 8% of IgM non-autoantibodies have been found to possess this type of L chains (2,9).

Based on these findings, we postulated that V_{kIIIb} L chains are the expression of a single V_k gene segment (6). This gene, Humkv325, has recently been isolated and sequenced (10). It encodes for the previously known "primary structure-dependent" idiotypes, PSL2 and PSL3, located on the second (CDR2) and third complementarity-determining regions (CDR3) of the L chains (11).

The considerable genetic homogeneity found among the L chains of human IgMk RFs and other autoantibodies and the demonstration of primary structure dependent idiotypy suggest a potential role in determining antibody specificity and idiotypic regulation.

To further analyze M autoantibodies and to determine the biological meaning and physiological regulation of these proteins we have studied IgM-RFs from essential mixed cryoglobulinemias, CAs from idiopathic cold agglutinin disease and chronic lymphocytic leukemias, and monoclonal autoantibodies with anti-LDL and anti-IF activity from lymphomas and other B-cell dyscrasiae. A common characteristic among these autoantibodies is that they are present, in low levels, in healthy individuals (12-14), and even after a monoclonal proliferation they do not produce a severe autoimmune pathology. However, their physicochemical ability to precipitate in the cold as immuno-complexes has helped to clinically diagnose them by the secondary effects they produce such as Raynaud's syndrome and hemolytic anemia.

II. MATERIALS AND METHODS

The methodologies for IgM autoantibody isolation, chemical and serological characterization, autoantibody activity determination, production and isolation of their L and H chains, amino acid sequence analyses and their idiotypic characterization with the PSL2 and PSL3 reagents were previously reported. (5,6,7,11)

III. RESULTS AND DISCUSSION

A. Structural similarities

The partial and/or complete amino acid sequence was determined for the L chains of 19 IgM-RF (proteins GLO, PAY,

Figure 1

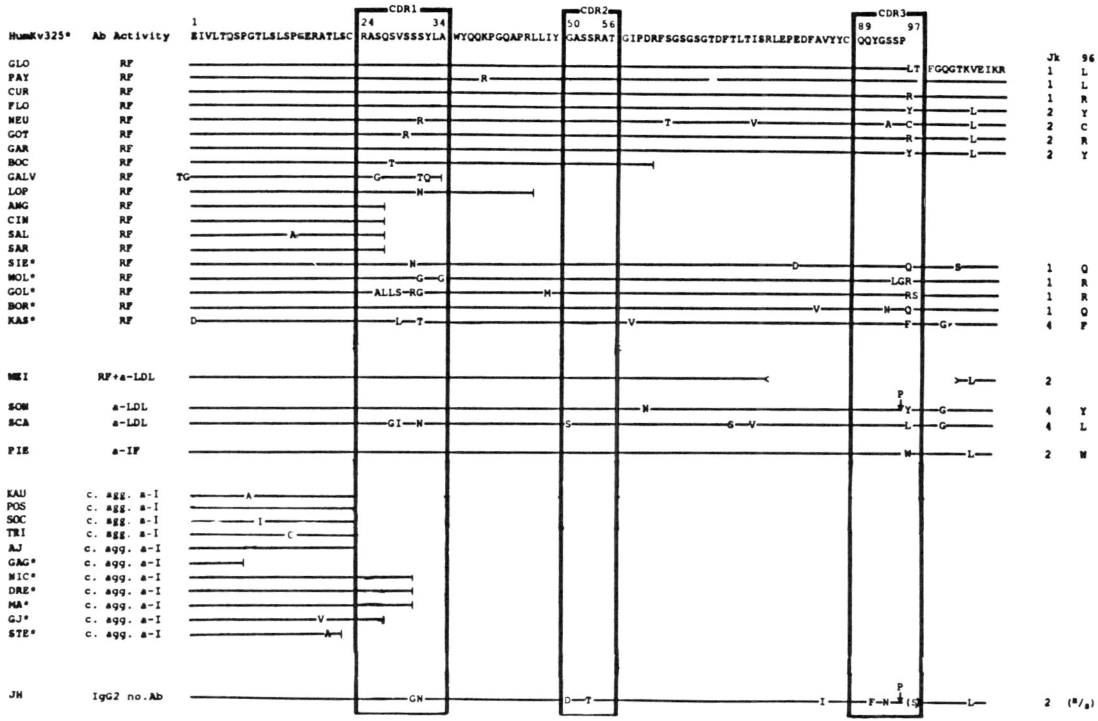

*: As per references 3,4,8,15,16.

CUR, FLO, NEU, GOT, GAR, BOC, GALV, LOP, ANG, CIN, SAL, SAR, CLA, SHE, LEW, JON and MIT), 1 IgM-RF that also has activity against LDL (protein WEI), 2 IgM anti-LDL (proteins SON and SCA), 1 IgM anti-IF (protein PIE), 5 IgM CA (proteins KAU, POS, SOC, and TRI, kindly provided by Dr. J. Oppenheim, NY Univ. Medical Center, and AJ, kindly provided by Dr. R. Williams) and 1 IgGk (protein JH) with unknown antibody activity.

The amino acid sequences of these proteins as well as previously reported data, are shown in Figure 1. Most of them belong to sub-subgroup kIIIb, although proteins CLA, SHE, LEW, JON and MIT belong to sub-subgroup kIIIa.

There is a remarkable homology among the L chains of these IgM autoantibodies. They seem to be derived from a single V_k gene (Humkv325), shown at the top of the figure. Very few amino acid changes are seen throughout the V_L segment; and they may be due to polymorphism of the V_k gene or to somatic mutation. Overall the framework (FR) residues are very conserved and most of the changes are seen in CDR1 and CDR3. In contrast the CDR2 appears to be remarkably stable.

Since different autoantibodies possess similar V_k segments its selection probably is not related to their specificities. However, the conserved structure of the Humkv325/KIIIb may insure a suitable framework for the three-dimensional position of autoreactive V_H regions and the basis for regulatory idiotypes. The amino acid changes more frequently seen in the CDR1, conformationally related to the active site, could contribute to the fine specificity and/or affinity of a particular antibody.

B. Specificity

Table I and Table II show the serological and chemical determination of the V_H usage by the different autoantibodies.

Sixty percent of the RFs use a V_{HI} and the rest is distributed between V_{HII} and V_{HIII} genes. It is not known if they correspond to a single gene or a family of related genes. Nevertheless, a certain restriction is seen in the V_H expression in RFs, restricted enough to insure the specificity and diversified enough to insure the reaction to the different epitopes present in the Fc portion of the four IgG subclasses.

A better correlation between V_H selection and specificity is seen with the CAs. The five CAs tested express a V_{HII} subgroup. This determination was done serologically with a reagent that could cross-react with V_{HIV} or V_{HVI} proteins.

Nevertheless, the V_H gene used appears to be specific in determining the activity against the I antigen present in red blood cells membranes.

The two anti-LDL and the anti-IF use similar V_{HIII} segments but the numbers are too small to attempt any correlation with the specificity.

TABLE I. Serological markers and gene segments present in the light and heavy chains of human monoclonal RF

		Serology						Sequence			V_H	
Name	Ab activity	Wa	Po	Bla	KIIIb	PSL2	PSL3	V_k	Jk	Km	ser	seq
GLO	RF	+		-	+	++	++	IIIb	1	3	III	III
PAY	RF				+	++	++	IIIb	1	3	III	
CUR	RF	+		-	+	++	++	IIIb	1	3	II	
FLO	RF				+	++	++	IIIb	2	3		
NEU	RF				+	++	+	IIIb	2	3	I	
GOT	RF	+		-	+	++	++	IIIb	2	3	II	II
GAR	RF	+		-	+	++	++	IIIb	2	3	I	I
BOC	RF				+	++	++	IIIb				
GALV	RF				+	+		IIIb				
LOP	RF					-	+	IIIb				
ANG	RF				+	++	++	IIIb			I	
BUS	RF				+	+	+				II	
CIN	RF				+	++	+	IIIb			I	
CSA	RF				+	+	+				II	
DAQ	RF				+	++	++				I	
SAL	RF				+	++	-	IIIb			I	
SAR	RF				+	++	+	IIIb			I	
SIE*	RF	+		-		++	++	IIIb	1		I	1
WOL*	RF	+		-		++	-	IIIb	1		I	I
COL*	RF	+				++	++	IIIb	1			
BOR*	RF	+				++	+	IIIb	1		I	I
KAS*	RF	+				+	++	IIIb	4		I	I
McD*	RF	+		-		++	++					

*As per references (3, 4, 15, 16, 17). The V_H serology was performed by G. Silverman, Scripps Clinic, and published elsewhere (22, 23).

C. Serological idiotypy

Kunkel and coworkers originally described the Wa CRI of RFs bearing K_{IIIb} L chains (1,2). Later, the Bla CRI for RFs cross-reacting with DNA-histone and some uncharacterized CRIs for the CAs were described (18-19). We recently succeeded in raising rabbit antisera that react with CAs-K_{IIIb} and another antiserum against the anti-LDL SON.

All these CRIs recognize K_{IIIb}-bearing proteins that have the same specificity, and they require assembly of the H and L chains for expression. Thus, the CRIs appear to be dependent on epitopes located on the V_H regions associated with structures provided by the K_{IIIb} chains. Therefore, they are quaternary structure-dependent and specificity-dependent CRIs.

On the other hand Solomon and McLaughlin (20) described an epitope that is privative to the K_{IIIb} chains, and we previously reported two primary structure-dependent idiotypes detected by antisera raised against synthetic peptides bearing the amino acid sequences of the L-CDR2 and L-CDR3 present in HumKv325/KIIIb proteins (11,21).

The relationship between these idiotypes and IgM-RF and other autoantibodies is shown in tables I and II.

Table II. Serological markers and gene segments present in the light and heavy chains of human monoclonal IgM autoantibodies

		Serology						Sequence			V_H	
Name	Ab activity	Wa	Po	Bla	KIIIb	PSL2	PSL3	V_k	Jk	Km	ser	seq
WEI	RF+a-LDL	+		-	+	++	++	IIIb	(2)	3		
SON	a-LDL	-		-	+	++	+	IIIb	4	1,2		III
SCA	a-LDL				+	++	++	IIIb	4	1,2		III
PIE	a-IF				+	++	++	IIIb	1	3		III
AJ*	CA a-I				+	+	-	IIIb			II	
GAG*	CA a-I					++	-	IIIb				
KAU	CA a-I				+	++	++	IIIb			II	
POS	CA a-I				+	+	++	IIIb			II	
SOC	CA a-I				+	++	-	IIIb			II	
TRI	CA a-I				+	++	+	IIIb			II	
JH(IgG)	none				+			IIIb	2	1,2	I	

*As per reference 8. The V_H serology was determined by G. Silverman, Scripps Clinics, and published elsewhere (22, 23).

There is a good correlation between the amino acid sequence and the expression of the K_{IIIb} determinant on all the IgM autoantibodies studied. More than 97% of IgM autoantibodies express the PSL2 idiotype whereas 90% of RFs and 70% of IgMs with other anti-self activities express the PSL3 idiotype. The PSL2 and PSL3 CRIs are genetically determined and preliminary studies on the secondary structure of K_{IIIb} proteins (not shown) show they are potential antigenic determinants in the intact molecule.

The existence of genetically determined epitopes shared by all IgM-K_{IIIb} autoantibodies but not present in other immunoglobulins suggests that the idiotype-antiidiotype network regulation of a whole family of IgMkIIIb autoantibodies could depend on structural features of their L chains.

D. Somatic mutation

Sequential structural studies were performed on completely reduced and alkylated L chains from protein GOT. They correspond to plasmaphereses collected from 1978 to 1982 (GOT'78, '79, '80, '81 and '82). All samples presented the same amino acid sequence through FR1. The L-CDR1, positions 24 to 34, sequenced as Arg-Ala-Ser-Gln-Ser-Val-Arg(29A)-Ser-Ser(31)-Tyr-Leu-Ala in GOT'78 and GOT'79 whereas in 10% of the molecules from GOT'80 it was found serine instead of arginine and asparagine instead of serine at positions 29A and 31, respectively. This ratio changed to 70%:30% in GOT'81 and reversed to 30%:70% on GOT'82, table III. No more specimens were available after 1982 and the patient eventually died in 1985. The complete amino acid sequence of the L chains from different years could not be completed due to lack of material, however, all samples tested positive for the PSL2 and PSL3 sequence dependent idiotypes indicating that all proteins should have identical or almost identical amino acid sequences on their CDR2 and CDR3 segments.

The sequential study of protein GOT suggests that during the lifespan of the disease, somatic mutation can occur in the V gene (HumKV325). Both amino acids, 29A and 31, were replaced at a similar ratio in the same years indicating that both changes occurred in only one cell at approximately the same time giving rise to a new subclone that in time replaced the original one. However, it cannot be ruled out

Table III. Amino acid variation at positions 29A and 31 in the sequential study of protein GOT L chain

	29A: Arg	Ser	31: Ser	Asn	PSL2	PSL3
GOT'78	100%	0%	100%	0%	+	+
GOT'79	100%	0%	100%	0%	+	+
GOT'80	90%	10%	90%	10%	+	+
GOT'81	70%	30%	70%	30%	+	+
GOT'82	30%	70%	30%	70%	+	+

that both clones were present at all times and were derived from independent recombinatorial events.

These preliminary results also show that L-CDR1 but not L-CDR2 and L-CDR3 is a "hot spot" for somatic mutation. In fact 60% of the changes observed in sequences of known Humkv325/KIIIb chains are present in the CDR1, Figure 1, followed by 19% in the CDR3 (the V_k-J_k recombination point, residue 96, was not considered). On the other hand the sequence of the CDR2 is remarkably conserved in all these proteins.

E. Switching

The presence of the KIIIb marker was originally detected on IgM autoantibody molecules. Serologically it is found in IgM producing cells and rarely less than 0.5%, in IgG or IgA producing cells (9). Thus, the switch from mu producing to gamma or alpha producing cells seems to be prevented when KIIIb is expressed.

From a large collection of monoclonal immunoglobulins we could find one IgG2K, protein JH (kindly provided by Drs. M. Cooper and H. Kubagawa), that chemically and serologically expresses a KIIIb molecule. So far this immunoglobulin has not been found to possess autoantibody activity (it was tested for RF, cold agglutinin activity, a-LDL, a-IF and normal cell components). Compared to the IgMkIIIb molecules the amino acid sequence of JH L chain (figure 1) shows very conserved FRs but a high number of changes present in the three CDRs, with the subsequent loss of the PSL2 and PSL3 idiotypes.

If as shown, KIIIb molecules usually possess some kind of autoantibody activity, the rare switch to IgG or IgA might be accompanied by somatic mutation that can eliminate the self-reactivity and the shared idiotypy.

IV. CONCLUSIONS

It is evident that a large proportion of human monoclonal IgM autoantibodies with different specificities are preferentially associated with kappa L chains, subgroup IIIb, encoded by a single V_k gene (HumKv325/K_{IIIb}). This gene appears to be very conserved through evolution and it is expressed, with rare somatic mutation, in the outbred human population. Although the selection/expression of the HumKv325/K_{IIIb} gene is unrelated to antibody specificity, it is preferentially associated with mu gene and has some kind of anti-self activity.

The V_{kIIIb} gene determines idiotypic sites that are shared by all these autoantibodies, and partially contributes, through its association to the V_H, to the specificity-dependent conformational idiotypes.

On the other hand, there is V_H selection related to the specificity of the autoantibody, but not as restricted as it is for the L chains.

The data points to the existence of a family of natural, genetically determined autoantibodies with specificities against conserved and widely distributed self-antigens. These autoantibodies can have physiological functions, i.e., the RFs can enhance the secondary and anamnestic immune response, while the CAs can bind senescent RBCs and newly formed neoplastic cells and be eliminated from the circulation. Natural autoantibodies may eventually remove from the circulation self-antigens that in certain conditions can elicit a pathological autoimmune response.

In sum, a family of natural autoantibodies of the $IgMk_{IIIb}$ type appears to be derived from a subset of B-cells, with particular genotypic and phenotypic expression. This B-cell subset could be part of a "physiological autoimmune system."

REFERENCES

1. Kunkel, H. G., Agnello, V., Joslin, F. G., Winchester, R. J. and Capra, J. D. (1973). J. Exp. Med. 137,131.
2. Kunkel, H. G., Winchester, R. J., Joslin. F. G. and Capra, J.D. (1974). J. Exp. Med. 139, 128.

3. Capra, J. D. and Kehoe, J. M. (1974). Proc. Natl. Acad. Sci. USA 71, 4032.
4. Andrews, D. W. and Capra, J. D. (1981). Proc. Natl. Acad. Sci. USA 78, 3799.
5. Ledford, D. K., Goñi, F. R., Pizzolato, M., Franklin, E. C., Solomon, A. and Frangione, B. (1983). J. Immunol. 131, 1322.
6. Goñi, F. R., Chen, P. P., Pons-Estel, B., Carson, D. A. and Frangione, B. (1985). J. Immunol. 135, 4073.
7. Pons-Estel, B., Goñi, F. R., Solomon, A. and Frangione, B. (1984). J. Exp. Med. 160, 893.
8. Capra, J. D., Kehoe, M., Williams, R. C. Jr., Feizi, T. and Kunkel, H. G. (1972). Proc. Natl. Acad. Sci. USA 69, 40.
9. Moynihan, J. A., Looney, R. J. and Abraham, G. N. (1985). Immunology 54, 207.
10. Chen, P. P., Albrandt, K., Kipps, T. J., Radoux, V., Liu, F. T. and Carson, D. A. (1987). J. Immunol. 139, 1727.
11. Chen, P. P., Goñi, F. R., Fong, S., Jirik, F., Vaughan, J. H., Frangione, B. and Carson, D. A. (1985). J. Immunol. 134, 3281.
12. Guilbert B., Dighiero, G. and Avrameas, S. (1982). J. Immunol. 128, 2779.
13. Kunkel, H. G., Posnett, D. N. and Pernis, B. (1983) Ann. N.Y. Acad. Sci. 418, 324.
14. Jenkins, W. J., Marsh, W. L., Noades, J, Tippet, P., Sanger, R. and Race, R. R. (1960). Vox Sang. 5, 97.
15. Newkirk, M., Chen, P. P., Carson, D., Posnett, D. and Capra, J. D. (1986). Mol. Immunol. 23, 239.
16. Newkirk, M., Mageed, R. A., Jefferis, R., Chen, P. P. and Capra, J. D. (1987). J. Exp. Med. 166, 550.
17. Agnello, V., Goñi, F. R., Barnes, J. L., de la Vega, M. T. and Frangione, B. (1987). J. Exp. Med. 165, 263.
18. Agnello, V., Arbetter, A., deKasep, G. I., Powell, R., Tan E. M. and Joslin, F. (1980). J. Exp. Med. 151, 1514.
19. Feizi, T., Kunkel H. G. and Roelcke, D. (1974). Clin. Exp. Immunol. 18, 283.
20. Solomon, A. and McLaughlin, C. L. (1971). J. Immunol. 106, 120.
21. Chen, P. P., Fong, S., Normansell, D., Houghten, R. A., Karras, J. G., Vaughan, J. H. and Carson, D. A. (1984). J. Exp. Med. 159, 1502.

22. Silverman, G., Goldfien, R., Chen, P. P., Mageed, R., Jefferis, R., Goñi, F. R., Frangione, B., Fong S. and Carson, D. A. (1988). J. Clin. Invest. 82, 469.
23. Silverman, G. J. Goñi, F. R., Fernandez, J., Chen, P. P., Frangione, B. and Carson, D. A. (1988). J. Exp. Med. 168, 2361.

MOLECULAR GENETICS OF HUMAN AUTOANTIBODIES

POJEN P. CHEN

Department of Molecular and Experimental Medicine
Scripps Clinic and Research Foundation
10666 North Torrey Pines Road
La Jolla, California 92037

I. INTRODUCTION

According to Ehrlich's concept of "horror autotoxicus", B cells with autoreactivities are aborted, deleted or tolerized during the development of B lymphocytes; and the "harmful" autoantibodies do not exist in normal conditions and appear only in pathologic situations. However, the presence of autoantibodies in normals has been clearly demonstrated in several instances. For example, although anti-IgG antibodies (rheumatoid factors, RFs) were initially discovered in patients with rheumatoid arthritis (RA), these autoantibodies have now been found in normal individuals (1-3). Immunochemical studies of the rheumatoid synovial fluid showed that they contained abundant aggregates of Ig, which are composed mainly of IgG and RFs. These findings suggested that RFs might contribute to immune complex formation and chronic tissue damage in the rheumatoid synovium (2). On the other hand, RF-producing cells were found in some apparently normal individuals; and RF precursor cells in normal subjects were shown to increase shortly after a booster immunization with tetanus toxoid (4). Similar observations have been made in

---

This is publication number 5629-BCR from the Research Institute of Scripps Clinic, La Jolla, California. Funding for this research supported in part by grants AR39039 and AR33489 from the National Institutes of Health.

mice (5,6). These results suggest that RFs may have some physiological functions in the immune system.

Idiotypes are the serologically defined individual antigenic determinants of antibody molecules. Among them, some are shared by different antibody molecules and are designated cross-reactive idiotypes (CRIs). Analyses of CRIs in "inbred" mice demonstrate that some CRIs are phenotypic markers for Ig variable region genes (7-9). Thus, anti-CRI antibodies have been very useful tools for delineating the genetic basis for murine antibody responses. Using this approach, we and others have defined some genetic components for human autoantibodies. Here, we shall review our studies in identifying and characterizing human Ig V gene segments for autoantibodies of various specificities.

II. IDENTIFICATION AND CHARACTERIZATION OF THE Humkv325 GENE

Among human monoclonal IgM RFs derived primarily from individuals with "mixed cryoglobulinemia", Kunkel et al. described two major CRIs, termed Wa and Po (10). The Wa CRI was expressed by 60% of human monoclonal IgM RFs. Importantly, they also noted that all Wa positive RFs contained light chains of the kIIIb sub-subgroup, which constitutes only about 13% of total Ig kappa chains (11). Subsequently, Capra and his coworkers showed that two Wa positive RFs (i.e. Sie and Wol) were extremely homologous in their light chain variable regions, but not in their heavy chain variable regions (12). Together, these data suggested that the Wa-CRI is associated mainly with RF light chains.

It is known that hypervariable regions (complementarity-determining regions, CDRs) are the structural correlates of many idiotypic determinants (7,8). Since the light chain variable regions of two Wa-positive RFs have an identical second CDR, a PSL2 peptide, corresponding to this CDR and the adjacent framework amino acids, was synthesized and used to immunize rabbits. The resultant anti-PSL2 antisera bound specifically to the RF Sie and its light chain, and the light chains of some human monoclonal IgM RFs (13,14). Importantly, antibody binding to these eight RF light chains was completely inhibited by the PSL2 peptide, but not by an unrelated control peptide (14). These data indicated that the anti-peptide antibody defined a RF light chain-associated CRI.

Similarly, antibodies were generated against the third CDR of the Sie light chain (PSL3). The anti-PSL3 antisera bound specifically to the intact Sie, the isolated Sie light chain and the light chains of many PSL2-positive human monoclonal RFs (15). To date, our accumulative data show that anti-PSL2 and anti-PSL3 react, respectively, with about 67% and 57% of human monoclonal IgM RFs from unrelated individuals (3,16). It should be noted that most PSL3 positive RFs express the PSL2-CRI marker; and that a majority of PSL2 positive monoclonal IgM RFs also react with a murine monoclonal anti-idiotype, termed 17.109 (16-18).

To delineate the genetic basis of the PSL2 and PSL3 CRIs, we compared the reported amino acid sequences of the CRI positive RFs and found that these sequences were extremely homologous in their variable regions, suggesting that most CRI positive light chains derived from a single germ-line gene, designated Vk(RF) (14). Thereafter, we screened a human fetal liver genomic library sequentially with a human VkIII cDNA probe NG9/3 and a human VkIII gene probe Humkv301.

Two interesting clones were isolated (19). Clone 321 contained a partial Vk gene (designated Humkv321). It encodes 54 amino acids, which correspond exactly to the postulated Vk(RF) sequence, from position 42 to 95. Clone 305 contained a Vk gene (designated Humkv305), which shares 92 of 96 amino acids with the postulated Vk(RF) gene. Importantly, Humkv305 and Humkv321 share 300 out of 303 base pairs (bp), and share nine out of ten restriction enzyme sites over a region of 14 kilobases (kb), indicating that these two genes are highly homologous (20).

Accordingly, we screened a human placenta DNA library with the Humkv305, and isolated the putative Vk(RF) gene (20,21). The cloned Vk gene, designated Humkv325, encodes exactly the 96 amino acid residues of the proposed Vk(RF) sequence, and is identical to Humkv321 in the overlapped area, indicating that Humkv325 is the full-length gene for Humkv321.

To date, the amino acid sequences of 12 PSL2-positive light chains have been reported (12,22-25). When these sequences were compared with the Humkv325 sequence, four are identical to Humkv325. The remaining 8 differs from the Humkv325 by 1-7 amino acid residues (Figure 1). Regarding the Jk gene usage, Humkv325 is joined to either Jk1, Jk2 or Jk4 gene segments, with different junctional amino acid residues for Jk1 and Jk2 (i.e., R,L,Q; and Y,R,C respectively). Collectively, these data demonstrate that a human Vk gene can encode RF light chains either with or without somatic changes; and that the Humkv325 is conserved among outbred populations, including normal subjects, as well as patients with autoimmune diseases.

In addition to RF light chains, the Humkv325 sequence is identical to the light chain variable region of an autoantibody (Pie) against intermediate filament (IF), and differs by only one amino acid residue from the light chain variable region of an autoantibody (Son) against low density lipoprotein (LDL) (Figure 1) (22). As expected, both Son and

```
            CRI                              -----CDR1----
         PSL2 PSL3  1                       24      30A  34
Humkv325            EIVLTQSPGT LSLSPGERAT LSCRASQSVS SSYLAWYQQK PGQAPRLLIY
RFs
1-4. CUR,FLO,GAR,GLO
5.  GOT   ++    ++  ---------- ---------- ---------R ---------- ----------
6.  PAY   ++    ++  ---------- ---------- ---------- ---------R ----------
7.  BOR   ++    +   ---------- ---------- ---------- ---------- ----------
8.  SIE   ++    ++  ---------- ---------- ---------- N--------- ----------
9.  NEU   ++    +   ---------- ---------- ---------- -R-------- ----------
10. WOL   ++    -   ---------- ---------- ---------- -G--G----- ----------
11. KAS   +     ++  D--------- ---------- --------L- -T-------- ----------
12. GOL   ++    ++  ---------- ---------- -----ALLS- RG-------- --------M-
Cold agglutinins
1.  AJ      nd      --------D- ---------- ---------- end of the published seq
2.  DRE     nd      ---------- ---------- ---------- ------end
3.  GJ      nd      ---------- --------V- ------end
4.  MA      nd      ---------- ---------- ---------- end
5.  NIC     nd      ---------- ---------- ---------- end
6.  PER     nd      -----Z---- ------Z--- ------Zend
7   STE     nd      ---------- ---------A --end
8.  TAK     nd      -----Z---- ------Z-V- ---------- ?----end
Anti-LDL antibody
1.  SON   ++    ++  ---------- ---------- ---------- ---------- ----------
Anti-IF antibody
1.  PIE   ++    ++  ---------- ---------- ---------- ---------- ----------
Anti-CMV antibody
1. EV1-15 ++    ++  ---------- ---------- ---------- -NE------- ---------S

                    -CDR2--                                   ----CDR3---/
                   50    56                                  89     95 96 Jk
Humkv325            GASSRATGIP DRFSGSGSGT DFTLTISRLE PEDFAVYYCQ QYGSSP
RFs
1-4. CUR,FLO,GAR,GLO                                     R 1, Y 2, Y 2, L 1
        DIFFERENCE
5.  GOT     1       ---------- ---------- ---------- ---------- ------  R  2
6.  PAY     1       ---------- ---------- ---------- ---------- ------  L  1
7.  BOR     2       ---------- ---------- ---------- ----V----- ---N--  Q  1
8.  SIE     2       ---------- ---------- ---------- -D-------- ------  Q  1
9.  NEU     4       ---------- ---T------ -----V---- ---------- ---A--  C  2
10. WOL     4       ---------- ---------- ---------- ---------- ----LG  R  1
11. KAS     5       --------V- ---------- ---------- ---------- ------  F  4
12. GOL     7       ---------- ---------- ---------- ---------- ------  R  1
Anti-LDL antibody
1.  SON     1       ---------- N--------- ---------- ---------- ------ PY  4
Anti-IF antibody
1.  PIE     0       ---------- ---------- ---------- ---------- ------  W  2
Anti-CMV antibody
1.  EV1-15  6       ---R------ ---------- ---------- -----M---- ----T-  R  1
```

FIGURE 1. Amino acid sequence comparison of Humkv325 and the kv325-encoded human antibodies, including their entire Vk gene-encoded regions (positions 1 to 95) and the VJ junctional amino acid residues (3,12,16,19-23,25,27,28). The Jk gene usage is indicated and the known PSL2 and PSL3 CRI expresssion of these antibodies are given. The deduced amino acid sequence of Humkv325 is given at the top. All the other sequences are first aligned for maximum homology, and the residues identical to kv325 are indicated by bars. The numbers after each antibody denote the number of residues by which the respective sequence deviates from kv325 sequence.

Pie are positive for the PSL2 and PSL3 CRIs. In addition, using these peptide-induced antiidiotypes, Agnello et al. showed that two cold agglutinins (i.e. Gag and Joh) expressed the PSL2 CRI (26). Similarly, in collaboration with Drs. F. Goni and B. Frangione, we found that anti-PSL2 antibodies reacted with 6/6 cold agglutinins, while anti-PSL3 antibodies reacted with only 3/6 cold agglutinins (16). Moreover, we noted that the partial amino acid sequences of 7 cold agglutinins (i.e. MA, NIC, DRE, PER, STE, GJ, TAK; from position 1 to position 22) all contained the diagnostic amino acid residues of the Humkv325 gene (i.e. Leu, Gly and Leu at positions 4, 9, and 13 respectively) (Figure 1) (16,27). Together, these data indicated that some cold agglutinins are encoded by the Humkv325.

Very recently, we found that both PSL2 and PSL3 CRIs were expressed by a human monoclonal antibody against cytomegalovirus (Ev1-15), suggesting that the anti-virus antibody used the Humkv325 gene for its light chain (16). This conclusion was indeed supported by the amino acid sequence of the Ev1-15 light chain (Figure 1) (28). Thus, although the Humkv325 is frequently used by autoantibodies of various specificities, it is also used by antibodies to foreign antigens.

III. IDENTIFICATION AND CHARACTERIZATION OF THE Humkv328 AND ITS HOMOLOGOUS GENES

Schrohenloher and Koopman generated a murine monoclonal anti-CRI (designated 6B6.6) which reacted with 7/22 (32%) RFs, but only 3/94 (3%) non-RFs (29,30). In addition, the anti-CRI bound to the separated light chains of the CRI-positive RFs, and the amino acid sequences of 3 6B6.6 positive RF light chains (i.e. Cla, Pom and Les) are homologous, suggesting that the 6B6.6 CRI may be the phenotypic marker of a single or a few human Vk genes (31,32).

To isolate this putative RF-associated Vk gene, we screened a genomic DNA library from the patient Les with the rearranged Les light chain gene, and characterized the positive clones (32,33). The results showed that two new Vk genes, designated Humkv328 and Humkv329, were isolated (33,34).

Humkv328 is most closely related to the Les light chain, sharing with ka3les 1315/1331 nucleotides at the DNA level, and 109/112 amino acid residues at the protein level (including the leader peptide) (Figure 2) (33,34). In addition, Humkv328 is identical to the Pom light chain from positions 44 to 95, and to the sequences of RFs Cla and She from positions 1 to 23/26 (33). Importantly, kv328 and most of

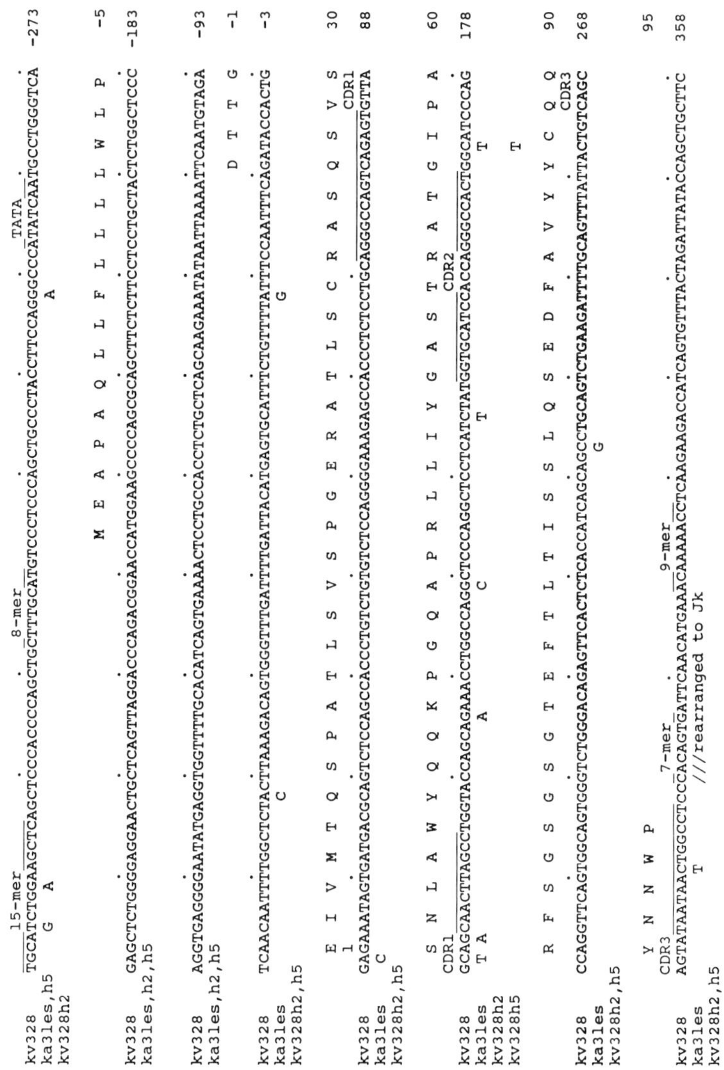

FIGURE 2. Genomic structures of four highly homologous human VkIII genes which are related to the 6B6.6 idiotype. All were sequenced from -922 to +430 (34). For simplicity, only nucleotides from -362 to +358 are expressed in the figure. The nucleotide and amino acid sequences of Humkv328 are given,

these light chains share the distinct characteristics of having respectively, Val, Glu and Ser (instead of Leu, Asp and Pro) at the positions 13, 70 and 80; and of lacking Tyr at the position 32 in the first CDR. Together, these data strongly suggest that kv328 is the corresponding germ-line gene for the rearranged Les light chain gene, as well as three other RF light chains; and that Humkv328 is the genetic basis for the 6B6.6 CRI in humans.

Humkv329 is highly homologous to kv328. First, restriction map analysis of clones containing these two genes revealed an identical pattern over a region of 13 kb long. Second, over a stretch of 1331 bp sequenced, kv328 and kv329 differed by only 3 bases (Figure 2). Among these 3 different bases, two were in the Vk-coding region and led to a Met/Thr substitution and a Trp/stop change at amino acid positions 5 and 94, respectively. The other different nucleotide was in the 3' flanking region (at nucleotide position 406).

Although the Pom light chain is most closely related to Humkv328, they differ from each other by 7/96 amino acid residues. To further define the genetic basis of the 6B6.6 CRI, it was important to determine whether the Pom light chain might be encoded by a VkIII germline gene other than Humkv328, or by various allelic forms of Humkv328. Our preliminary studies of polymorphisms in human Vk genes (including Humkv305, 325 and 328) failed to reveal any restriction fragment length variability (unpublished data). These results suggested that Vk genes from outbred human populations are relatively conserved, and that there may be only microscopic differences, if any, among corresponding Vk genes from different people. Accordingly, we decided to isolate the Humkv328-corresponding gene(s) and/or Vk genes that are very closely related to Humkv328 from an unrelated individual.

The results showed that two new Vk genes, designated Hah2 and Hah5, were isolated (34). Hah2 differs from kv328 by only one base (at nucleotide position -753), while Hah5 differs from kv328 by 6 nucleotides (at nucleotide positions -673, -439, -376, -372, -313 and +174) (Figure 2). Interestingly, the deduced amino acid sequences of Hah2 and Hah5 are identical

---

FIGURE 2. (con't)
whereas sequences of other genes are given only at the positions where they differ from the kv328 sequence. All sequences were first aligned for maximum homology. To reduce the complexity of the figure, nucleotide sequences of different genes are listed together in one line when they are identical over that specific region.

with that of kv328. Thus, Hah2 and Hah5 were renamed Humkv328h2 and Humkv328h5.

There are several possible relationships among these four highly homologous human Vk genes. They could represent alleles of a single Vk gene locus, or, alternatively different

```
             G6  CRI                                       CDR 1            CDR2
RFs               1                                       31--35             50-
1. BOR        +   <EVQLVQSGAE VKKPGSSVKV TCKASGDTFS SSAISWVRQA PGQGLEWMGG
2. KAS        +   --H------- ---------- S-----G--- -Y-------- ----------
3. SIE        +   ---------- --------R- ---T--G--- GYT------- --R----V-S
4. WOL        +   ----M----- --------R- S--T--G--V DYKGL----- --K----V-Q
Vh cDNA
1. 51P1       nd  Q--------- ---------- S-----G--- -Y-------- ----------
Rearranged Vh gene
1. 783        nd  Q--------- ---------- S-----G--- -Y-------- ----------
Germline Vh genes
1. hv1263     nd  Q--------- ---------- S-----G--- -Y-------- ---------R
2. 21-2       nd  Q--------- -----A---- S-----Y--T -YYMH----- ---------I
3. HG3        nd  Q--------- -----A---- S-----Y--N -YYMH----- ---------I
4. 7-2        nd  QM-------- ---T------ S-----Y--T YRYLH----- ---A-----W

                  CDR2
RFs               ---------------66                                  98
1. BOR            IIPIFGTPNY AQKFQGRVTI TTDESTSTAY MEVSSLRSED TALYYCAR
2. KAS            ------QA-- ---------- -A----N--- --LR----D- --M----K
3. SIE            PAKWTDPFQG VYIKWE---V SLKP-FNQ-- --LVN-FN-- G-V-----
4. WOL            -PLR-NGEVK NPGSVV--SV SLKP-FNQ-H --L---F--- --V-----
          DIFFERENCE
Vh cDNA
1. 51P1       8   -------A-- ---------- -A-------- --L------- --V-----
Rearranged Vh gene
1. 783        9   -------A-- ---------- -A-------- --L------- --V----K
Germline Vh genes
1. hv1263    12   ----L-IA-- ---------- -A-K------ --L------- --V-----
2. 21-2      22   -N-SG-STS- ---------M -R-T----V- --L------- --V-----
3. HG3       22   -N-SG-STS- ---------M -R-T----V- --L------- --V-----
4. 7-2       24   -T-FN-NT-- -----D---- -R-R-M---- --L------- --M-----
```

FIGURE 3. Amino acid sequence comparison of four Wa- and G6-positive RF heavy chains (Bor, Kas, Sie and Wol), one Vh1 cDNA (51P1), one Vh1 rearranged gene (783) and all known human Vh1 germline genes (12,25,38-43). The Bor heavy chain sequence is given at the top, whereas other sequences are given only at the position where they differ from the Bor sequence. All sequences are first aligned for maximum homology, and the residues identical to Bor are indicated by bars. The numbers after each sequence denote the number of amino acid residues which the respective sequence deviates from RF Bor heavy chain.

Vk genes from two separate Vk gene loci in the haploid human genome. Zachau and colleagues have characterized the human Vk gene locus extensively, and identified about 80 different Vk genes, spread over 3000 kb upstream of the Jk-Ck region, in the order of centromere- Vk- Jk- Ck- telomere on chromosome 2 (35,36). Detailed analysis of these genes revealed that they could be divided into two similar sets which probably were generated by a very recent gene duplication (36,37). In addition, two highly homologous VkI genes (termed Vb and Vb''), which encode an identical variable region amino acid sequence, were found to come from the different set of the duplicated Vk genes, and thus were non-allelic (37). In light of these observations, the exact relationship among the four currently isolated Vk genes remains unclear. To address this question will require both family and population analyses, that are currently in progress.

IV. DEFINING A Vh GENE FOR HUMAN RHEUMATOID FACTORS

Recently, Mageed et al., generated a murine monoclonal anti-CRI antibody (designated G6), which reacted with the heavy chains of many human monoclonal IgM RFs. Subsequently, Capra and colleagues showed that the heavy chains of two G6-positive RFs (i.e. Bor and Kas) were homologous to each other and to a rearranged Vh gene, termed 783 (Figure 3) (25). In addition, we noted that a Vh1 cDNA clone 51P1 differed from Bor and Kas by only 8 residues each (Figure 3) (38-41). Accordingly, we screened a human genomic library separately with both 783 and 51P1, and the strong positive clones were isolated and characterized by restriction mapping and sequence analysis. The results showed that one isolate contained a human Vh1 gene, designated Humhv1263, which was highly homologous to 51P1, and to 783 in the coding region, but not in the 5' flanking region (42).

The 783 gene was isolated from a chronic lymphocytic leukemia (CLL), termed LR (43), and its DNA sequence (designated Humighaa) was deposited by Ravetch and Leder in GenBank. The observation that Humhv1263 was highly homologous to Humighaa in the coding region, but not in the upstream flanking region suggested that there may be some sequence errors in the deposited sequence of Humighaa. Accordingly, we re-sequenced a 366 bp fragment (BamHI-BamHI) of the 783/Humighaa gene. We found that our DNA sequence of 783 differs from the deposited 783 sequence by 27 bases, and that the revised 783 sequence is identical to the 51P1 sequence, except one difference near the VD junction (Figure 3) (42). Since 783 and 51P1 were isolated from two unrelated individuals (38,43), these results indicated that, up to the A nucleotide at the amino acid position 98, the 783 sequence is likely to be the unmutated form of its corresponding germline Vh gene.

```
                                 M  E  F  G  L  S  W  L  F  L  V  A  I     -7
                   .         .         .         .         .         .
VH26      GGACTGAACAGAGAGAACTCACCATGGAGTTTGGGCTGAGCTGGCTTTTTCTTGTGGCTA   -124
30P1      ------------------------------------------------------------

            L  K                                                           -5
                   .         .         .         .         .         .
VH26      TTTTAAAAGGTAATTCATGGAGAAATAGAAAAATTGAGTGTGAATGGATAAGAGTGAGAG    -64
30P1      ---------...................................................

                                                              G  V  Q      -2
                   .         .         .         .         .         .
VH26      AAACAGTGGATACGTGTGGCAGTTTCTGACCAGGGTTTCTTTTTGTTTGCAGGTGTCCAG     -4
30P1      ....................................................--------

           C  E  V  Q  L  L  E  S  G  G  G  L  V  Q  P  G  G  S  L  R     19
              1    .         .         .         .         .         .
VH26      TGTGAGGTGCAGCTGTTGGAGTCTGGGGGAGGCTTGGTACAGCCTGGGGGGTCCCTGAGA     57
30P1      ------------------------------------------------------------
18/2      ...---------------------------------------------------------

           L  S  C  A  A  S  G  F  T  F  S  S  Y  A  M  S  W  V  R  Q     39
                   .         .         .   _____CDR1______  .         .
VH26      CTCTCCTGTGCAGCCTCTGGATTCACCTTTAGCAGCTATGCCATGAGCTGGGTCCGCCAG    117
30P1      ------------------------------------------------------------
18/2      ------------------------------------------------------------

           A  P  G  K  G  L  E  W  V  S  A  I  S  G  S  G  G  S  T  Y     59
                   .         .         .__________________________CDR2
VH26      GCTCCAGGGAAGGGGCTGGAGTGGGTCTCAGCTATTAGTGGTAGTGGTGGTAGCACATAC    177
30P1      ------------------------------------------------------------
18/2      ------------------------------------------------------------

           Y  A  D  S  V  K  G  R  F  T  I  S  R  D  N  S  K  N  T  L     79
          CDR2________________         .         .         .         .
VH26      TACGCAGACTCCGTGAAGGGCCGGTTCACCATCTCCAGAGACAATTCCAAGAACACGCTG    237
30P1      ------------------------------------------------------------
18/2      ------------------------------------------------------------

           Y  L  Q  M  N  S  L  R  A  E  D  T  A  V  Y  Y  C  A  K        98
                   .         .         .         .         .         .
VH26      TATCTGCAAATGAACAGCCTGAGAGCCGAGGACACGGCCGTATATTACTGTGCGAAAGAC    297
30P1      ---------------------------------------------------------/rearranged
18/2      ---------------------------------------------------------/rearranged
```

FIGURE 4. The nucleotide sequences of the VH26 gene, the cDNA 30P1 and the 18/2 Vh sequence, isolated from a 16/6-CRI positive anti-DNA antibody (38,48-50). The deduced amino acid sequence of VH26 is shown. Dots between the leader and leader' regions of the 30P1 sequence denote the gap which is deleted during mRNA processing. The CDR and conserved nucleotide sequences for splicing and rearrangement, including GT/AG, heptamer and nonamer, are marked.

When the deduced amino acid sequences of hv1263, 783 and all other reported human Vh1 genes were compared with the heavy chains of RFs Bor and Kas, 783 is the most closely related one. It differs from Kas and Bor by only 7 and 9 residues, respectively (Figure 3). In contrast, germline gene hv1263 differs from Kas and Bor by 11 and 12 residues, respectively; while all other Vh1 germline genes each differs from both RFs by 22-40 residues (Figure 3). Detailed molecular analyses of CRIs in mice reveal that variant antibody molecules deviate from their respective germline genes by up to 8 amino acid residues, and that the extent of somatic diversifications on the heavy chain and light chain of a variant antibody molecule is correlated to each other (44,45). The latter phenomena are called "parallel diversifications". A comparison of Bor and Kas light chains with all human Vk germline genes shows that both are encoded by Humkv325 with 2 and 5 amino acid substitutions, respectively. Combined, these data show that the putative "783 Vh gene" is the Vh gene for the heavy chains of Bor and Kas, and is the genetic basis for the G6 CRI.

V. MOLECULAR BASIS OF THE HUMAN ANTI-DNA ANTIBODY-ASSOCIATED 16/6 CRI

During the past decade, Schwartz, Stollar and their associates have studied intensively the anti-DNA antibodies in patients with systemic lupus erythematosus (SLE) (46-48). They analyzed a CRI, termed 16/6, that occurs in about 50% of patients with active SLE (46,47). To define the genetic basis of this CRI, the nucleotide sequence of heavy chain mRNA from hybridomas secreting 16/6-positive anti-DNA antibodies was determined. The results revealed that the Vh sequences of the 16/6-positive heavy chains were homologous to a human Vh germline gene, VH26 (48,49). They differ from the germline sequence by one amino acid residue at the protein level, and by two bases over a region of 294 bp at the DNA level. However, it was unclear whether the differences reflected somatic changes and/or allelic variation in the human Vh gene repertoire. Thus, we decided to isolated and characterized some Vh genes which are closely related to VH26.

In order to obtain a specific probe, we first sequenced a large segment of the VH26 gene. The results showed that our sequence of the VH26 gene differs from the reported VH26 sequence at four positions (50). When compared with the 16/6-positive Vh sequence from cell line 18/2, our VH26 sequence is identical in the entire Vh gene coding region (Figure 4). These data thus demonstrate that a human germline Vh gene encodes directly the heavy chain variable region of an anti-DNA antibody without any somatic mutation. In addition, the revised VH26 sequence shares 351/351 bp with another heavy chain cDNA sequence (30P1) that was isolated from fetal liver (38). Collectively, these results show that this autoantibody-associated Vh gene is conserved in outbred human populations.

VI. DISCUSSION

As reviewed here, idiotypic and molecular analyses of human monoclonal autoantibodies have led to the identification and characterization of 4 autoantibody-related Ig V genes: Humkv325, Humkv328, Vh783, and VH26. In particular, Humkv325 is shown to encode, with or without mutation, the light chains of various autoantibodies and one anti-virus antibody. All 4 V genes are conserved in outbred human populations. Others have similar observations that autoantibody-associated V genes are conserved in humans (48,51). Together, these observations indicate that human autoantibody-associated Ig V genes are preserved by the evolution pressure, and thus suggest that they may have some important physiological roles (16,42,50,51).

The fact that human autoantibody-associated Ig V genes are conserved stands in marked contrast to the reported Ig V gene polymorphisms in humans (52-54). To discern whether this human Ig V gene conservation is restricted only to autoantibody-associated V genes, we characterized some additional human V genes. Among them, one Vh3 gene, designated Humhv3033, contains a stop codon at the amino acid position 59, and thus is a pseudogene. When hv3033 was compared with all the reported human Vh3 nucleotide sequences, it was found that hv3033 is completely identical to the 2-3 Vh3 gene in a overlapped region of 422 bases, from positions -78 to 344 (Figure 5). Since this one pseudogene is also conserved in humans, it should be cautious in concluding that the human autoantibody-associated V gene conservation implies their physiological importance. Further investigation regarding the conservation of additional human V pseudogenes is required to clarify this issue.

Although at the gross level there is no unique restriction fragment length polymorphism in the Ig V genes of autoimmune mouse strains, these studies do not exclude the possibility that microscopic sequence variation in the *cis*-regulatory elements of some critical Ig V genes of autoimmune mice may predispose them to disease. Maniatis et al., demonstrated that a single base change in the beta-globin promoter region can decrease drastically the transcription level of beta-globin gene (55). In light of this observation, it is noteworthy that 2 of 6 bases that distinguish kv328h5 from kv328 are in the conserved pentadecanucleotide region (at positions -380 to -366), which was shown by Zachau and colleagues to be important in transcription of a human k light chain gene (56). A

```
                     .         .         .         .         .         .
hv3033      GGATAAGAGTGAGAGAAACAGTGGATACGTGTGGCAGTTTCTGACCAGGGTTTCTTTTTG   -19
2-3         ------------------------------------------------------------

                  G  V  Q  C  E  V  Q  L  V  E  S  G  G  G  L  V  Q  P     14
                     .        1.         .         .         .         .
hv3033      TTTGCAGGTGTCCAGTGTGAGGTGCAGCTGGTGGAGTCTGGGGGAGGCTTGGTACAGCCT    42
2-3         ------------------------------------------------------------

            G  G  S  L  R  L  S  C  A  A  S  G  F  T  F  S  Y  Y  Y  M     34
                     .         .         .         .      31_______CDR1
hv3033      GGGGGGTCCCTGAGACTCTCCTGTGCAGCCTCTGGATTCACCTTCAGTTACTACTACATG   102
2-3         ------------------------------------------------------------

            S  G  V  R  Q  A  P  G  K  G  L  E  W  V  G  F  I  R  N  K     54
        CDR1         .         .         .         .    50__________CDR2
hv3033      AGCGGGGTCCGCCAGGCTCCCGGGAAGGGGCTGGAATGGGTAGGTTTCATTAGAAACAAA   162
2-3         -NN---------------------------------------------------------

            A  N  G  G  T  T  E  *  T  T  S  V  K  G  R  F  T  I  S  R     74
            CDR2________________61________________68         .         .
hv3033      GCTAATGGTGGGACAACAGAATAGACCACGTCTGTGAAAGGCAGATTCACAATCTCAAGA   222
2-3         ------------------------------------------------------------

            D  D  S  K  S  I  T  Y  L  Q  M  K  S  L  K  T  E  D  T  A     94
                     .         .         .         .         .         .
hv3033      GATGATTCCAAAAGCATCACCTATCTGCAAATGAAGAGCCTGAAAACCGAGGACACGGCC   282
2-3         ------------------------------------------------------------

            V  Y  Y  C  S  R                                              100
                     .         .*7-mer*  .  23 bp spacer     .**9-mer**.
hv3033      GTGTATTACTGTTCCAGAGACACAGTGAGGGGAGGTCAGTGTGAGCCCGGACACAAACCT   342
2-3         ------------------------------------------------------------


                     .         .         .         .         .         .
hv3033      CCCTGCAGGGGCGCGCGGGGCCACCAGGGGGCGCTAGGGACCCACTGAGGGCGGGACAGG   402
2-3         --/// end of the published sequence


                     .         .         .         .         .         .
hv3033      AGCAGGTGCCGGGAGAGGTTTCCTTTCTCCTCAGCTGGAAAAGTCAGGTTTGTGTTTGCC   462
hv3033      GGACTCTGGAGCTTTCTAGGCTGTGACGTTTTATTACTTGTGTTTATTATGAATTTATTA   522
                     .         .         .         .         .         .
hv3033      TCGTTAGTATTTAAATTTTAGTAATTTAAAAATTATATATATATGTTTACACTTTAATGA   582
hv3033      AATAAGCATTCCTATTTGCACCGATTCTTCCAGAGTTTTATTAACATTTGTTGACGTCAG   642
                     .         .         .         .         .         .
hv3033      CAGCTACGAAGCTATAGGGACATAAATTTATAACCATAGAAAGATGTATAGGCCAGGCGC   702
hv3033      GGTGGCTCACGCATGTAATCCCAGCACGTTGGAAGCCATAGGTGGGTGATC            753
```

FIGURE 5. Conservation of the human Vh3 pseudogenes, Humhv3033 and 2-3 (41). The nucleotide and amino acid sequcnces of hv3033 are shown at the top. With the exception of two uncertain bases in 2-3, hv3033 is identical to 2-3 in an overlapped region of 422 bp. The CDR and the conserved heptamer and nonamer are marked.

comparison of these two Vk genes by an in vitro transcription assay shall reveal the significance, if any, of their microsequence difference, and could provide some clue toward understanding the role of Ig V gene repertoire in human autoantibody production.

It is clearly established that some monoclonal IgM antibodies against different autoantigens are encoded by Ig V genes without somatic mutation. However, it should be noted that most of these antibodies react with multiple antigens. In contrast, among 82 monoclonal Igs bearing the 3I CRI, that has been associated with the kappa light chains of anti-DNA antibodies in patients with SLE, reactivity with double stranded DNA was mainly found in IgG proteins (57). These experiments suggested that somatic changes were important in generating the 3I-positive anti-DNA antibodies. We have shown that the PSL3 CRI, but not the PSL2 CRI, is lacking on the IgM RF from patients with established rheumatoid arthritis (3). In mice, Shlomchik et al., found that mitogen-induced RFs, or RFs occurring during secondary immune responses in normal mice, were mainly of the IgM isotype and were probably encoded directly by germline V genes with no or little mutations (58). In contrast, spontaneously occurring RFs in autoimmune mice were mainly of the IgG isotype and contained many somatic changes due to antigen selection (59). Taken together, it can be concluded that somatic mutation, as well as the recruitment of multiple B cell clones, must contribute significantly toward the generation of both IgM and IgG autoantibodies in disease states. However, autoantibodies of IgM isotype, that may be found in both patients and normals, can be encoded by germline V genes with no or little somatic change.

In mice, studies of their Vh genes show that Vh genes of each different families are clustered together with minimal interspersion, and that the 7183 family locates most closely to the Jh locus (60,61). Moreover, it was found that Vh genes of the 7183 family were preferentially expressed during the early developmental stage (61,62), and were also preferentially used by antibodies reactive against self determinants (63-65). These data suggest that autoreactive clones arise early in ontogeny, and may contribute significantly toward generating the functional antibody repertoire.

In humans, Vh genes of different families are interspersed extensively (40,41). Recently, Perlmutter and coworkers found that human fetus preferentially express a restricted set of Vh genes (38). Among them, 2 (51P1, 20P3), 5 (56P1, 30P1, 38P1, 60P2, and 20P1), 1 (58P2) and 1 (15P1) genes belong, respectively, to the Vh1, 3, 4 and 6 families. As discussed earlier, 30P1 is identical to the revised sequence of the VH26 gene and to the heavy chain of an anti-DNA antibody (18/2);

and 51P1 is almost identical to the 783 Vh gene, which encodes the heavy chains of two RFs (48,50). Taken together, these findings indicate that, similar to murine studies, some human autoantibodies are encoded by a restricted set of Ig V genes which are expressed more frequently during early ontogenic development, and that such autoreactive antibodies may be of physiological importance. If substantiated, then it is the abnormal expression of these antibodies, in term of their quantity and quality, which is responsible for the pathology of various autoimmune diseases.

ACKNOWLEDGMENTS

I greatly appreciate the constant support and encouragement by Dr. D.A. Carson in my study of human autoantibodies, and his critical review of this manuscript. I gratefully acknowledge the significant contributions from my collaborators: Drs. J.D. Capra, J.J. Crowley, S. Fong, B. Frangione, F. Goni, T.J. Kipps, W.J. Koopman, M. Liu, M.M. Newkirk, D.L. Robbins, and R.E. Schrohenloher. I thank the excellent technical assistance of S. Sinha, and the secretarial assistance of Ms. Nancy Noon and the BCR Word Processing Center in the preparation of this manuscript.

REFERENCES

1. Carson, D. A., Chen, P. P., Fox, R. I., Kipps, T. J., Jirik, F., Goldfien, R. D., Silverman, G., Radoux, V., and Fong, S. (1987). Annu. Rev. Immunol. 5, 109.
2. Carson, D. A. (1985). In "Textbook of Rheumatology" (W. J. Kelley, E. D. Jr. Harris, S. Ruddy and C. B. Sledge, ed.), 2nd Ed., p. 664. W.B.Saunders, Philadelphia.
3. Chen, P. P., Fong, S., and Carson, D. A. (1987). Rheum. Dis. North Am. 13(3), 545.
4. Welch, M. J., Fong, S., Vaughan, J. H., and Carson, D. A. (1983). Clin. Exp. Immunol. 51, 299.
5. Coulie, P., and Van Snick, J. (1983). Eur. J. Immunol. 13, 895.
6. Nemazee, D. A., and Sato, V. L. (1983). J. Exp. Med. 158, 529.
7. Rajewsky, K., and Takemori, T. (1983). Annu. Rev. Immunol. 1, 569.
8. Rudikoff, S. (1983). Contemp. Top. Mol. Immunol. 9, 169.
9. Capra, J. D., and Fougereau, M. (1983). Immunol. Today 4, 177.

10. Kunkel, H. G., Agnello, V., Joslin, F. G., Winchester, R. J., and Capra, J. D. (1973). J. Exp. Med. 137, 331.
11. Kunkel, H. G., Winchester, R. J., Joslin, F. G., and Capra, J. D. (1974). J. Exp. Med. 139, 128.
12. Andrews, D. W., and Capra, J. D. (1981). Proc. Natl. Acad. Sci. USA 78, 3799.
13. Chen, P. P., Fong, S., Normansell, D., Houghten, R. A., Karras, J. G., Vaughan, J. H., and Carson, D. A. (1984). J. Exp. Med. 159, 1502.
14. Chen, P. P., Goni, F., Fong, S., Jirik, F., Vaughan, J. H., Frangione, B., and Carson, D. A. (1985). J. Immunol. 134, 3281.
15. Chen, P. P., Goni, F., Houghten, R. A., Fong, S., Goldfien, R., Vaughan, J. H., Frangione, B., and Carson, D. A. (1985). J. Exp. Med. 162, 487.
16. Chen, P. P., Fong, S., Goni, F., Silverman, G. J., Fox, R. I., Liu, M. -F., Frangione, B., and Carson, D. A. (1988). Springer Semin. Immunopathol. 10, 35.
17. Carson, D. A., and Fong, S. (1983). Mol. Immunol. 20, 1081.
18. Fong, S., Chen, P. P., Gilbertson, T. A., Fox, R. I., Vaughan, J. H., and Carson, D. A. (1985). J. Immunol. 135, 1955.
19. Chen, P. P., Albrandt, K., Orida, N. K., Radoux, V., Chen, E. Y., Schrantz, R., Liu, F. -T., and Carson, D. A. (1986). Proc. Natl. Acad. Sci. USA 83, 8318.
20. Chen, P. P., Albrandt, K., Kipps, T. J., Radoux, V., Liu, F-T., and Carson, D. A. (1987). J. Immunol. 139, 1727.
21. Radoux, V., Chen, P. P., Sorge, J. A., and Carson, D. A. (1986). J. Exp. Med. 164, 2119.
22. Pons-Estel, B., Goni, F., Solomon, A., and Frangione, B. (1984). J. Exp. Med. 160, 893.
23. Goni, F., Chen, P. P., Pons-Estel, B., Carson, D. A., and Frangione, B. (1985). J. Immunol. 135, 4073.
24. Newkirk, M., Chen, P. P., Carson, D. A., Posnett, B., and Capra, J. D. (1986). Mol. Immunol. 23, 239.
25. Newkirk, M. M., Mageed, R. A., Jefferis, R., Chen, P. P., and Capra, J. D. (1987). J. Exp. Med. 166, 550.
26. Agnello, V., Goni, F., Barnes, J. L., de la Vega, M. -T., and Frangione, B. (1987). J. Exp. Med. 165, 263.
27. Kabat, E. A., Wu, T. T., Reid-Miller, M., Perry, H., and Gottesman, K. S. (1987). Sequences of proteins of immunological interest. U.S. Dept. of Health and Human Services.
28. Newkirk, M. M., Gram, H., Heinrich, G. F., Ostberg, L., Capra, J. D., and Wasserman, R. L. (1988). J. Clin. Invest. 81, 1151.
29. Schrohenloher, R. E., and Koopman, W. J. (1986). Arthritis Rheum. 29, S28.

30. Crowley, J. J., Goldfien, R. D., Schrohenloher, R. E., Spiegelberg, H. L., Silverman, G. J., Mageed, R. A., Jefferis, R., Koopman, W. J., Carson, D. A., and Fong, S. (1988). J. Immunol. 140, 3411.
31. Capra, J. D., and Klapper, D. G. (1976). Scand. J. Immunol. 5, 677.
32. Jirik, F. R., Sorge, J., Fong, S., Heitzmann, J. G., Curd, J. G., Chen, P. P., Goldfien, R., and Carson, D. A. (1986). Proc. Natl. Acad. Sci. USA 83, 2195.
33. Chen, P. P., Robbins, D. L., Jirik, F. R., Kipps, T. J., and Carson, D. A. (1987). J. Exp. Med. 166, 1900.
34. Liu, M. -F., Robbins, D. L., Crowley, J. J., Sinha, S., Kozin, F., Kipps, T. J., Carson, D. A., and Chen, P. P. (1989). J. Immunol. 142, 688.
35. Klobeck, H., Zimmer, F., Combriato, G., and Zachau, H. G. (1987). Nucleic Acids Res. 15, 9655.
36. Lorenz, W., Straubinger, B., and Zachau, H. G. (1987). Nucleic Acids Res. 15, 9667.
37. Pech, M., Smola, H., Pohlenz, H-D, Straubinger, B., Gerl, R., and Zachau, H. G. (1985). J. Mol. Biol. 183, 291.
38. Schroeder Jr. , H. W., Hillson, J. L., and Perlmutter, R. M. (1987). Science 238, 791.
39. Takahashi, N., Noma, T., and Honjo, T. (1984). Proc. Natl. Acad. Sci. USA 81, 5194.
40. Kodaira, M., Kinashi, T., Umemura, I., Matsuda, F., Noma, T., Ono, Y., and Honjo, T. (1986). J. Mol. Biol. 190, 529.
41. Berman, J. E., Mellis, S. J., Pollock, R., Smith, C. L., Suh, H., Heinke, B., Kowal, C., Surti, U., Chess, L., Cantor, C. R., and Alt, F. W. (1988). EMBO J. 7, 727.
42. Chen, P. P., Liu, M. -F., Glass, C. A., Sinha, S., Kipps, T. J., and Carson, D. A. (1989). Arthritis Rheum. 32, 73.
43. Ravetch, J. V., Siebenlist, U., Korsmeyer, S., Waldmann, T., and Leder, P. (1981). Cell 27, 583.
44. Perlmutter, R. M., Crews, S. T., Klotz, J., Livant, D., Siu, J., and Hood, L. (1984). Ann. Immunol. (Inst. Pasteur) 135C, 83.
45. Gearhart, P. J. (1984). Ann. Immunol. (Inst. Pasteur) 135C, 137.
46. Shoenfeld, Y., Isenberg, D. A., Rauch, J., Madaio, M. P., Stollar, B. D., and Schwartz, R. S. (1983). J. Exp. Med. 158, 718.
47. Isenberg, D. A., Shoenfeld, Y., Madaio, M. P., Rauch, J., Reichlin, M., Stollar, B., and Schwartz, R. S. (1984). Lancet 2, 417.
48. Dersimonian, H., Schwartz, R. S., Barrett, K. J., and Stollar, B. D. (1987). J. Immunol. 139, 2496.
49. Matthyssens, G., and Rabbitts, T. H. (1980). Proc. Natl. Acad. Sci. USA 77, 6561.

50. Chen, P. P., Liu, M., Sinha, S., and Carson, D. A. (1988). Arthritis Rheum. 31, 1429.
51. Makar, R., Sanz, I., Thomas, J. W., and Capra, J. D. (1988). Ann. Immunol. (Inst. Pasteur) 139, 651.
52. Johnson, M. J., Natali, A. M., Cann, H. M., Honjo, T., and Cavalli-Sforza, L. L. (1984). Proc. Natl. Acad. Sci. USA 81, 7840.
53. Turnbull, I. F., Sriprakash, K. S., and Mathews, J. D. (1987). Immunogenetics 25, 193.
54. Turnbill, I., Bernard, O., Sriprakash, K. S., and Mathews, J. D. (1987). Immunogenetics 25, 184.
55. Maniatis, T., Goodbourn, S., and Fischer, J. A. (1987). Science 236, 1237.
56. Falkner, F. G., and Zachau, H. G. (1984). Nature 310, 71.
57. Davidson, A., Preud'Homme, J-L., Solomon, A., Chang, M-D. Y., Beede, S., and Diamond, B. (1987). J. Immunol. 138, 1515.
58. Shlomchik, M., Nemazee, D., Van Snick, J., and Weigert, M. (1987). J. Exp. Med. 165, 970.
59. Shlomchik, M. J., Marshak-Rothstein, A., Wolfowicz, C. B., Rothstein, T. L., and Weigert, M. G. (1987). Nature 328, 805.
60. Brodeur, P. H., and Riblet, R. (1984). Eur. J. Immunol. 14, 922.
61. Alt, F. W., Blackwell, T. K., DePinho, R. A., Reth, M. G., and Yancopoulos, G. D. (1986). Immunol. Rev. 89, 5.
62. Perlmutter, R. M., Kearney, J. F., Chang, S. P., and Hood, L. E. (1985). Science 227, 1597.
63. Monestier, M., Manheimer-Lory, A., Bellon, B., Painter, C., Dang, H., Talal, N., Zanetti, M., Schwartz, R., Pisetsky, D., Kuppers, R., Rose, N., Brochier, J., Klareskog, L., Holmdahl, R., Erlanger, B., Alt, F., and Bona, C. (1986). J. Clin. Invest. 78, 753.
64. Holmberg, D. (1987). Eur. J. Immunol. 17, 399.
65. Bona, C. A. (1988). Arthritis Rheum. 6, 327.

MOLECULAR CHARACTERIZATION OF HUMAN ANTI-DNA ANTIBODIES

Katherine A. Siminovitch[1]

Department of Medicine
Toronto Western Hospital
University of Toronto
Toronto, Ontario, Canada

I. INTRODUCTION

It is now well established that the presence of antibodies directed against self-components represents a major feature of a broad spectrum of human disease. Not surprisingly, therefore, the study of the immunochemical properties and the clinical relevance of such antibodies has received considerable attention over the past few decades. Particular emphasis has been placed on anti-DNA antibodies which are virtually a hallmark of the prototype autoimmune disease, systemic lupus erythematosus (SLE). The tendency of anti-DNA antibodies to fluctuate with disease activity and to deposit in areas of tissue damage, has led to the suggestion that such molecules represent not only disease markers, but may contribute directly to tissue injury in lupus. More recently, however, it has become increasingly apparent that anti-DNA immune responses occur in the absence of concomitant disease and can, in fact, be detected or elicited in normal mice or healthy individuals (1,2). The existence of naturally occurring anti-DNA antibodies implies that the genetic elements encoding autoreactive immune

[1]Supported by Grant No. 7-288-86 from the Arthritis Society of Canada and by an Ontario Ministry of Health, Career Scientist Award and the Canadian Life & Health Insurance Association Medical Scholarship.

responses are present in the general "healthy" population and are not restricted to individuals with autoimmune disease, a hypothesis which has been borne out by molecular studies of rheumatoid factors (3,4). Determining whether these physiologic or natural autoantibodies can be distinguished serologically or structurally from disease-associated or "pathogenic" autoantibodies, as well as their relevance to immune regulation and repertoire generation, has emerged as a central issue to developing an understanding of autoimmunity.

The recent generation of both murine and human monoclonal antibodies expressing autoreactive specificities has provided extremely useful reagents for probing the genetic mechanisms underlying the formation of autoantibodies, both natural and disease-associated. Over the past few years, my research has centered largely on human natural autoimmune responses and, in particular, the structural and immunochemical characterization of monoclonal autoantibodies of normal (non-autoimmune) tonsillar origin. As previously reported by my colleagues (2,5) and others, these natural autoantibodies exhibit antigen reactivities and idiotypic specificities closely resembling those of SLE patient anti-DNA antibodies. Sharing of these serologic properties implies structural relatedness of natural and lupus-associated autoantibodies and their utilization of common genetic elements. To directly address this issue as well as others concerning the genetic basis of anti-DNA immune responses, we initiated structural analyses of the genes encoding monoclonal autoantibodies secreted by selected natural hybrid clones. In this paper, I describe results in which the heavy (V_H) and light (V_L) chain variable region nucleotide sequences of the anti-DNA antibody secreted by a representative natural hybrid clone, KIM4.6, are related to corresponding sequences previously reported for four other human anti-DNA antibodies. By comparing the V gene elements used by these antibodies, insights are provided into the V gene repertoire of the anti-DNA immune response and the structural basis for expression of DNA-binding specificity. Our data indicate that anti-DNA immune responses are genetically heterogeneous and suggest that the genetic elements and molecular mechanisms which engender these reponses are essentially the same among natural and pathogenic autoantibodies.

II. VARIABLE REGION GENES ENCODING ANTI-DNA IMMUNE RESPONSES

A. Genetic Diversity of V_H and V_L Genes Used by Anti-DNA Antibodies

Among the many insights gained by structural analysis of V region genes has been the realization that expression of the available V gene repertoire can be non-stochastic and that restricted patterns of V_H and V_L gene utilization occur consistently within certain contexts. A skewing of the expressed B cell repertoire, for example, toward use of the most 3′ located V_H genes has been observed in murine (6) and human (7) foetal pre-B cells and has been ascribed to early ontogenic restriction of the immune repertoire and possible developmental programming of V_H gene rearrangement. Genetic restriction also occurs in many immune responses, particularly those involving haptenic antigens, although this finding most likely reflects stringency of the structural requirements for antigen binding. Recent data from numerous studies which show restrictive kappa variable gene usage among rheumatoid factors (3,4), and possible preferential utilization of 3′ mapping V_H gene families in murine anti-DNA antibodies (8,9), are particularly intriguing with respect to the elucidation of the genetic basis for autoimmune responses. These data provide incentive for further investigation of V gene usage in specific autoimmune responses and prompted our comparison of V_H and V_L genes employed among five human anti-DNA antibodies.

Among our natural anti-DNA antibodies, the IgM lambda autoantibody secreted by the normal tonsillar-derived KIM4.6 hybridoma (2), was selected for these analyses because it represents a prototype autoantibody which was used to define a cross-reactive idiotype found frequently in lupus sera and on paraproteins from patients with B lineage malignancies (5). Similarly, a second anti-DNA antibody considered in our analysis, the lupus-associated 18/2 IgMk monoclonal autoantibody, expresses a public idiotypic marker which occurs on both the anti-DNA antibodies of lupus sera as well as on Waldenstrom's and myeloma paraproteins (10). For these comparisons we have also included the IgMk antibody of another lupus-derived cell line, 21/28 (10), an IgMk antibody secreted by a leprosy patient-derived clone, 8E10 (10), and one other natural autoantibody, an IgMk protein secreted by clone C6B2 (11). We hypothesized that examination of the V region elements of these anti-DNA antibodies would provide information pertaining not only to the structural basis of specificity but also with regard to the sequences which influence idiotype expression.

Sequence comparisons of the V_H genes encoding the five anti-DNA antibodies revealed their use of V_H genes from three of the six major V_H germ-line gene families described most recently by Berman and Alt et al. (12). As detailed elsewhere (13), the KIM4.6 rearranged V_H segment (shown in figure 1) is identical in nucleotide sequence with a germ-line V_H gene, designated V_H 1.9 III, and assigned to the V_H3 gene family (12). The V_H gene expressed in hybridoma 18/2 (figure 1) exhibits 90% nucleotide sequence similarity with that of KIM4.6, reflecting their derivation from the same V_H gene family, V_H3. By contrast, a V_H1 gene segment is used in the heavy chains secreted by 21/28 and 8E10 and the C6B2 antibody contains a V_H gene from the

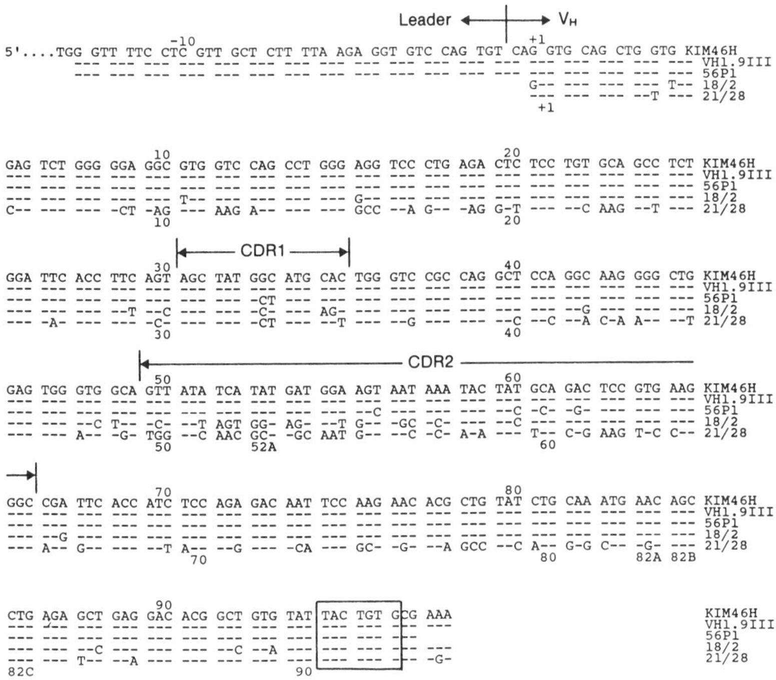

Figure 1. Nucleotide sequences of the rearranged 56P1, 18/2 and 21/28 V_H gene segments and the germ-line $V_H1.9III$ gene compared to the $KIM4.6V_H$. 56P1 is a foetal-derived and 18/2 and 21/28 are lupus-derived clones. The dashes indicate nucleotides identical to those in the $KIM4.6V_H$.

recently delineated V_H4 family (14). Therefore, five anti-DNA antibodies for which sequence data can be compared use four different V_H genes belonging to three different V_H families.

Just as the anti-DNA antibodies produced by these hybridomas contain a variety of V_H gene segments, heterogeneity is also evident with regard to their use of heavy chain joining (J_H) genes (Table I). The KIM4.6 antibody has been shown previously (13) to use the J_H6 gene segment, whereas 18/2 uses the J_H5 germ-line gene (10), 21/28 and 8E10 use J_H4 (10) and the C6B2 V_H recombined to a J_H3 segment (11). Thus four of the six functional human J_H germ-line segments appear in this small sample of antibodies.

Table I. Genetic characteristics of five monoclonal IgM anti-DNA antibodies

Clone[a]		V_H gene family	J_H	V_L subtype and family
KIM4.6	(13)	3	6	λ1
18/2	(10)	3	5	k1
21/28	(10)	1	4	k2
8E10	(10)	1	4	k[b]
C6B2	(11)	4	3	k[b]

[a] Reference sources for sequence data are indicated in parentheses.
[b] Information on V gene family not available.

Comparisons of the light chains employed in the anti-DNA antibodies (Table I) again reveals diversity with regard to V gene usage. The KIM4.6 antibody differs from the others in using a lambda light chain and of the four kappa secreting antibodies, at least two employ V_k genes from different V_k families (15). Previous studies in our lab indicate a correlation between the use of a λI V gene segment and expression of an anti-DNA defined specific idiotype by the KIM4.6 and other antibodies and suggest that V_L gene sequences play a major role in the formation of this idiotypic determinant (13).

Taken together, the sequence data indicate that human anti-DNA immune responses are genetically heterogeneous and that several different combinations of V_H and V_L segments can encode DNA-binding specificity. While further sequence information is required to ascertain the full extent of diversity in this autoantibody response, the present conclusion is consistent with the results of more extensive analyses in the murine system (16). The latter data also indicate a lack of obvious correlation between V gene utilization and expression of anti-DNA autoreactivity.

B. Preferential V_H Gene Utilization and Anti-DNA Antibodies

While human anti-DNA antibodies appear heterogeneous with respect to V gene usage, in considering the limited amount of available sequence data pertaining to this response, some bias in V gene selection cannot be excluded. Restricted V_k gene utilization in both murine and human rheumatoid factors has been well-documented (3,4) and, based on their frequent use of V_H genes from the 7183 and Q52 V_H gene families, preferential use of specific V_H genes has been postulated to occur in anti-DNA antibodies of MRL-lpr/lpr mice (8). The suggestion of non-random selection of genes from these particular families is intriguing as they represent the most J_H-proximal gene families and their preferential rearrangement has been previously observed among foetal pre-B cells (6). In this context, it is noteworthy that both the natural KIM4.6 and the lupus-associated 18/2 anti-DNA antibodies utilize V_H genes which closely resemble gene segments found in an unusually high proportion of the rearranged alleles in human foetal B cells (7). The KIM4.6V_H differs from one such segment, 56P1, by only five nucleotides, while the sequence of the 18/2 V_H is identical with a second foetal-associated V_H segment, 30P1 (7). A foetal pattern of V_H gene usage in anti-DNA antibodies might reflect their derivation from an immature population of B cells or alternatively may represent the consequence of overly-rapid expansion of the preimmune repertoire due to the breakdown of regulatory mechanisms which normally shape the expressed B cell repertoire. While proof of this hypothesis requires more extensive information on V_H gene usage in human anti-DNA antibodies as well as other immune responses, if verified, the finding of foetal-like restriction of autoimmune responses would have important implications for defining the processes which lead to pathogenic versus normal evolution of anti-DNA immune responses.

C. Germ-line V_H Genes in IgM Anti-DNA Antibodies

The relative contribution of germ-line and somatic events to the evolution of anti-DNA immune responses represents another issue of importance to understanding the genetic origin of natural anti-DNA antibodies and their relationship to disease-associated autoantibodies. Somatic mutation has been demonstrated in IgG anti-DNA autoantibodies of autoimmune mice (17), and it has been argued by some that mutation events might be a prerequisite for expression of DNA-binding properties or might render these autoantibodies "pathogenic". The former supposition is clearly incorrect as both the KIM4.6 and 18/2 anti-DNA antibodies are encoded by non-mutated V_H genes. However, determination of the extent to which somatic mutation occurs among human anti-DNA antibodies and how such mutation affects their role in disease pathogenesis will require sequence analysis of DNA-binding antibodies of the IgG isotype, since the latter are considered the most relevant with regard to tissue damage in lupus.

The finding that several V_H genes derived from different individuals are identical in nucleotide sequence is somewhat surprising considering the high level of V_H polymorphism found among mouse strains. Similar observations have, however, been reported by Sanz and Capra (18) based on their analysis of V_H gene usage in several human autoantibodies. The preservation of these V_H genes in outbred populations may simply reflect a relative lack of polymorphism of human V_H genes or may indicate an important physiologic role for the V_H genes which are used in autoimmune responses.

III. THE STRUCTURAL BASIS FOR DNA-BINDING SPECIFICITY

A. Relatedness of the V_H Subregions of Anti-DNA Antibodies

One of our objectives in comparing anti-DNA antibody primary sequences was to ascertain the structural basis for the binding properties of these antibodies. Data from X-ray crystallographic analyses of antibodies (19) have implicated the heavy chain hypervariable or complementarity determining regions (CDRs) in the generation of the antigen-combining site. This is supported by the finding in a number of antigenic systems of highly restricted usage of V region elements and conservation of the V_H CDR primary sequences among antibodies which share specificities. Thus, despite the heterogeneity of V_H gene usage in the anti-DNA antibodies, in an attempt to localize sites which might engender antigen binding and/or specificity, we have analyzed the relatedness of their subsegments. To this end, the deduced amino acid sequences for each of the KIM4.6V_H subregions (two complementarity determining, CDR, and three framework, FR regions) have been compared in terms of percent homologies with those of the other human as well as murine anti-DNA antibodies, in addition to antibodies with other specificities.

As can be discerned from the eight representative examples presented in Table II, the KIM4.6V_H subsegments are no more similar to those of the other human anti-DNA antibodies (exemplified by 18/2, C6B2 and 21/28) than to those comprising other V_H3-encoded antibodies. The IgM paraprotein CAM (20), for example, shares more CDR residues with the KIM4.6V_H than do any of the DNA-binding antibodies. Although not shown here, this was true for a number of other V_H3-encoded myeloma proteins. Similarly, segmental comparisons of the human KIM 4.6V_H with the deduced amino acid sequences encoding the V_H segments of murine anti-DNA antibodies, represented in the table by MRLDNAIO (21), and U4 (22), reveal no greater CDR1 and CDR2 sequence similarities than are detected in comparisons with murine antibodies encoding other specificities which utilize V_H genes from families related to V_H3. The murine monoclonal antibody, NL-1 (23), for example, which is V_H7183-encoded, exhibits greater overall CDR homology (73%) with KIM4.6 than do the human anti-DNA antibodies (50-67%), yet the NL-1 specificity is directed against a tumour-related cell membrane protein, the common acute lymphoblastic leukemia antigen. While it is possible that antibodies, such as CAM or NL-1, have DNA-binding specificity which might account for their CDR sequence similarities to KIM4.6, this seems unlikely, since the data in Table 1 are representative of an analysis which includes data from all previously reported V_H genes.

TABLE II. Amino Acid Homology Between the KIM4.6V_H and Eight other Antibody V_H Subregions

		Percent Homology[a]						
Segments	Family	FR1[b]	CDR1[c]	FR2	CDR2	FR3	FRs	CDRs
HUMAN								
18/2	3	87	60	93	69	100	93	67
CAM	3	93	60	93	75	88	91	68
POM	3	87	40	100	44	76	88	42
C6B2	4	47	40	79	60	63	63	50
21/28	1	60	80	71	24	63	65	52
MURINE								
MRLDNA10	J558	57	40	64	24	56	59	32
NL-1	7183	83	80	93	65	81	86	73
U4	S107	87	40	86	35	78	84	22

[a] Values represent summation of the number of amino acid similarities between the five V_H regions of KIM4.6V_H and each of the other V_H genes divided by the number of amino acids in each region. The names of the amino acid sequences are listed on the left.

[b] FR, framework region

[c] CDR, complementarity determining region

Overall, these data indicate relatively little correlation between primary CDR1 and CDR2 sequence and expression of DNA-binding specificity, and imply that residues other than, or at least in addition to, those contained in the first two V_H CDRs must be involved in defining this reactivity. Not surprisingly, the same conclusion is evident from framework region comparisons. As shown in Table II, for example, there is no significant difference in the percent of homology between the KIM4.6V_H FRs and either the DNA-binding 18/2 V_HFRs (93%) or the V_HFRs encoding the unrelated CAM myeloma (91%) and POM rheumatoid factor (88%) heavy chain proteins.

Finally, alignment of the V_H gene sequences discussed above reveals that the KIM4.6 as well as the murine and other human anti-DNA antibodies all have a tyrosine residue at position 32 or 33 in CDR1 and at position 59 in CDR2. KIM4.6 and 18/2 display an additional tyrosine residue at position 58. Since tyrosine residues are thought to facilitate antigen-binding (24), their conservation at these positions among anti-DNA antibodies may be of some functional significance. It is unlikely, however, that these residues are relevant to specificity in anti-DNA antibodies, as they can also be found at these positions in antibodies of different specificities. Thus, it appears that no simple correlation exists between V_H genes, their subregion sequences and anti-DNA reactivity.

B. Diversity Gene Usage in Anti-DNA Antibodies

In contrast to the results obtained by V_H segment and V_H subregion comparisons between the anti-DNA antibodies, a striking structural feature emerges from examination of the diversity (D) gene segments (figure 2A). Although varying both in length and nucleotide sequence, the CDR3 regions of four of the five DNA-binding antibodies contain a conserved core of sixteen nucleotides and appear to have arisen from a common germ-line D segment, designated DXP'1 (25). The leprosy-associated 8E10 antibody represents an exception and contains an entirely different D segment (10). The use of the DXP'1 gene in four of five anti-DNA antibodies is intriguing, particularly in the context of recent evidence indicating that the human D_H germ-line genes are highly complex (25). Determination of whether human anti-DNA antibodies are genetically restricted with regard to D gene usage will require more information on D gene utilization in both anti-DNA and other immune responses, but demonstration that such restriction does occur would implicate the CDR3 segment in defining DNA-binding specificity.

Since little is known with regard to correlations between D segment utilization and specific immune responses in humans, the human anti-DNA antibody D segments have also been compared with those employed in murine antibodies. Interestingly, the translated amino acid sequence of the 16 base pair core conserved among the human autoantibodies (figure 2B), although actually expressed in a different reading frame in C6B2 shares an identical four amino acid stretch, Tyr-Tyr-Gly-Ser, with the murine anti-DNA antibody, U4, as well as a murine germ-line D segment, DFL16.1 (26).

A.

```
          Val Arg Glu Tyr Tyr Tyr Gly Ser Gly Thr Thr Thr Lys Arg Gly Leu Thr
KIM46H    GTA AGG GAG TAT TAC TAT GGT TCG GGG ACT ACT ACT AAA CGG GGG CTC ACA

DXP'1               - --- --- --- --- --- --- -G- TA- TA- --C

18/2      -GG CAA -T- -TG --- --- --- --- --- -G- TA-
21/28           - --  GG- --- --- --- --- --- -GC
C6B2        G --- AGC A-- --- --- --- --- --- -T- TA- TT- CTG G-- CTT T-G -T- TC

U4                        --- --C --- AGT A-C
B1.8              T-C G-- --- --- --- AGT A-C
DFL16.1            TT --- --- --C --- AGT A-C
```

B.

```
KIM46H      E  Y | Y  Y  G  S | G

DXP'1          - | -  -  -  - |
18/2        V  L | -  -  -  - | -
21/28          G | -  -  -  - | -
C6B2           N | -  -  -  - | -
U4               | -  -  -  - | -
B1.8        Y  D | -  -  -  - | S
DFL16.1        - | -  -  -  - | S
```

Figure 2. Diversity segments of human anti-DNA antibodies 18/2, C6B2 and 21/28 and germ-line gene DXP'1 and murine antibodies U_4 (anti-DNA) and B1.8 (anti-NP) and germline gene DFL16.1 compared to the KIM4.6D_H. A. The nucleotide sequences are aligned to maximize homology. Dashes indicate nucleotide identity to KIM4.6 and a conserved 16 base pair core is shown in between the lines. B. The deduced amino acid sequences corresponding to the conserved core four amino acid residues.

The latter D segment is used almost exclusively in a number of murine anti-hapten responses, including that directed against 4-hydroxy 3 nitrophenylacetyl (NP), an immunogen with which some monoclonal anti-DNA antibodies cross-react (27). Thus the murine NP-binding B1.8 antibody expresses a D segment with the same four amino acid stretch conserved among the anti-DNA antibody CDRs (27).

Polyreactivity of anti-DNA antibodies is a well recognized phenomenon, but the structural basis for binding both a spectrum of autoantigens as well as exogenous antigens, such as the NP hapten, is poorly understood. The pattern of cross-reactivity can be distinctly different among different monoclonal anti-DNA antibodies, and based on this finding as well as data from competitive binding studies (27), these cross reactivities appear to reflect immunochemical specificity and suggest sharing of certain epitopes among seemingly unrelated antigens. While the nature of the epitope shared by DNA and a synthetic hapten such as NP is unclear, the finding that human anti-DNA antibodies utilize a specific D segment which appears to be particularly important in defining NP-binding in anti-NP antibodies as well as the DNA-binding specificity of anti-DNA antibodies, argues strongly that the cross-reactivity reflects a response to an antigenic determinant shared by DNA and NP. In a sense, these findings are analagous to the observed utilization of the identical V_H segments to encode antigen binding sites in apparently unrelated immune responses, such as to GAT and alprenolol (28). Although more extensive genetic analysis of human anti-DNA antibodies are required to verify the role of the D segment in determining antigenic specificity in anti-DNA antibodies, these data provide a structural basis for the cross-reactivity of anti-DNA antibodies with the hapten NP and imply their origins from the same germ-line elements encoding anti-NP reactivity.

IV. SUMMARY

In an attempt to elucidate the molecular mechanisms involved in the development of autoimmune disease, we have used monoclonal anti-DNA antibodies as a model system for investigating the genetic origins and structural basis of human autoimmune responses. Comparison of V gene utilization in five human anti-DNA antibodies reveals their use of a variety of V_H and V_L gene segments, suggesting that anti-DNA immune responses are genetically heterogeneous. Analysis of the variation between the anti-DNA antibody V_H gene subregion sequences and corresponding sequences of unrelated antibodies indicates relatively little correlation between primary CDR1 and CDR2 sequence and expression of DNA-binding specificity. In contrast, the use of the same germ-line diversity segment, DXP'1, by four of five human DNA-binding antibodies, suggests an important role for the heavy chain CDR3 segment in defining antigen-selectivity of anti-DNA antibodies and provides a molecular explanation for their frequently observed cross-reactivity with the NP hapten. Finally, based on the present analysis, it appears that anti-DNA antibodies, while diverse in terms of V gene utilization, may exhibit a bias toward rearrangement of V_H genes that are over-represented in the foetal immune repertoire. This pattern of V gene usage among anti-DNA antibodies suggests that anti-DNA immune responses originate in the normal preimmune repertoire, as is consistent with their idiotypic connectivity to paraproteins and the hypothesis that autoreactivity plays a major role in shaping the normal immune repertoire.

ACKNOWLEDGMENTS

It is a pleasure to acknowledge the assistance of P. Kwong, V. Misener, E. Cairns and P. Ip and to thank D. Bell for providing KIM4.6.

REFERENCES

1. Dighiero, G., Lymberi, P., Holmberg, D., et al. (1985). J. Immunol. 134, 765.
2. Cairns, E., Block, J., and Bell, D.A. (1984). J. Clin. Invest. 74, 880.
3. Shlomchik, M., Nemazee, D., van Snick, J., and Weigert, M. (1987). J. Exp. Med. 165, 970.
4. Carson, D.A., Chen, P.P., Kipps, T.J., et al. (1987). Arth. Rheum. 30, 1321.
5. Bell, D.A., Cairns, E., Cikalo, K., et al. (1987). J. Rheum. 14, 127.
6. Yancopoulos, G.D., Desiderio, S.V., Paskind, M., et al. (1984). Nature 311, 727.
7. Schroeder, H.W., Hilson, J.L., and Perlmutter, R.M. (1987). Science 238, 791.
8. Trepicchio, W., and Barrett, K.J. (1987). J. Immunol. 138, 2323.
9. Monestier, M., Manheimer-Lory, A., Bellon, B., et al. (1986). J. Clin. Invest. 78, 753.
10. Dersimonian, H., Schwartz, R.S., Barrett, K.J., and Stollar, B.D. (1987). J. Immunol. 139, 2496.
11. Hoch, S., Schwaber, J. (1987). J. Immunol. 139, 1689.
12. Berman, J.E., Mellis, S.J., Pollack, R., et al. (1988). Embo. J. 7, 727.
13. Cairns, E., Kwong, P.C., Misener, V., et al. (1988). Submitted manuscript.
14. Lee, K.H., Matsuda, F., Kinashi, T., et al. (1987). J. Mol. Biol. 195, 761.
15. Atkinson, P.M., Lampman, G.W.,Furie, B.C., et al. (1985). J. Clin. Invest. 75, 1138.
16. Kofler, R., Dixon, F.J., and Theofilopoulos, A.N. (1987). Imm. Today 8, 374.

17. Shlomchik, M.J., Aucoin, A.H., Pisetsky, D.S., and Weigert, M.G. (1987). Proc. Natl. Acad. Sci. USA 84, 9150.
18. Sanz, I., and Capra, J.D. (1988). J. Immunol. 140, 3283.
19. Saul, F.A., Amzel, L.M., and Poljack, R.J. (1978). J. Biol. Chem. 253, 585.
20. Lehman, D.W., and Putnam, F.W. (1980). Proc. Natl. Acad. Sci. USA 77, 3239.
21. Kofler, R., Noonan, D.J., Levy, D.E. et al. (1985). J. Exp. Med. 161, 805.
22. Giusti, A.M., Chien, N.C., Zack, D.J. et al. (1987). Proc. Natl. Acad. Sci. USA 84, 2926.
23. Kudo, A., Nishimura, Y., and Watanabe, T. (1985). J. Immunol. 135, 642.
24. Cebra, J.J., Koo, P.H., and Ray, A. (1974). Science 186, 263.
25. Ichihara, Y., Abe, M., Yasui, H., et al. (1988). Eur. J. Immunol. 18, 649.
26. Landolfi, N.E., Capra J.D., and Tucker, P.W. (1986). J. Immunol. 137, 362.
27. Zouli, M.P., Migliorini, P., and Stollar, D.B. (1987). Eur. J. Immunol. 17, 509.
28. Nahmias, C., Strosberg, D., and Emorine, L. J. (1988). J. Immunol. 140, 1304.

FROM IDIOTYPIC EXPRESSION OF LUPUS ANTI-DNA ANTIBODIES TO DIVERSIFICATION OF Ig VARIABLE REGION GENES

Moncef ZOUALI[1,2]

Department of Biochemistry, Tufts University, Medical School, Boston, MA 02111

At the end of the XIX century, while the concept of self-recognition was foreseen by Metchnikoff and demonstrated in experimental animals by Metalkinoff, Ehrlich's competing view maintained that the immune system does not have the potential to react against its own components. This dogma, also known as the suggestive term of "Horror Autotoxicus" prevailed for many decades. However, with the passing of time it has been challenged by many experimental findings which led to the realization that autoreactivity is of central importance for the immune system. There is strong evidence that self-recognition and self-non-self-discrimination play important roles in regulation of the immune system : T cells are selected for self-MHC restriction, B cells from normal individuals express receptors for autoantigens, and immunoglobulins isolated from normal persons have been shown to bind autoantigens. According to this emerging view, autoimmune diseases would result from an exaggerated expression of events that occur normally within the immune system.

Systemic lupus erythematosus (SLE) is an autoimmune disease associated with the presence of a wide variety of autoantibodies, including antibodies to DNA, RNA, ribonucleoproteins and histones. Despite considerable efforts, only a few aspects of SLE are clearly known. It is generally accepted that anti-DNA antibodies are involved, at least in part, in the pathogenesis of the disease, that assays of serum antibodies to DNA improve the diagnosis, and that immunosuppressive drugs and plasmapheresis are useful for the treatment. Advances in the study of the binding specificity of murine and human anti-DNA

---

1 Supported by a National Institutes of Health John F. Fogarty International Award, and by a Senior Research Research Fulbright Grant

2 Present address : Immunogénétique Cellulaire, Institut Pasteur, 28 rue du Docteur Roux, 75724 Paris Cédex 15, France

antibodies has permitted much greater definition of the epitopes recognized (reviewed in ref. 1). Progress in cellular immunology is allowing more incisive studies of the clonal interactions involved in anti-DNA hyperproduction.

However two major aspects of SLE remain mysterious : how is the hyperautoimmune response initiated and sustained ? How can this abnormal production of autoantibodies be specifically suppressed ? There are multiple approaches to this problem. They include examining genetic -MHC- factors, abnormalities stemming from malfunction of the immune system, elements related to pathogens and environmental agents, abnormal expression of self components, and changes associated with physiological factors such as aging and hormones. In this communication, the view that analysis of clonal and molecular diversity of anti-DNA antibodies may lead to a better understanding of the mechanisms responsible for the development of this disease will be adopted.

ANTI-DNA IDIOTYPIC RECURRENCY

Idiotopes represent molecular finger-prints of the variable region of antibody molecules, and as such, they offer unique probes to explore the diversity of anti-DNA antibodies. Initially, the availability of experimental models of SLE in various inbred strains of mice allowed significant progress in this respect. Hybridomas constructed from the splenocytes of lupus-prone mice were used to build a library of autoantibodies. Such anti-DNA antibodies, which exhibit a pattern of paratope reactivity similar to human lupus antibodies, were reported to share cross-reactive idiotopes (2,3). It was then found that human polyclonal (4,6) and monoclonal (7,8) anti-DNA antibodies express a restricted set of idiotopes. Even more significant was the demonstration that this anti-DNA idiotypic recurrency crosses the species --common idiotypic determinants were described on murine and human (9,10), and on canine and murine (11) antibodies to DNA.

An intriguing open question relates to the mechanism responsible for this apparent idiotypic dominance among lupus anti-DNA antibodies. It seems conceivable that this phenomenon is mediated by idiotype anti-idiotype interactions.However it might be explained just as well by preferential rearrangements of V genes. Alternatively, antigen-driven selection could account for the expression of a selected repertoire. Future experiments will certainly resolve this important issue. In evolutionary terms, these observations showing that a restricted idiotypic repertoire is used in response to phylogenetically highly conserved epitopes on the DNA molecule suggest that ancestral V genes have been evolutionarily selected for this autoantibody response.

An important issue stemming from auto-antibody idiotypic cross-reactivity relates to the functional relevance of anti-DNA recurrent idiotopes. Shared idiotypy among paratopically related and unrelated antibodies allows connection of lymphocyte clones that are individually specific for structurally similar and distinct epitopes. This phenomenon is reminiscent of the network concept formulated by Jerne (12). According to this hypothesis, the immune system may be regarded as comprising a series of idiotypic interactions between many cell types through complementary variable region receptors which dynamically stimulate and regulate clonal expansion. This innovative view has been supported by several lines of evidence (reviewed in ref. 13). This autoantibody idiotypic recurrency may reflect an important regulatory function for immune network-mediated regulation of the autoimmune response. Support for this notion comes from experimental evidence accumulated in various systems. First, auto anti-idiotypic clones against self-epitopes are detectable in the normal human repertoire (14,15). Second, when anti-idiotype-containing human immunoglobulins isolated from normal blood donors are injected in patients with autoimmune disorders, clinical improvement and/or decrease in autoantibody titres have been reported in idiopathic autoimmune thrombocytopenic purpura, in autoimmune neutropenia, autoimmune red cell aplasia, myasthenia gravis, chronic inflammatory demyelinating neuropathy, and in anti-factor VIII autoimmunization (16). Third, anti-idiotypes to anti-DNA autoantibodies are present in SLE (17-19) and even more convincingly a reciprocal behaviour of anti-DNA antibody oscillatory levels and of the corresponding autologous anti-idiotype was observed (18).

Among the various implications of this high idiotypic recurrency, attention has been paid to the potential use of idiotypic manipulation as a specific means of autoimmune modulation. However the applicability of this strategy has been challenged by other observations. For example, immunoglobulins from normal individuals express autoantibody-related idiotopes, thus suggesting that cross-reactive idiotope-carrying antibodies and self-binding antibodies are overlapping populations, and that autoantibody related genes are not restricted to autoimmune conditions (8,13,20). Other results indicate that administration of anti-idiotypes to autoimmune mice may produce opposite effects : suppression (21) or exacerbation (22) of the anti-DNA idiotype. In several systems, anti-idiotypic antibodies carrying the internal images of antigen were shown to mimic the effects of the nominal antigen (23). These observations, together with other results, give rise to cautious optimism with regard to the potential use of passive anti-idiotypic immunity for medical purposes in autoimmune conditions (24).

Another implication of the phenomenon of anti-DNA idiotypic restriction relates to the origin of the genes encoding lupus autoantibody variable regions. Several questions are of central importance to this issue. Are there major alterations of organization of immunoglobulin gene loci in autoimmune conditions ? What are the relative contributions of germline, combinational and somatic variation mechanisms to generation of a functional autoantibody molecule ? Are autoantibody variable regions related to other V gene families, or do they constitute a unique restricted variable gene subgroup ? Are there molecular constraints on the assembly of variable gene elements expressed by autoantibodies, or do these genes recombine randomly ? Is the process of somatic diversification of variable genes actively engaged in generation of anti-self specificities, or are the corresponding V genes derived from genes in a germline configuration ? Is there a molecular connection between antibodies to self and those to exogenous antigens ? These and related questions will certainly cast some light on the mechanisms that shape the human B cell repertoire, and may provide clues to the origin of anti-DNA hyperproduction in lupus.

THE Vκ LOCUS IN HUMAN LUPUS

A prominent feature of SLE is the hyperproduction of autoantibodies. It is theoretically possible that this abnormality results from major alterations of the immunoglobulin V gene loci. To exclude this possibility and to accurately compare the size and characteristics of the human germline Vκ gene repertoire, germline DNAs from normal individuals and from SLE patients were probed with cDNA probes corresponding to the 4 different human Vκ families and shown in Fig. 1. VκI probe was cloned in EMBL3 from Burkitt lymphoma-derived Walker cell line (25) and subcloned in pCK19. VκII probe was cloned in Charon 30 from a normal individual (26) and subcloned in pCK19. VκIII probe was cloned in EMBL3 from IARC-BL41 cell line (27) and subcloned in M13-mp10. VκIV probe was cloned from the cell line JM and subcloned in pCK19 (28). The genomic Southern blots of human germline DNA revealed between one and fifteen hybridizing fragments (29). Because the Vκ genes appear to be separated by an average distance of 7 Kb (30), it is likely that some of these fragments contain more than one Vκ gene. Two conclusions may be drawn from this analysis. First, the restriction site polymorphism among human Vκ genes is limited. Because some of the V gene segments detected by hybridization correspond to pseudogenes that cannot be productively rearranged, or are not transcribed in populations of B cells, it seems that the repertoires of both expressed Vκ genes and Vκ pseudogenes are conserved in humans. Second, Vκ genes are apparently not missing from the SLE genome as indicated by genomic blotting analysis, although mutations not revealed by this limited analysis could prevent the gene from undergoing productive rearrangement or transcription. Within the limitations of this technique, it seems therefore reasonable to conclude that SLE is not associated with altered

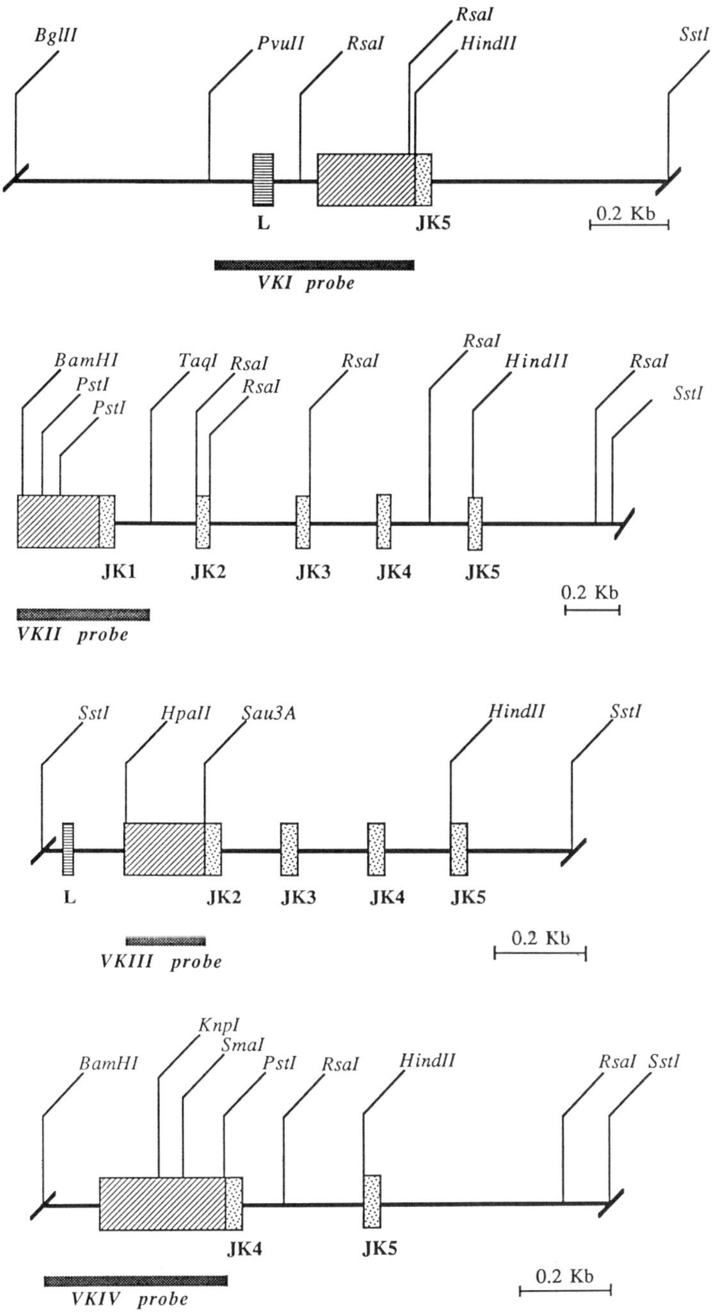

Fig. 1. Restriction maps of the human VK-gene family probes used.

gene location, gene dosage due to duplications or deletions within the VK gene cluster. Following a similar approach, Kofler et al. (31) reached similar conclusions for the VK locus in murine lupus.

VK FAMILY GENE UTILIZATION IN AUTOANTIBODY PRODUCING CELLS

While the experiments described above and those of Kofler et al. (31) suggest that in lupus there is no major alteration of the structure, the size or the organization of the VK locus, little is known about the VK genes expressed in the human disease. Differentiation of a normal antibody-producing cell is associated with a number of molecular choices. In humans, there is a hierarchy of constant region gene rearrangements in which the process is ordered so that the heavy chain is expressed before the light chain, and the light chain gene assembly usually progresses from the K to the λ genes (32). V gene segments are also sequentially assembled during B cell development : D to JH joining precedes VH to DJH rearrangements (33). Members of the different V gene families are also expressed in a developmentally ordered fashion. The most proximal VH genes - VH6 family in human and VH7183 family in mice - are rearranged early in foetal life and normalization occurs in adult life (33, Alt, personal communication). How these tightly programmed phenomena are regulated remains an extremely interesting but unanswered question.

An important question is how the library of V gene segments is utilized by B cells to generate autoantibody specificities. Are some families preferentially selected, or does B cell expression reflect the relative importance of the genes in the potential repertoire ? In the case of murine autoantibodies, this question has consumed the attention of many investigators (reviewed in ref. 34). In the human system, it was recently addressed in a study in which VK-gene family expression by a panel of EBV-transformed B cell clones and B hybridomas from SLE patients was compared to that of a panel of corresponding cells from normal individuals (35). When RNAs extracted from these cells were tested by Northern blot analysis using probes corresponding to the 4 human VK-gene families, it was found that autoantibody VK genes originated from the 4 VK gene families, and no restricted VK distribution could be seen. These results must be considered in light of recent data on the human VK locus. This cluster, which is located on chromosome 2, encompasses approximately 900 Kb of DNA, with at least 100 non-allelic VK genes distributed in 4 VK families. Members of these families are interspersed on the chromosome, and some of them are pseudogenes (25-28). More recent evidence indicates that some of the VK genes are located outside chromosome 2, and that the VK locus has been, at least in part, duplicated (30). Given this high intermingling of members of VK-gene families, it may not be too surprising that no preferential Vκ family utilization is seen (35). This apparent random expression of the Vκ gene families does not militate in favour of a conventional specific triggering of the autoantibody response in human lupus.

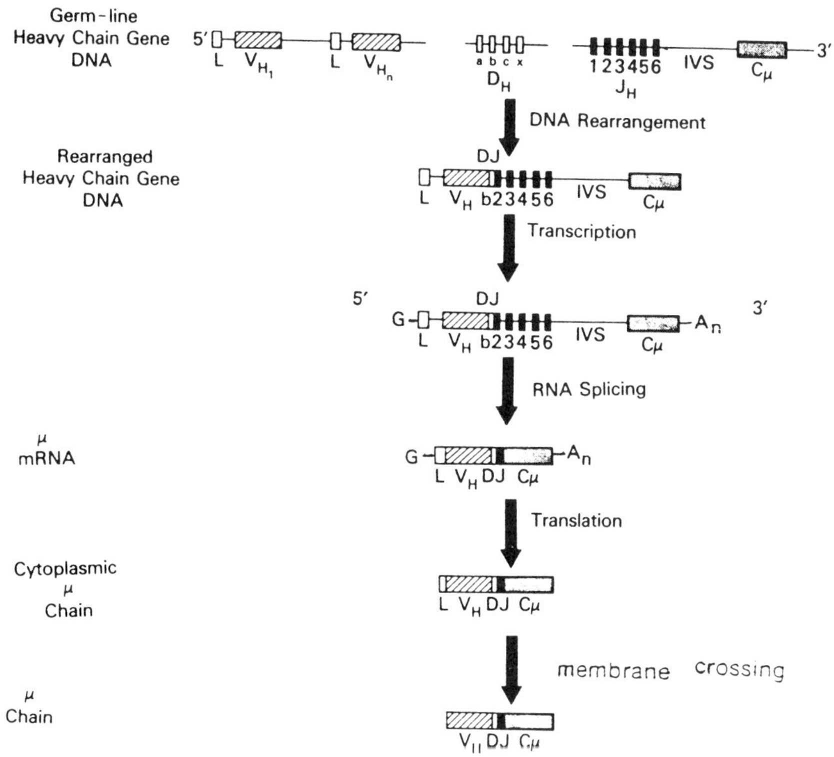

Fig. 2. Germline organization and somatic assembly of human Ig heavy chain variable genes

MOLECULAR CONFIGURATION OF ANTI-SELF-RELATED V GENES

The initial observations of lupus anti-DNA antibody binding degeneracy (1) and idiotypic recurrency led to the proposition that the variable regions genes utilized by these autoantibodies are essentially in an unmutated form (6-8). In humans, this assumption may be approached by examining the variable gene segments expressed by anti-DNA-producing B cell clones and hybridomas.

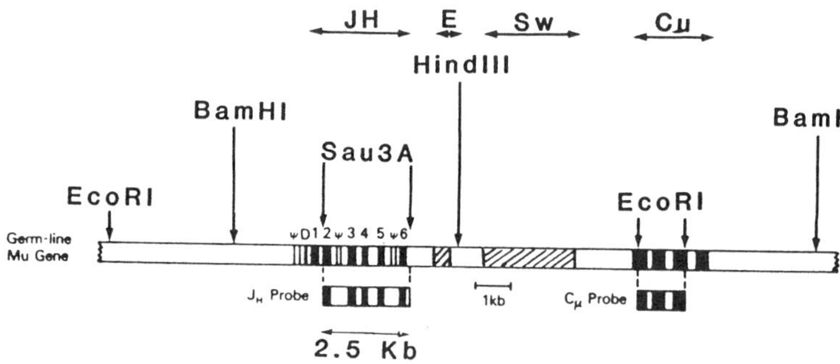

Fig. 3. Human embryonic JH probe (ref. 38) used to detect germline and rearranged VH genes.

Using Southern blot hybridization of DNA extracted from B cells with an embryonic JH probe, it is possible to see how V gene rearrangements are related. This strategy is based on the mechanisms of joining and assembly of the heavy chain gene segments as outlined in Fig.2. In man, upstream of the C-region genes are located nine JH genes -three of which are pseudogenes-, at least six D gene segments, and six VH families comprising about 100 non-allelic genes, with a high proportion of pseudogenes (36,37). DNA extracted from human B cells were probed with a human JH embryonic probe (Fig.3) capable of detecting germline and rearranged V gene segments. Fig.4 shows that B cells not producing autoantibodies exhibit unrelated pairs of restriction fragments, reflecting the expression of different VH genes. Five of the lupus-derived hybridomas shown in Fig.5 possess a common restriction band of approximatively 5 Kb, the other band being derived from the fusion partner GM-4672 that was used to generate these hybridomas (7). Nucleotide sequence analysis revealed that the VHDJH gene segments utilized by these hybridoma cells are identical (39), implying that these cells are clonaly related. More importantly, it was found that the consensus sequence expressed by these anti-DNA-producing lupus hybridomas is identical to that of a germline gene cloned from human liver (39), and to that of a VH gene expressed by a preB clone isolated from human foetal liver (40). The Southern blot shown in Fig.6 as well as analysis using other restriction

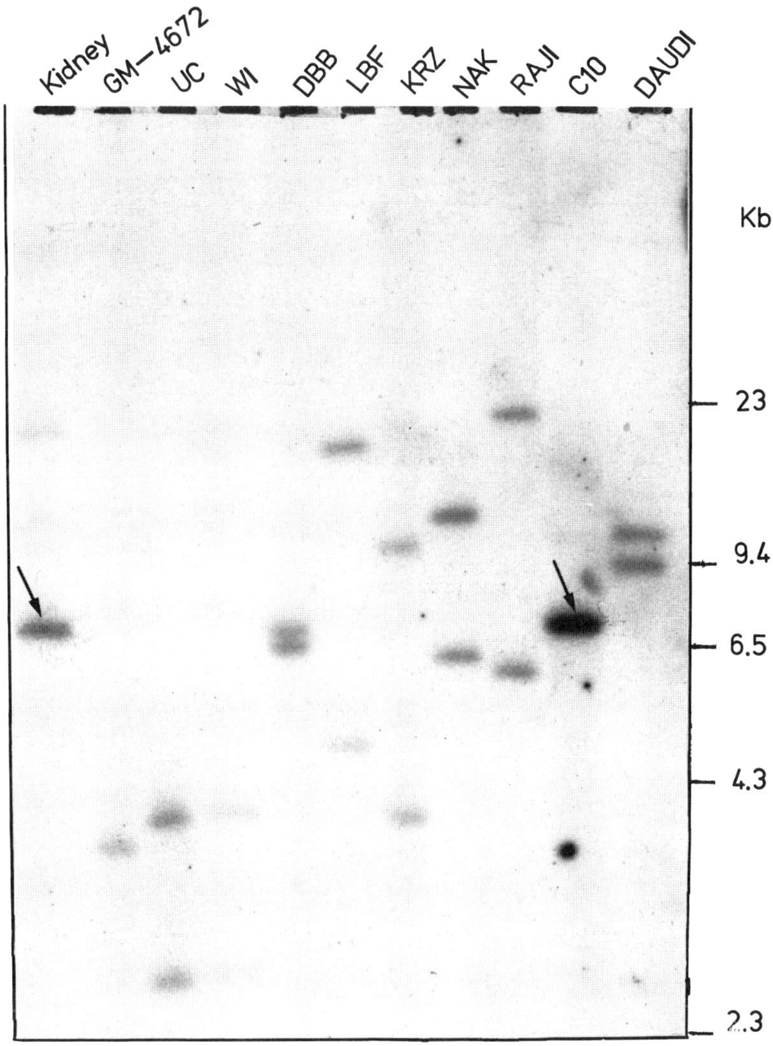

Fig.4. Southern blot analysis of human DNAs extracted from various origins, digested with BamHI and HindIII restriction enzymes and hybridized to the human JH probe shown in Fig. 3. The germline configuration of the VH locus is present in human Kidney, and in the human cell line C10. The corresponding restriction band is denoted by an arrow. All other DNAs were from human B lymphoblastoid cell lines. Positions of the molecular weight markers are also shown. Experimental conditions were as described elsewhere (29), and the filter was washed at a final stringency of 2 X SSC at 68°C.

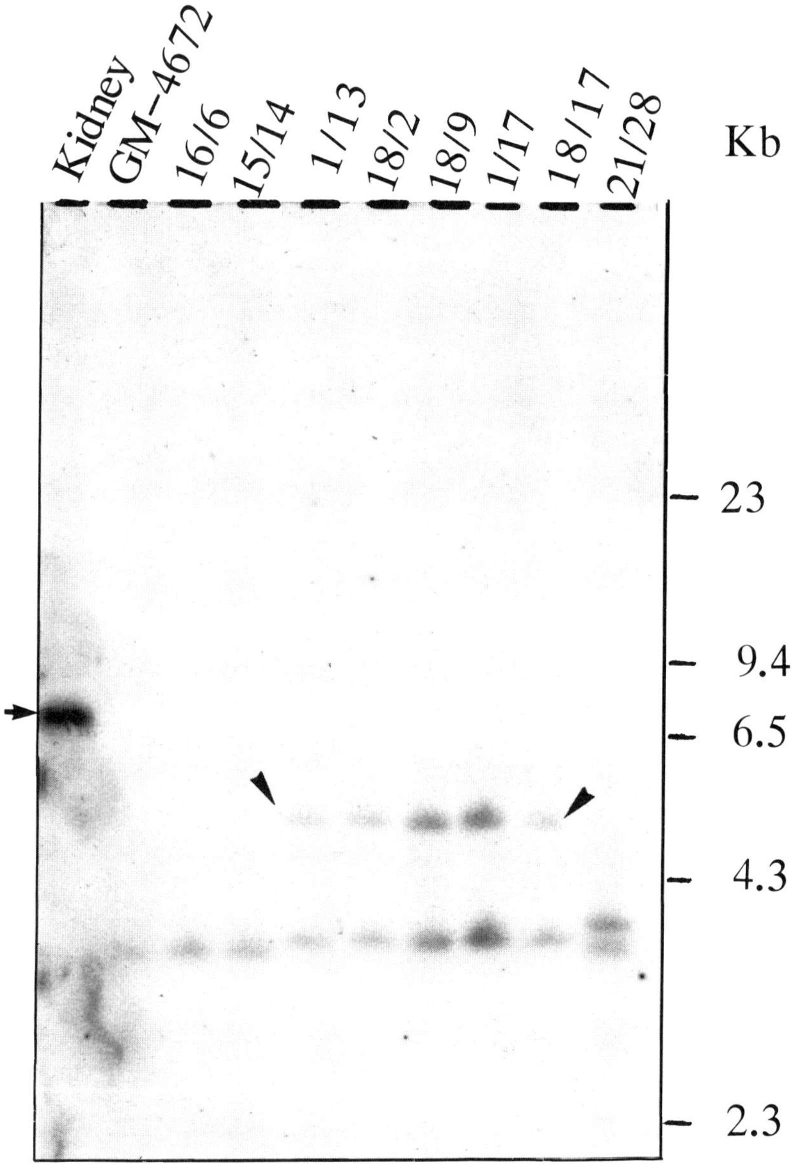

Fig. 5 Southern blot analysis of human DNAs. Experimental conditions are those indicated in legend to Fig.4. GM4672 is the lymphoblastoid cell line used to derive the B cell hybridomas 16/6, 15/14, 1/13, 18/9, 18/17, 18/2, 18/9 and 21/28 from 2 SLE patients. The arrowheads denote the common restriction band discussed in the text.

enzymes, revealed that the 2 anti-DNA-producing hybridoma lines 21/28 and 8E10, derived from 2 unrelated individuals, exhibit a similar restriction fragment. Further studies confirmed this analysis by showing that the VH genes expressed by these cells are completely identical (39). In an independent study, another lupus-derived human hybridoma was found to utilize a VH gene identical to a gene expressed by a human preB cell clone (Siminovitch et al., personal communication).

AUTOANTIBODIES, GERMLINE GENES AND THE PREIMMUNE REPERTOIRE

These findings together with related evidence (39-43) suggest that autoantibody variable region genes may be expressed in an unmutated configuration. It is therefore tempting to speculate that autoantibody B clonotypes are precursors of clones with an anti-exogenous specificity, that the preimmune repertoire is essentially composed of anti-self specificities, and that the corresponding V regions are germline-encoded (44). Within this conceptual framework, antibodies to exoantigens are somatically diversified from this V gene pool by affinity maturation processes.

However, in certain circumstances autoantibodies were found to be derived from mutated V region genes (45,46). Although this may seem an apparent contradiction of the model discussed above and elsewhere (44), the two possibilities may be accommodated in the following fashion. During the processes of gene duplication and expansion of the potential repertoire, germline V genes with primordial combining sites may be selected for specificity for self-antigens, so that self-non-self discrimination becomes an essential feature of the germline repertoire. Somatic diversification mechanisms then predominate to generate an antibody repertoire able to cope with the various intruders and with the rapidly changing epitopic make-up of pathogens, such as the influenza virus, the African trypanosome, or the human immunodeficiency virus. Because the rate of somatic mutation occuring in the variable genes of Ig is relatively high (10^{-4}-10^{-3}/bp/generation), it seems inevitable that during this somatic stage, an anti-self specificity is produced from another anti-self-related germline V gene.

Of central importance towards understanding the cause of SLE are the pathogeneic roles of the array of autoantibodies found in the sera of patients with lupus (1,13,44). The data concerning their specific involvement in tissue injury are scanty. Are the human autoantibodies analyzed in different systems those involved in the disease ? Are "aggressive" autoantibodies and harmless autoantibodies generated by similar germline and/or somatic molecular processes ? Are they

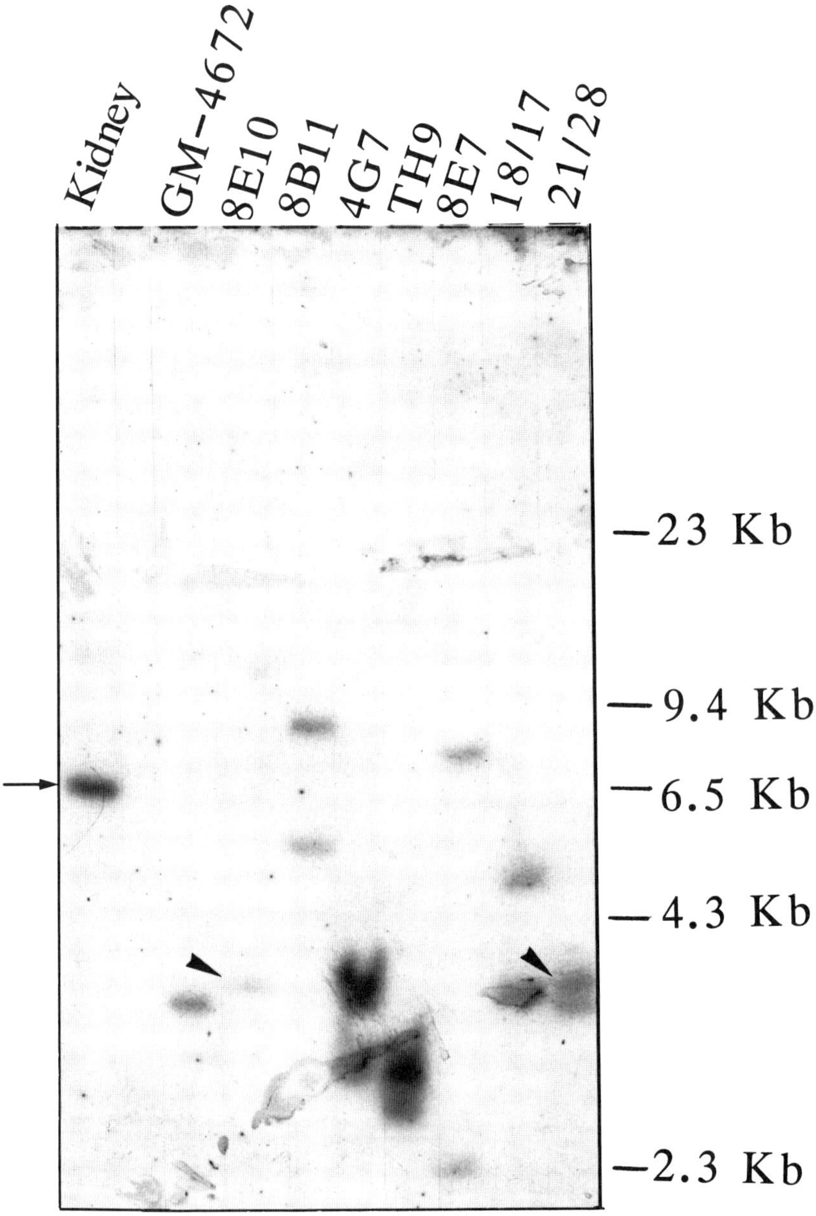

Fig. 6. Southern blot analysis of human DNAs. Conditions were as described in legends to Fig.4 and Fig.5. 18/17 and 21/28 are human B hybridomas of lupus origin. 8E10, 8B11, 4G7, TH9 and 8E7 are B hybridomas from lepromatous leprosy origin. The arrowheads mark the position of the common restriction band discussed in the text.

products of different clonotypes, or do they derive from related clones at different developmental stages ? The schema proposed recently (44) and discussed above offers a working hypothesis to further define the molecular events required to generate an "autoaggressive" antibody.

ACKNOWLEDGMENTS

I am indepted to B. David Stollar for invaluable involvement in some of these studies and continuing encouragements, and to Robert S. Schwartz for support and fruitful discussions.

I wish to thank Drs. H.G. Zachau, H.G. Klobeck, P. Leder, T. Logtenberg, R. Canoso, M. Madaio for generosity in providing probes and other valuable reagents, Dr. P. Brodeur for advice and stimulating discussions, Dr. K. Barrett for helpful comments, and Diane Arsenault for excellent technical assistance.

REFERENCES

1. Stollar, B.D. (1986) Antibodies to DNA. *CRC Crit. Rev. Biochem.* **20**,1

2. Rauch, J., Murphy, E., Roths, J.B., Stollar, B.D., and Schwartz, R.S. (1982) A high-frequency idiotypic marker of anti-DNA autoantibodies in MRL-lpr/lpr mice. *J. Immunol.* **129**, 236

3. Marion, T.N., Lawton, A.R., III, Kearney, J.F., and Briles, D.E. (1982) Anti-DNA autoantibodies in (NZB x NZW) F1 mice are clonally heterogenous but the majority share a common idiotype. *J. Immunol.* **128**, 668

4. Solomon, G., Schiffenbauser, J., Keiser, H.D., and Diamond, B. (1983) Use of monoclonal antibodies to identify shared idiotypes on human antibodies to native DNA from patients with SLE. *Proc. Natl. Acad. Sci. USA* **80**, 850

5. Zouali, M., and Eyquem, A. (1984) Idiotype restriction in human autoantibodies to DNA in systemic lupus erythematosus. *Immunol. Lett.* **7**, 187

6. Isenberg, D.A., Shoenfeld, Y., Madaio, M.P., Rauch, J., Reichlin, M., Stollar, B.D. and Schwartz, R.S. (1984) Anti-DNA antibody idiotypes in systemic lupus erythematosus. *Lancet* **2**, 418

7. Shoenfeld, Y., Isenberg, D.A., Rauch, J., Madaio, M., Stollar, B.D., and Schwartz, R.S. (1983) Idiotypic cross-reactions of monoclonal human autoantibodies. *J. Exp. Med.* **158**, 718

8. Zouali, M., Fine, J.M., and Eyquem, A. (1984) Anti-DNA autoantibody and idiotypic relationships of human monoclonal proteins. *Eur. J. Immunol.* **14**, 1085

9. Eilat, D., Fischel, R., and Zlotnick, A. (1985) A central anti-DNA idiotype in human and murine systemic lupus erythematosus. *Eur. J. Immunol.* **15**, 368

10. Morgan, A., Isenberg, D.A., Napartsek, Y., Rauch, J., Duggan, R., Staines, N.A., and Schattner, A. (1985) Shared idiotypes are expressed on mouse and human anti-DNA autoantibodies. *Immunology.* **55**, 393

11. Zouali, M., Migliorini, P., Mackworth-Young, C., and Stollar, B.D. (1988) Nucleic acid binding specificity and idiotype expression of canine lupus antibodies. *Eur. J. Immunol.* **18**, 923

12. Jerne, N.K. (1984) Idiotypic networks and other preconceived ideas. *Immunol. Rev.* **79**, 5

13. Burdette, S., and Schwartz, R.S. (1987) Idiotypes and idiotypic networks. *N. Eng. J. Med.* **317**, 219

14. Zouali, M., and Eyquem, A. (1983) Expression of anti-idiotypic clones against auto-anti-DNA antibodies in normal individuals. *Cell. Immunol.* **76**, 137

15. Zouali, M., Fine, J.M., and Eyquem, A. (1984) A human monoclonal IgG1 with anti-idiotypic activity against anti-human thyroglobulin autoantibody. *J. Immunol.* **133**, 190

16. Sultan, Y., Rossi, F., Kazatchkine, M.D. (1987) Recovery from anti-VIII:c (anti-hemophilic factor) autoimmune disease is dependent on generation of anti-idiotypes against anti-VIII:c autoantibodies. *Proc. Natl. Acad. Sci. USA* **84**, 828

17. Abdou, N.I., Wall, H., Lindsey, H.B., Halsey, J.F., and Suzuki, T. (1981) Network theory in autoimmunity. In vitro suppression of serum anti-DNA antibody binding to DNA by anti-idiotypic antibody in systemic lupus erythematosus. *J. Clin. Invest.* **67**, 1297

18. Zouali, M., and Eyquem, A. (1983) Idiotypic/antiidiotypic interactions in systemic lupus erythematosus : demonstration of oscillatory levels of anti-DNA autoantibodies and reciprocal antiidiotypic activity in a single patient. *Ann. Immunol. (Paris)* **134C**, 377

19. MacKworth-Young, C.G., and Schwartz, R.S. (1988) *Clin. Exp. Immunol.* **77**, 56

20. Datta, S.K., Stollar, B.D., and Schwartz, R.S. (1983) Normal mice express idiotypes related to autoantibody idiotypes of lupus mice. *Proc. Natl. Acad. Sci. USA* **80**, 2723

21. Hahn, B.H. (1984) Suppression of autoimmune diseases with anti-idiotypic antibodies : murine lupus nephritis as a model. *Springer Semin Immunopathol.* **7**, 25

22. Teitelbaum, D., Rauch, J., Stollar, B.D., and Schwartz, R.S. (1984) In vivo effects of antibodies against a high frequency idiotype of anti-DNA antibodies in MRL mice. *J. Immunol.* **132**, 1282

23. Essani, K., Srinivasappa, J., McClintock, P.R., Prabhakar, B.S., and Notkins, A.L. (1986) Multiple organ-reactive IgG antibody induced by an antiidiotypic antibody to a human monoclonal IgM autoantibody. *J. Exp. Med.* **163**, 1355

24. Zouali, M., Jolivet, M., Leclerc, C., Ravisse, P., Audibert, F., Eyquem, A., and Chedid, L. (1985) Suppression of murine lupus autoantibodies to DNA by administration of muramyl dipeptide and syngenic anti-DNA IgG. *J. Immunol.* **135**, 1091

25. Klobeck, H., Combriato, G., and Zachau, A. (1984) Immunoglobulin genes of the κ light chain type from two human lymphoid cell lines are closely related. *Nucleic Acids Res.* **12**, 6995

26. Klobeck, H.G., Solomon, A., and Zachau, H.G. (1984) Contribution of human VκII germ-line genes to light-chain diversity. *Nature* **309**, 73

27. Klobeck, H.G., Meindl, A., Combriato, G.,Solomon, A., and Zachau, H.G. (1985) Human immunoglobulin κ light chain genes of subgroups II and III. *Nucleic Acids Res.* **13**, 6499

28. Klobeck, H.G., Bornkamm, G.W., Combriato, G., Mocikat, R., Pohlenz, H.D., and Zachau, H.G. (1985) Subgroup IV of human immunoglobulin κ light chains in encoded by a single germline gene. *Nucleic Acids Res.* **13**, 6515

29. Zouali, M., Madaio, M.P., Canoso, R., and Stollar, B.D. Restriction fragment length polymorphism analysis of the Vκ locus in human lupus ; in preparation

30. Straubinger, B., Huber, E., Lorenz, W., Osterholzer, E., Pargent, W., Pech, M., Pohlenz, H., Zimmer, F., and Zachau, H.G. (1988) The human Vκ locus. Characterization of a duplicated region encoding 28 different immunoglobulin genes. *J. Mol. Biol.* **199**, 23

31. Kofler, R., Strohal, R., Balderas, R.S., Johnson, M.E., Noonan, D.J., Duchosal, M.A., Dixon, F.J., and Theofilopoulos, A.N. (1988) Immunoglobulin κ light chain variable region gene complex organization and immunoglobulin genes encoding anti-DNA autoantibodies in lupus mice. *J. Clin. Invest.* **82**, 852

32. Hieter, P.A., Korsmeyer, S.J., Waldmann, T., and Leder, P. (1981) Human immunoglobulin κ light chain genes are deleted or rearranged in λ producing B cells. *Nature* **290**, 368

33. Yancopoulos, G.D., and Alt, F.W. (1986) The regulation of variable region gene assembly. *Ann. Rev. Immunol.* **4**, 339

34. Bona, C.A. (1988) V genes encoding autoantibodies : molecular and phenotypic characteristics. *Ann. Rev. Immunol.* **6**, 327

35. Zouali, M., Logtenberg, T., Young, F., and Stollar, B.D. Vκ gene utilization in human autoantibody-producing cells. In preparation

36. Kodaira, M., Kinashi, T., Umemura, I., Matsuda, F., Noma, T., Ono, Y., and Honjo, T. (1986) Organization and evolution of variable region genes of the human immunoglobulin heavy chain. *J. Mol. Biol.* **190**, 529

37. Berman, E., Mellis, S.J., Pollock, R., Smith, C.L., Suh, H., Heinke, B., Kowal, C., Surti, U., Chess, L., Cantor, C.R. and Alt, F.W. (1988) Content and organization of the human Ig VH locus : definition of three new VH families and linkage to the Ig CH locus. *EMBO J.* **7**, 727

38. Ravetch, J.V., Siebenlist, U., Korsmeyer, S., Waldmann, T., and Leder, P. (1981) Structure of the human immunoglobulin μ locus : characterization of embryonic and rearranged J and D genes. *Cell* **27**, 583

39. DerSimonian, H., Schwartz, R.S., Barrett, K.J., and Stollar, B.D. (1987) Relationship of human variable region heavy chain (VH) germline genes to genes encoding anti-DNA autoantibodies. *J. Immunol.* **139**, 2496

40. Schroeder, H.W., Jr., Hillson, J.L., and Perlmutter, R.M. (1987) Early restriction of the human antibody repertoire. *Science* **238**, 791

41. Chen, P.P., Albrandt, K., Orida, N.K., Radoux, V., Chen, E.Y., Schrantz, R., Liu, F. T., and Carson, D.A. (1986) Genetic basis for the cross-reactive idiotypes on the light chains of human IgM anti-IgG autoantibodies. *Proc. Natl. Acad. Sci. USA* **83**, 8318

42. Reininger, L., Ollier, P., Poncet, P., Kaushik, A., and Jaton, J.C. (1987) Novel V genes encode virtually identical variable regions of six murine monoclonal anti-bromelain-treated red blood cell autoantibodies. *J. Immunol.* **138**, 316

43. Naparstek, Y., André-Schwartz, J., Manser, T., Wysocki, T., Breitman, L., Stollar, B.D., Gefter, M., and Schwartz, R.S. (1986) A single germ line VH gene segment of normal A/J mice encodes autoantibodies characteristic of systemic lupus erythematosus. *J. Exp. Med.* **164**, 614

44. Zouali, M., Stollar, B.D., and Schwartz, R.S. (1988) Origin and diversification of anti-DNA antibodies. *Immunol. Rev.* **105**, 137

45. Diamond, B., and Scharf, M. (1984) Somatic mutation of the T15 heavy chain gives rise to an antibody with autoantibody specificity *Proc. Natl. Acad. Sci. USA* **81**, 5841

46. Shlomchik, M.J., Marshak-Rothstein, A., Wolfowicz, C.B., Rothstein, T.L., and Weigert, M.G. (1987) The role of clonal selection and somatic mutation in autoimmunity. *Nature* **328**, 805

MURINE AUTOANTIBODIES SPECIFIC FOR BROMELINIZED RED BLOOD CELLS USE A RESTRICTED SET OF GENETIC ELEMENTS AND THEIR HEAVY CHAINS DEFINE A NOVEL VH FAMILY[1]

Jean-Claude Jaton[2]
Luc Reininger[3]

Departments of Medical Biochemistry[2] and Pathology[3],
Medical Center of the University of Geneva,
CH-1211 Geneva 4, Switzerland.

The nucleotide sequences of the variable (V) regions of anti-bromelinized mouse red blood cells (BrMRBC) monoclonal autoantibodies were determined. Identical combinations of VH-VCP12, diversity-DSP2 (5,7 or 8) and joining-JH1 genes for the H chains, and Vκ-9-Jκ2 (or Jκ4) gene segments for the L chains were identified in 3 NZB-, 3 CBA/J- and one BALB/c derived hybridomas. The BALB/c VCP12 (BrMRBC) nucleotide sequence was less than 80% homologous to members of the ten known VH families, and the genomic restriction fragments detected under moderate stringency conditions with the radiolabeled cDNA probe, did not correspond to those obtained with probes of the most homologous VH families (7183 and X24).

The results indicate that the VCP12 gene defines a new VH gene family which we propose to designate **VH11**. The observation of 1, 2 or 3 genomic restriction fragments at the most, with mice bearing the Igh-$V^{d \text{ or } j}$, Igh-$V^{a \text{ or } b}$ or Igh-V^{c} haplotypes, suggests the existence of a few **VH11** related genes.

---

[1]Supported in part by grant No. 3.342-0.86 from the Swiss National Foundation for Scientific Research.

We gratefully acknowledge Ms. Thi Nha Huynh for typing the manuscript.

INTRODUCTION

Diseases associated with autoimmune phenomena are regarded as a consequence of the presence of auto-reactive antibodies. The diseases are distributed within a large spectrum since antibodies may be directed against one organ resulting in an invasive destructive lesion or, against endogeneous antigens throughout the body with the lesions characteristic of the diseases widely disseminated (1). At the same time, the presence of autoantibodies in apparently healthy animals and men is now well established (2-6). These autoantibodies may play a significant physiological role, e.g., resistance to bacterial infection (7,8), clearance of senescent cells and damaged tissue (9) or their possible involvment in the idiotypic network (1,10). However, in contrast to autoimmune diseases associated with autoantibodies, their self-reactivity is apparently not associated with pathogenicity.

The autoantibodies against bromelain-treated mouse red blood cells (BrMRBC) are reactive towards hidden self-antigens since they recognize a cryptic antigen exposed after proteolytic treatment of mouse erythrocytes with the enzyme, bromelain. The high frequency of cells secreting anti-BrMRBC antibodies among B cells in the peritoneal cavity has been observed by several groups (2,11,12,13). Several IgM-secreting hybridomas have been established by fusions of peritoneal cells from several NZB or CBA/J mice with myelomas and used to characterize their antigen-binding specificity, and structural relatedness. These monoclonal autoantibodies were shown to comprise a family of highly related molecules based on homology in partial N-terminal amino acid sequences and the presence of a common cross-reactive idiotype (14).

The structural comparison between autoantibodies and antibodies raised against exogeneous antigens has stimulated much work in recent years because little was known about the V region gene repertoire of autoantibodies (15) and natural antibodies (16). In particular, it was of major interest to know whether the autoantibodies from autoimmune-prone mice were similar to those expressed by non-autoimmune mice, and whether the genetic elements encoding these autoantibodies were common to antibodies directed against exogeneous antigens, as suggested by recent studies (17,18,19).

In this paper, we will review mRNA sequences encoding the heavy (H) and light (L) chain variable (V) regions of 3 NZB, 3 CBA/J and one Balb/c anti-BrMRBC monoclonal antibodies. A restricted combination of VH (BrMRBC), DSP2 (5,7 or 8) and JH1 genes for the H chain and Vκ9 (BrMRBC) and Jκ2 or Jκ4 genes for the L chain, likely in a germ-line configuration, was observed for all of the autoantibodies. It is noteworthy that the VH (BrMRBC) gene could not be classified with more than 80% of nucleotide homology in any of the ten known VH families (20,21,22); we report here the restriction fragment length polymorphism (RFLP) patterns of genomic murine DNA detected by a specific VH (BrMRBC) cDNA probe, as compared to those defined by the most homologous VH families, 7183 and X24. The data suggest that the VH (BrMRBC) gene segment defines a new, small, VH family.

MATERIALS AND METHODS

Hybridomas

Hybridomas CP4 12-18, CP4 9-9 and CP3 23-24 were prepared from the NZB strain, CP5 B5-3, CP5 A23-3 and CP5 A21-1, from the CBA/J strain (14) and hybridoma CP8 B3-D3 was derived from BALB/c mice (23). They all have been shown to secrete an IgM, κ monoclonal antibody reacting with BrMRBC (14,23).

Direct mRNA nucleotide sequencing

This was carried out according to Hamlyn et *al*. (24), as adapted from Sanger et *al*. (25), using oligonucleotide primers as described in details elsewhere (26).

cDNA cloning

Double stranded cDNA from H chain-enriched mRNA encoding BALB/c CP8 B3-D3 antibody was prepared, as described (27). One of the recombinant plasmids, pCP12, containing a 500 bp-long insert corresponding to the entire VH region, was characterized (27).

Southern blot analysis

Digestions of high Mr mouse liver DNA by EcoRI, BamHI, or HindIII, electrophoresis, blotting and hybridizing conditions were detailed elsewhere (27). The VH DNA probes used in this study were a 950 bp EcoRI-BamHI fragment isolated from plasmid pVH SAPC15 (20,28) for the 7183 family, a 252 bp HindIII-BglII fragment isolated from plasmid pVH XRPC24 (20, 29) for the X24 family, and a 261 bp DraI-PstI fragment from plasmid pCP12 for the VH (BrMRBC) family (27).

RESULTS

The VH nucleotide sequences of seven anti-BrMRBC hybridomas are virtually identical

The mRNA sequences encoding the VH regions of monoclonal anti-BrMRBC autoantibodies derived from BALB/c, NZB and CBA/J strains are illustrated in Fig.1. The hybridomas were prepared from 4 independent cell fusions, each carried out with pooled peritoneal cells from several mice. Such conditions rule out the possibility that hybridomas were derived from the same cell clone.

The VH sequence of CP8 B3-D3 antibody was also confirmed by the characterization of a cDNA recombinant plasmid, designated pCP12, which was found to contain a 500 bp-long insert corresponding to the entire variable region including part of the 5' untranslated region, the leader sequence (L), the variable (VH), the diversity (D) and part of the joining (JH) segments (27). Two additional sequences from hybridomas CP4 9-9 and CP3 23-24 (NZB) and CP5 A23-3 and CP5 A21-1 (CBA/J) were found identical to those of CP4 12-18 and CP5 B5-3, respectively (26). The VH nucleotide sequences (Fig.1) of one BALB/c antibody, three NZB and three CBA/J antibodies are almost identical except for a few undetermined bases and for base substitutions distributed throughout the V region within codons numbered -13, -1, 13, 27, 66, 84, 96 and 105. The nucleotide differences observed for codons -1, 13, 96 and 105 lead to amino acid substitutions, i.e., Cys for Gly, Gln for Pro, Gly for Ser and Ala for Thr, respectively, whereas changes at the third base of codons 27, 66 and 84 as well as in the first base of codon -13 remain silent. These base changes present uniformly in all sequences most probably reflect allelic variations of the same gene among the different strains of mice.

Whereas the 3' ends of most VH genes encode the classical Cys-Ala-Arg sequence (positions 92-94), the sequence Cys-**Met**-Arg is observed in all seven anti-BrMRBC antibodies (Fig.1). Met-93 has not previously been recorded among murine VH regions (35) and may constitute a marker for that family of antibodies.

The seven antibodies exhibit D regions of the same length (positions 95-97). The diversity D segment derives from either the SP 2.5, the SP 2.7 or the SP 2.8 germ-line D gene segment (30) by the deletion of 5 and 3 nucleotides at the 5' and 3' boundaries, respectively. At codon 96, a transition (G for A) is observed between BALB/c and NZB, on one hand, and CBA/J antibodies, on the other. The allelic variation in the D region (residue 96 is substituted by either glycine or serine), although localized in a complementarity determining region, does not appear to affect the specificity of the antibodies.

The JH segment of anti-BrMRBC antibodies from the three strains is identical with the JH1 germ-line gene segment of the BALB/c strain (31) except for a silent substitution at the third base of codon 111 (C for T). The NZB-derived JH1 segment displays another substitution in the first base of codon 105 as compared to the BALB/c JH1 sequence (G for A). For the seven antibodies studied here, the JH1 segment is used in its entirety. Thus the VH regions of anti-BrMRBC antibodies, independently of their origin, are encoded by the highly conserved combination, VH(BrMRBC)-D SP2 (5,7 or 8)-JH1 genes.

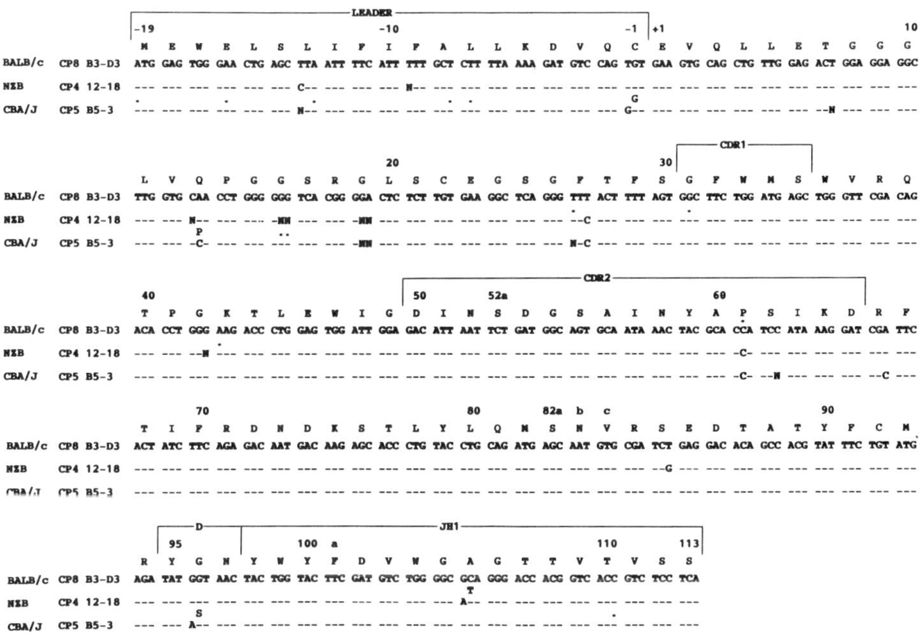

Fig. 1. Nucleotide sequences of the VH regions of anti-BrMRBC IgM hybridomas from BALB/c, NZB and CBA/J strains. The sequence of CP8 B3-D3 between codon -19 and 110 was derived by sequencing the cDNA insert of clone pCP12, and for codon -6 to 113, by direct mRNA sequencing (27). The protein sequence in the one-letter code is indicated above the nucleotide sequence. Two other VH sequences from hybridomas CP4 9-9 and CP3 23-24 (NZB) and from hybridomas CP5 A23-3 and CP5 A21-1 (CBA/J) are identical to those of CP4 12-18 and CP5 B5-3, respectively (26). N, undetermined base; a dot indicates the probable base at that position. Numbering corresponding to codons is according to Kabat et al. (35).

The Vκ domains are likely encoded by the association of the same Vκ9 gene with either the Jκ2 or Jκ4 joining segment

The portions of mRNAs encoding L chain V regions have been completely sequenced except for codons 87-95 of NZB-derived antibodies (Fig.2). The mRNA sequences corresponding to the Vκ domains are probably identical across the 3 strains with the exception of a few nucleotide ambiguities in the 5' end of the message. In NZB-derived autoantibodies, from codons 95 onwards, a double nucleotide sequence was encountered due to the presence of the contaminating MOPC-21 encoding Vκ mRNA from the fusion partner genome (26). To circumvent this difficulty, a Vκ1 primer complementary to codons 89-93 of antibody CP5-B5-3 was synthesized and used successfully to resume sequencing. As the Vκ regions from codons 88-95 could not be determined for NZB-derived antibodies, their homology with the prototype CP5 B5-3 sequence, was estimated by a comparison of the melting profiles of hybrids formed between L chain enriched-mRNAs and the Vκ1 primer. The data were consistent with a very high degree of sequence homology between the mRNAs compared over codons 89-93 (26).

The comparison of the primary structures deduced from the nucleotide sequences (Fig.2) with all of the published Vκ sequences revealed 97% homology within the N-terminal 35 amino acids of the L chain derived from RPC5 myeloma (secreting a IgG2a,κ protein of unknown specificity) which is a member of the Vκ9 subgroup (32). One unique Lys (AAA) to Asn (AAT/AAC) substitution at position 30 distinguishes anti-BrMRBC Vκ from RPC5 Vκ region. It is, therefore, possible that the Vκ regions of myeloma RPC5 and anti-BrMRBC antibodies originate from closely related Vκ genes.

The three CBA/J-derived antibodies and the three NZB-derived antibodies use the Jκ2 segment which corresponds exactly to the germ-line Jκ2 gene of BALB/c mice (33) and is used without deletion. In contrast, the Vκ region of the BALB/c-derived antibody CP8 B3-D3 is associated with the Jκ4 segment in its unmutated form (33). This is of interest as the Jκ4 segment has been reported to be 5-10 times less frequently used that Jκ1 or Jκ2 segments (34). Thus, the Vκ domains of the seven antibodies are likely constituted by the association of the same Vκ gene with either the Jκ2 or the Jκ4 joining segment in the case of the BALB/c autoantibody.

```
                    1                                   10                                      20                          ┌────────CDR1────────
                    D   I   K   M   T   Q   S   P   S   S   M   Y   A   S   L   G   E   R   V   T   I   T   C │ K   A   S   Q   D
BALB/c CP8 B3-D3   GAC ATC AAG ATG ACC CAG TCT CCA TCC TCC ATG TAT GCA TCG CTG GGA GAG AGA GTC ACT ATC ACT TGC AAG GCG AGT CAG GAC
NZB    CP4 12-18   --- --- --- --- --- --- --- --- --- --- --- --- --- --- --- --- --- --- --- --- --- --- --- --- --- --- --- -A-
CBA/J  CP5 B5-3    --- --- --- --- --- --- --- --- --- --- --- --- --- --- --- --- --- --- --- --- --- --- --- --- --- --- --- ---

                   ─────────────────────┐                                                     ┌────────CDR2────────────┐
                       30                    │                    40                                              │50                      │
                    I   K   S   Y   L   S │ X   Y   Q   Q   K   P   W   K   S   P   K   T   L   I   Y │ Y   A   T   S   L   A   D
BALB/c CP8 B3-D3   ATT AAA AGC TAT TTA AGC TNG TAC CAG CAG AAA CCA TGG AAA TCT CCT AAG ACC CTG ATC TAT TAT GCA ACA AGC TTG GCA GAT
                                           W
NZB    CP4 12-18   --- --- --- --- --- --- -G- --- --- --- --- --- --- A-- --- --- --- --- --- --- --- --- --- --A --- --- --- ---
                                           W                           X
CBA/J  CP5 B5-3    --- --- --- --- --- --- -G- --- --- --- --- --- --- N-- --- --- --- --- --- --- --- --- --- --A --- --- --- ---

                                    60                                      70                                      80
                    G   V   P   S   R   F   S   G   S   G   S   G   Q   D   Y   S   L   T   I   S   S   L   E   S   D   D   T   A
BALB/c CP8 B3-D3   GGG GTC CCA TCA AGA TTC AGT GGC AGT GGA TCT GGG CAA GAT TAT TCT CTA ACC ATC AGC AGC CTG GAG TCT GAC GAT ACA GCA
NZB    CP4 12-18   --- --- --- --- --- --- --- --- --- --- --- --- --- --- --- --- --- --- --- --- --- --- --- --- --- --- --- ---
CBA/J  CP5 B5-3    --- --- --- --- --- --- --- --- --- --- --- --- --- --- --- --- --- --- --- --- --- --- --- --- --- --- --- ---

                                                                ┌──────────────────────JK──────────────────────┐
                                   ┌───────────CDR3──────────┼─────────┐                                      │
                                   │   90                                 │       100                            │
                    T   Y   Y   C │ L   Q   H   G   E   S   X   F   T │ F   G   S   G   T   K   L   E   I   K
BALB/c CP8 B3-D3   ACT TAT TAC TGT CTA CAG CAT GGT GAG AGC CNA TTC ACG TTC GGC TCG GGG ACA AAG TTG GAA ATA AAA
                            X                                   Y               G
NZB    CP4 12-18   --- --- -                                   -A- --- --- --A GG- --C --C --- C-- --- --- ---
                                                            P   Y               G
CBA/J  CP5 B5-3    --- --- --- --- --- --- --- --- --- --- -CT -A- --- --- --A GG- --- --C --- C-- --- --- ---
```

Fig.2. Nucleotide sequences of the Vκ regions of anti-BrMRBC hybridomas from BALB/c, NZB and CBA/J strains. The sequences were derived by direct mRNA sequencing (26,37). They are all virtually identical except that the hybridoma CP8 B3-D3 from BALB/c strain uses the Jκ4 segment instead of Jκ2 in the other strains. Two additional Vκ sequences from NZB (CB4 9-9 and CP3 23-24) and CBA/J (CP5 A23-3 and CP5 A21-1) origin were identical to their respective consensus sequence shown here (26). See also legend to Fig.1.

By the criterion of nucleotide sequence homology, the VH segment encoding anti-BrMRBC antibodies does not fit in any of the ten known VH families

As arbitrarily defined, the percentage of homology between VH members of the same family is usually greater than 80% at the nucleic acid level. The VH genes most similar to the BrMRBC VH segment (Table 1) were found among members of the 7183 and X24 families, where only 75.8 and 75.1% homology respectively, were observed with the 50.1 and 55.1 VH genes (26,27).

TABLE 1. Comparison of nucleic acid sequences from members of the ten known Igh-V families with VCP12

Igh-V Family				Homology[d]
No	Name	Complexity[a]	Gene[c]	%
1	J558	60[b]	J558	58.5
2	Q52	15	VH101	57.1
3	36-60	5	36-60	56.8
4	X24	2	55.1	75.1
5	7183	12	50.1	75.8
6	J606	10	V22	65.3
7	S107	4	V11	68.0
8	3609	9	V31	51.3
9	VGAM3.8	5	VMU1	55.7
10	DNA4	3	DNA4	64.0

_a_ The estimated number of genes within each family in BALB/c mice is based on Southern blot analysis.

_b_ It has been also suggested that the J558 family may contain 500-1000 members.

_c_ J558 (BALB/c), VMU1 (BALB/c), and DNA4 (MRL) are rearranged; all others are germ-line genes from BALB/c origin.

_d_ The percentages of homology were calculated from codon 1 to codon 94.

Hybridization of genomic DNA with a BrMRBC VH-encoding DNA fragment defines a new RFLP pattern

A 261 bp-long DraI-PstI sub-fragment derived from the pCP12 cDNA clone encoding the VH region of BALB/c hybridoma CP8 B3-D3 was used as a specific VH (BrMRBC) probe (27). Successive hybridizations of the VCP12 VH probe, SAPC15 VH probe (VH family 7183) and XRPC24 VH probe (VH family X24) to digested mouse genomic DNA, were carried out in an attempt to assign the VCP12 gene to one of the two closest VH families, 7183 and X24. Since inbred strains of mice show extensive polymorphism over the Igh-V locus (20), several Igh-V haplotypes were used to facilitate the comparison between the VCP12 gene and other VH genes. Accordingly, Southern blots of digested genomic DNAs were hybridized to VCP12, 7183 and X24 VH probes, and washed under moderate stringency conditions (Fig.3).

The general RFLP patterns defined by the VCP12 probe was different from those defined by the closest VH probes 7183 and X24, in EcoRI, BamHI or HindIII digested DNA (Figs. 3A, B and C respectively) among various strains of mice, differing by the Igh-V haplotype (haplotypes a, b, c, d and j; lanes 1 to 5). For instance, in BALB/c DNA (lane 1 of Fig.3A), the VCP12 cDNA probe hybridized to two EcoRI fragments (8.1 and 8.7 kb), while the 7183 probe hybridized to twelve fragments. Moreover, even though the smaller 8.1 kb fragment was nearly superimposable to one of the restriction fragments detected by the 7183 VH probe, the larger 8.7 kb fragment was clearly undetectable by the 7183 VH probe (indicated by an arrow). Similarly, the upper VCP12-hybridzing fragment in EcoRI digest of C57BL/6 DNA (lane 2 of Fig.3A), and the upper and lower VCP12-hybridizing fragments in EcoRI digest of DBA/2 DNA (lane 3 of Fig.3A), indicated by arrows, were not detected by the 7183 VH probe.

The X24 VH probe hybridized very strongly to a monomorphic 0.5 kb EcoRI fragment and weakly to 8-10 larger fragments (Fig. 3A). The upper fragments of BALB/c (lane 1), C57BL/6 (lane 2) and DBA/2 (lane 3), and the lower fragment of DBA/2 DNA digests (indicated by arrows), which hybridized to the VCP12 VH probe, did not so with the X24 VH probe. Actually, two VH genes comprised in the 0.5 kb EcoRI fragment are true members of the X24 VH family. Other VH genes present in some of the cross-hybridizing larger fragments have been shown to belong to other VH families, i.e., J606 and 7183 (29).

When the VCP12, 7183 and X24 VH probes were hybridized either to BamHI or HindIII digested genomic DNA (Fig.3B or 3C), markedly different RFLP patterns and unshared fragments

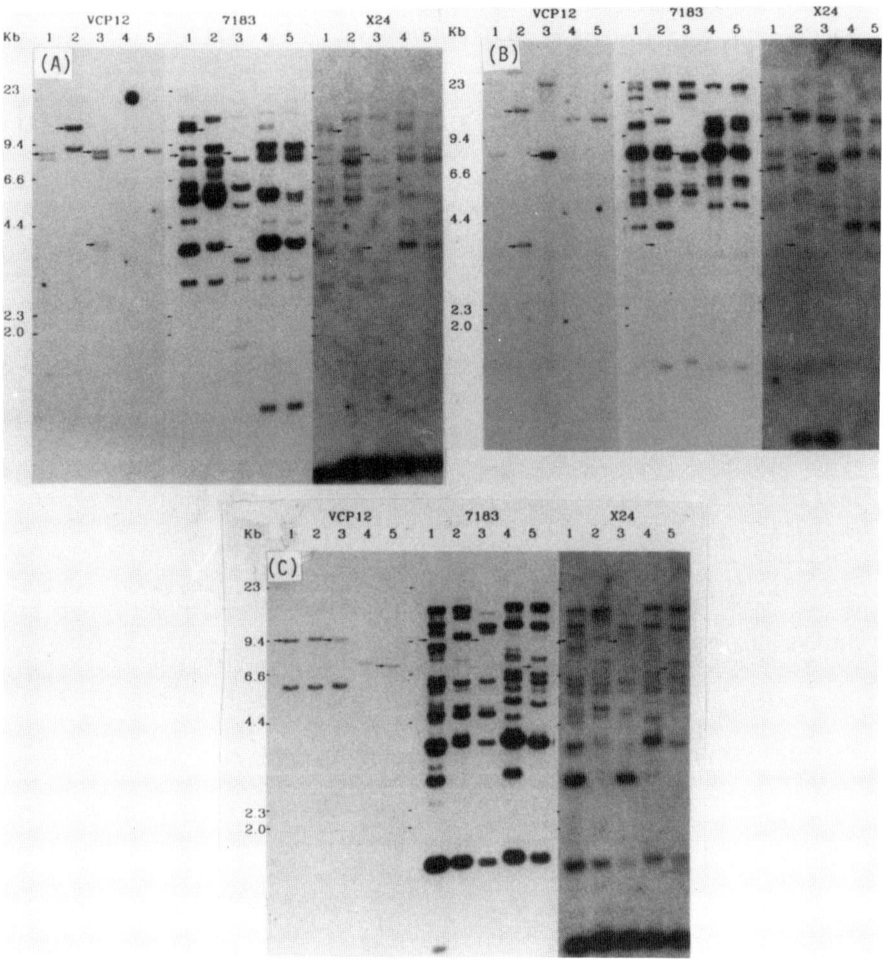

Fig.3. Southern blot hybridizations of VH probes to mouse genomic digested DNA. The VH probes VCP12, 7183 and X24 were hybridized to A) EcoRI digested DNA, B) BamHI digested DNA, and C) HindIII digested DNA. The filters were washed under moderate stringency conditions. See (27) and Materials and Methods, for details. Lanes 1 = BALB/c (Igh-V^{a}), 2 = C57BL/6 (Igh-V^{b}), 3 = DBA/2 (Igh-V^{c}), 4 = NZB (Igh-V^{d}), and 5 = C3H (Igh-Vj).

(indicated by arrows) were again observed. According to the mouse strains and the restriction enzymes considered, excepted for the NZB strain, at least one if not two VCP12-hybridizing fragments were detected neither by the 7183 VH probe nor by the X24 probe. Thus, the genes contained in such fragments belong to a novel VH family.

A few genes could account for the anti-BrMRBC VH repertoire

Under moderate stringency conditions, the VCP12 probe was found to hybridize to one, two or three EcoRI restriction fragments, depending on the mouse strain considered : one in NZB (Igh-V^d) and C3H (Igh-V^J) mice, two in BALB/c (Igh-V^a) and C57BL/6 (Igh-V^b) mice, and three in DBA/2 (Igh-V^c) mice (Fig.3A). The analysis of two other enzymatic digests (Figs. 3B and 3C) did not change the number of fragments identified for any strain tested except for the DBA/2 strain, where one fragment was lost. However, in the BamHI digest (Fig.3B, lane 3), the increased intensity of the hybridization signal with the low Mr fragment (indicated by an arrow) is consistent with the presence in the same band of at least two genes. Therefore, the three fragments at the most detected here likely represent the upper number of genes closely related to the VCP12 probe.

DISCUSSION

The fusion of peritoneal cells from LPS-stimulated BALB/c mice and unstimulated NZB and CBA/J mice with myeloma cells led to the insolation of seven hybridomas secreting anti-BrMRBC monoclonal antibodies (14,26,27). The structure of their VH and Vκ regions was found to be virtually identical (Fig.1 and 2), thus supporting the germ line feature of V genes encoding BrMRBC antibodies. Since the seven antibodies originate from four independent fusion events and from three different strains of mice, they likely reflect the anti-BrMRBC antibody VH repertoire.

Although genetic restriction in the VH and Vκ gene usage in anti-hapten antibodies as well as in rheumatoid factors or anti-DNA autoantibodies was noted (reviewed in 36), the extremely high homogeneity of the anti-BrMRBC V regions is one of the most striking observations. Indeed, the anti-BrMRBC reactivity was found to be encoded by a single VCP12-D SP2 (5,7 or 8)-JH1 gene combination for the H chain and two possible Vκ9-Jκ2 or Jκ4 gene combinations for the L chain. This result is consistent with the idiotypic analysis of natural anti-BrMRBC antibodies (14,26), which has shown that a major idiotype is highly conserved, although other possible V-D-J combinations cannot be excluded. Some nucleotide substitutions observed among seven anti-BrMRBC monoclonal antibodies are most likely related to the strain considered rather than to particular hybridomas (26), and in agreement with the determination of the murine Igh-V and Igh-D haplotypes (20,37), they reflect the Ig gene polymorphism rather than somatic mutations. In addition, almost all of the anti-BrMRBC antibodies belong to the IgM class. This observation is consistent with the finding that IgM rheumatoid factors and IgM anti-DNA antibodies are encoded by germ-line genes (38,39,40). This is not a general rule, however, as some autoantibodies may acquire self-reactivity after somatic mutational events (41,42). The absence of immune maturation of the anti-BrMRBC antibody "response", even though the total number of anti-BrMRBC secreting cells increases with age (14), could be explained by the lack of participation of T helper cells in this particular autoimmune response. In fact, previous attempts at self immunization of mice with BrMRBC have failed to yield IgG anti-BrMRBC antibodies (A. Bussard, personal communication), a finding consistent with the observation that the large majority of IgM autoantibodies do not switch to other isotypes (43).

Whereas most of the genetic elements in autoantibodies are identical with, or closely related to, those expressed by non-autoantibodies (36), the VH gene of anti-BrMRBC has not yet been found expressed in responses to exogeneous antigens : the VCP12 BrMRBC encoding gene could not be clearly assigned to any of the ten known VH families, both by the criteria of nucleotide sequence homology and Southern blot RFLP patterns (Fig.3). Consequently, the VCP12 related genes likely belong to a new VH family, which we tentatively designate **VH11**. Our results differ from RNA dot blot analyses of anti-BrMRBC hybridomas, which have led the authors to propose a 7183 VH family assignement (15). The analysis of VH families from LPS-induced polyclonal antibody responses has demonstrated that the VH family frequencies appear to correlate with the size of the families (44). It could be predicted that VH families, which have not been identified so far, are made up of only a few members. Accordingly, the last two described VH families, VH10 (22) and VH11 (this paper) exhibit a low degree of complexity since 3 (36) and 2 genes in the BALB/c mouse respectively, have been estimated. Alternatively, the few remaining VH families to be described may have a size larger than that of VH10 and VH11 and may be composed mostly of pseudogenes, a significant proportion of which constituting the Ig-V gene repertoire (45).

Almost all anti-BrMRBC producing cells may belong to a unique subpopulation of B cells expressing the Ly-1 antigen (46). Apparently, the Ly-1$^+$ B cells constitute a particular B cell subset which produce most of the autoantibodies even though not exclusively (48), but fail to respond to some exogeneous antigens in T-dependent and T-independent immunizations (46,47), suggesting that Ly-1$^+$ B cells may express a restricted Ig-V gene repertoire. This is consistent with the fact that the new **VH11** family described here is apparently not represented among the VH gene repertoire known to encode antibodies induced by immunization with foreign antigens. Thus, it is possible that this VH family is largely represented in the Igh-V gene repertoire of the Ly-1$^+$ B cells. Indeed, recent work has shown that Ly-1$^+$ B cell lymphomas of the CH series express a restricted repertoire of VH and VL region genes, that are essentially unmutated. This restriction was not due to the preferential usage of any particular VH or VL gene family. Among ten CH lymphomas, three expressed VH genes identical to VCP12 gene studied here (49).

The VCP12 related genes were recently mapped into the 3609-J558 gene cluster (J.D. Capra et al., personal communication), which was reported to be more DH distal than originally thought (50). Evidence for the preferential rearrangement of VH segments most proximal to the rearranged DH-JH segments (e.g.X24, Q52, 7183 gene cluster (50)) is controversial (28, 51); this observation may be associated, in part, with the existence of certain B cell subsets which predominate in the fetal liver (pre-B cells) but represent a minor population in adult mice. The preferential D-proximal VH gene utilization does not appear to be specific for autoantibodies derived from normal mice.

REFERENCES

1. Shoenfeld, Y., and R.S. Schwartz. 1984. N. Engl. J. Med. 311: 1019.
2. Pages, J.M., and A.E. Bussard. 1975. Nature 257:316.
3. Dighiero, G., P. Lymberi, J.C. Mazié, S. Rouyre, G.S., Butler-Browne, R.G. Whalen, and S. Avrameas. 1983. J. Immunol. 131:2267.
4. Avrameas, S., G. Dighiero, P. Lymberi, and B. Guilbert. 1983. Ann. Immunol. (Inst. Pasteur) 134D:103.
5. Prabhakar, B.S., J. Saegusa, T. Onodera, and A.L. Notkins. 1984. J. Immunol. 133:2815.
6. De Maeyer-Guignard, J., and E. De Maeyer. 1986. J. Immunol. 136: 1708.
7. Carroll, P., D. Stafford, R.S. Schwartz, and B.D. Stollar. 1985. J. Immunol. 135:1086.

8. Naparstek, Y., D. Duggan, A. Schattner, M.P. Madair, F. Goni, B. Frangione, B.D. Stollar, E.A. Kabat, and R.S. Schwartz. 1985. J. Exp. Med. 161:1525.
9. Grabar, P. 1983. Immunology Today 4:337.
10. Holmberg, D., G. Wennerstrom, L. Andrade, and A. Coutinho. 1986. Eur. J. Immunol. 16:82.
11. Lord, E., and R.W. Dutton. 1975. J. Immunol. 115:1199.
12. Steele, E.J., and A.J. cunningham. 1978. Nature 274:483.
13. Cox, K.O., D. Evans, D. Brooks, and D.A. Cunliffe. 1979. J. Immunol. 38:355.
14. Poncet, P., H.P. Kocher, J.M. Pages, J.C. Jaton, and A.E. Bussard. 1985. Mol. Immunol. 22:541.
15. Painter, C., M. Monestier, B. Bonin, and C.A. Bona. 1986. Immunol. Rev. 94:77.
16. Holmberg, D., A.A. Freitas, D. Portnoï, F. Jacquemart, S. Avrameas, and A. Coutinho. 1986. Immunol. Rev. 93: 147.
17. Eilat, D., M. Hochberg, J. Pamphrey, and S. Rudikoff. 1984. J. Immunol. 133:489.
18. Diamond, B., and M.D. Scharff. 1984. Proc. Natl. Acad. Sci. USA 81:5841.
19. Kofler, R., D.J. Noonan, D.E. Levy, M.C. Wilson, N.P.H. Möller, F.J. Dixon, and A.N. Theofilopoulos. 1985. J. Exp. Med. 161:805.
20. Brodeur, P.H., and R. Riblet. 1984. Eur. J. Immunol. 14: 922.
21. Winter, E., A. Radbruch, and U. Krawinkel. 1985. EMBO J. 4:2861.
22. Kofler, R. 1988. J. Immunol. 140:4031.
23. Kaushik, A., A. Lim, P. Poncet, X.-R. Ge, and G. Dighiero. 1988. Scand. J. Immunol. (In press).
24. Hamlyn, P.H., G.G. Brownlee, C.C. Cheng, M.J. Gait, and C. Milstein. 1978. Cell 5:1067.
25. Sanger, F., S. Niclen, and A.R. Coulson. 1977. Proc. Natl. Acad. Sci. USA 74:5463.
26. Reininger, L., P. Ollier, P. Poncet, A. Kaushik, and J.-C. Jaton. 1987. J. Immunol. 138:316.
27. Reininger, L., A. Kaushik, S. Izui, and J.-C. Jaton 1988. Eur. J. Immunol. 18:1521.
28. Wu, G.E., and C.J. Paige. 1986. EMBO J. 5:3475.
29. Hartman, A.B., and S. Rudikoff. 1984. EMBO J. 3:3023.
30. Kurosawa, Y, and S. Tonegawa. 1982. J. Exp. Med. 155: 201.
31. Sakano, H., R. Maki, Y. Kurosawa, W. Roeder, and S. Tonegawa. 1980. Nature 286:676.
32. Potter, M., J.B. Newel, S. Rudikoff, and E. Haber. 1982. Mol. Immunol. 19:1619.

33. Sakano, H., K. Huppi, G. Heinrich, and S. Tonegawa. 1979. Nature 280:288.
34. Wood, D., and C. Coleclough. 1984. Proc. Natl. Acad. Sci. USA 81:4756.
35. Kabat, E.A., T.T. Wu, M. Reid-Miller, H.M. Perry, and K.S. Gottesman. 1987. Sequences of Proteins of Immunological Interest, 4th Ed. US Dept of Health and Human Services. NIH, Bethesda.
36. Kofler, R., F.J. Dixon, and A.N. Theofilopoulos. 1987. Immunol. Today 8:374.
37. Trepicchio, W.J., and K.J. Barrett. 1985. J. Immunol. 134:2734.
38. Shlomchik, M.J., D.A. Nemazee, V.L. Sato, J. Van Snick, D.A. Carson, and M.G. Weigert. 1986. J. Exp. Med. 164: 407.
39. Naparstek, Y., J. André-Schwartz, T. Manser, L.J. Wysocki, L. Breitman, B.D. Stollar, M. Gefter, and R.S. Schwartz. 1986. J. Exp. Med. 164:614.
40. Trepicchio, W.J., A. Maruya, and K.J. Barrett. 1987. J. Immunol. 139:3139
41. Diamond, B., and M.D. Scharff. 1984. Proc. Natl. Acad. Sci. USA 81:5841.
42. Giusti, A.M., N.C. Chien, D.J. Zack, S-U. Shin, and M.D. Scharff. 1987. Proc. Natl. Acad. Sci. USA 84:2926.
43. Manser, T.,L.J. Wysocki, M.N. Margolies, and M.L. Gefter. 1987. Immunol. Rev. 96:141.
44. Dildrop, R., U. Krawinkel, E. Winter, and K. Rajewsky. 1985. Eur. J. Immunol. 15:1154.
45. Rechavi, G., D. Ram, L. Glaser, R. Zakut, and D. Givol. 1983. Proc. Natl. Acad. Sci. USA 80:855.
46. Hayakawa, K., R.R. Hardy, M. Honda, L.A. Herzenberg, A.D. Steinberg, and L.A. Herzenberg. 1984. Proc. Natl. Acad. Sci. USA 81:2494.
47. Förster, I., and K. Rajewsky. 1987. Eur. J. Immunol. 17: 521.
48. Conger, J.D., B.L. Pike, and G.J.V. Nossal. 1987. Proc. Natl. Acad. Sci. USA 84:2931.
49. Pennell, C.A., L.W. Arnold, G. Haughton, and S.H. Clarke. 1988. J. Immunol. 141:2788.
50. Rathbun, G.A., J.D. Capra, and P.W. Tucker. 1987. EMBO J. 6:2931.
51. Schultze, D.H., and G. Kelsoe. 1987. J. Exp. Med. 166: 163.

MOLECULAR ANALYSIS OF MURINE LUPUS-ASSOCIATED HUMORAL ANTI-SELF RESPONSE[1]

Reinhard Kofler

Institute for General and Experimental Pathology
University of Innsbruck, Medical School
Innsbruck, Austria
and
Department of Immunology
Research Institute of Scripps Clinic
La Jolla, California

Frank J. Dixon
Argyrios N. Theofilopoulos

Department of Immunology
Research Institute of Scripps Clinic
La Jolla, California

I. INTRODUCTION

The genetic origin of autoantibodies, particularly those associated with, and possibly responsible for, systemic lupus erythematosus (SLE) and other autoimmune diseases, has attracted considerable interest over the last years. Corresponding studies have become possible by the advent of molecular techniques and address a variety of important problems related to disease etiology, pathogenesis, and novel therapeutic approaches (reviewed in 1). To this end, Ig gene loci in autoimmune states, and possible

[1]This is Publication Number 5743IMM from the Department of Immunology , Research Institute of Scripps Clinic, 10666 North Torrey Pines Road, La Jolla, CA 92037, The work reported herein was supported, in part, by NIH grants AR31203, AR33826, AI07007, AG01743, the Keck Foundation and the Austrian Research Council Project S-41/06.

genetic, structural and clonotypic restriction of autoantibodies and their primary structure have been investigated in great detail both in the human and murine system. Perhaps the most relevant question asked in such studies is whether abnormalities in the genes and complex mechanisms generating antibody diversity (reviewed in 2,3) contribute to autoantibody formation and disease.

Our laboratory has studied the genetic origin of the murine lupus-associated anti-self response and has taken 2 basic approaches to address the above issue: First, we have investigated whether murine lupus is associated with abnormalities in Ig gene loci and, since these loci exhibit considerable polymorphism (4-6), whether this disease is restricted to a particular Ig heavy or kappa light chain gene haplotype. Second, we have employed cDNA cloning, nucleic acid sequencing, and other molecular techniques to characterize the gene segments that encode spontaneously arising autoantibodies from lupus mice.

II. IG GERMLINE GENES IN MURINE LUPUS

A. Ig Heavy Chain Gene Loci

Murine Ig heavy chain variable (V_H) genes are organized in at least 11 multigene families with related members that exhibit extensive genetic polymorphism among inbred strains of mice defining several Ig heavy chain variable region gene (Igh-V) haplotypes [(4,7-9), and J.-C. Jaton, these proceedings]. The complexity of individual families varies considerably, with 1 family (J558) comprising the majority of the entire repertoire (10). To address possible V_H germline gene defects or Igh-V haplotype associations with autoantibody production and lupus disease, we analyzed restriction fragment length polymorphisms (RFLPs) in DNA from all major lupus strains, mice carrying the *lpr* (lymphoproliferation) gene (which induces autoantibody expression on various genetic backgrounds), their respective ancestors, and non-autoimmune controls using DNA probes corresponding to 9 V_H gene families (11,12; data not shown). This analysis defined the Igh-V haplo-types of all major lupus strains (Table I) and revealed that murine lupus is not associated with a particular Igh-V haplotype.

Lupus mice with known genetic derivation (MRL, BXSB) and mice congenic for the *lpr* gene have inherited the Igh-V loci apparently unaltered from their non-autoimmune ancestral strains. NZW and NZB lupus mice, with unknown genetic

Table I. Igh and Igk Haplotypes[a] of Lupus Mice and Their Ancestors

Lupus Strain	Igh-V	Igk	Ancestors[b]	Igh-V	Igk
MRL	j	a	LG (75%)	j	h
			AKR (12.6%)	d	a
			C3H (12.1%)	j	c
			C57BL/6 (0.3%)	b	c
BXSB	b	c	C57BL/6 (50%)	b	c
			SB (50%)	b	c
NZB	d	b	unknown		
NZW	d	c	unknown		

[a]Igh-V and Igk haplotypes according to refs. (4) and (5), respectively.
[b]Percent estimated contributions of ancestors to the genome of the respective lupus strain are given in parenthesis.

derivation, have Igh-V loci almost indistinguishable from those of non-autoimmune AKR mice. These observations strongly suggested that the V_H germline gene repertoires of lupus mice may be normal, a conclusion also drawn by Treppicchio et al. (13) and subsequently by others (14).

Since murine lupus shows a good correlation between disease onset and switch of polyclonal and autoantibody Ig from predominantly IgM to predominantly IgG, and since IgG autoantibodies have an excellent predictive value for disease expression, and are found in eluates from diseased kidneys (15), we investigated the genomic organization of Ig heavy chain switch regions of the various murine Ig isotypes by RFLP analysis with appropriate probes. No evidence for gross abnormalities was detected (16), suggesting that enhanced switching may occur under the influence of abnormal levels of, or in response to, T cell-derived factors, as we have already suggested (17,18). To investigate the possibility of subtle, but functionally significant, abnormalities in Ig regulatory sequences that may have escaped detection by RFLP analyses, we cloned and sequenced the Igh enhancer region in 2 strains that develop lupus early in life (BXSB and MRL-*lpr/lpr*)(16). The reference BALB/c sequence was identical to that of BXSB, and the MRL-*lpr/lpr* Igh enhancer differed by a single nucleotide. This possibly allelic difference resides outside of the enhancer core regions (19,20) and is, therefore, probably functionally irrelevant.

B. Ig Kappa Light Chain Loci

Polymorphism, organization and complexity of the murine Igk gene complex has recently been investigated in greater detail in M. Potter's and our laboratory (5,6). To this end, 17 DNA probes corresponding to 15 previously defined (21) and 2 novel V_k protein groups along with probes for the kappa joining (J) and constant (C) gene segments have been used to explore the Igk gene complex in some 50 inbred strains of mice. These studies have revealed considerable polymorphism of this locus, and have defined 9 murine Igk haplotypes. Complexity approximations have been provided for the investigated V_k gene families, and the total number of V_k genes in the murine genome may not exceed 150 by much. In our study (5), considerable overlaps were observed between certain V_k gene families (*i.e.*, DNA probes corresponding to different V_k protein groups hybridized to partly overlapping sets of V_k genes). This observation somewhat distinguishes V_k from V_H gene families and has important implications for V_k gene usage determinations by nucleic acid hybridization techniques.

To address whether the Igk gene complex in lupus mice harbors abnormalities that might contribute to autoantibody formation, and to determine possible associations of murine lupus with a particular Igk haplotype, we subjected genomic DNA from all major lupus strains and their progenitors (as far as known) to RFLP analysis with our probe panel (V_k1, 2, 4-5, 8, 9, 10, 11, 12-13, 14, 19, 21, 22, 23, 24, 28, V_kRF, and J_k/C_k). As exemplified in Fig. 1A and 1B for probes corresponding to 12 V_k gene families, the V_k loci of autoimmune mice with known genetic derivations appear essentially identical to those of their non-autoimmune ancestral strains, *i.e.*, MRL and BXSB lupus mice derived their V_k locus essentially unaltered from their AKR (haplotype "a") and C57BL/6 or SB (both haplotype "c") progenitors, respectively. NZW mice with unknown genetic derivation share their V_k locus with normal mice of the Igk^c haplotype (such as BALB/c and C57BL/6). Only NZB revealed an unusual, possibly recombinant, Igk haplotype, termed Igk^b: ten of their analyzed V_k families (V_k5,8,10,12-13,14,19,21,22,23,

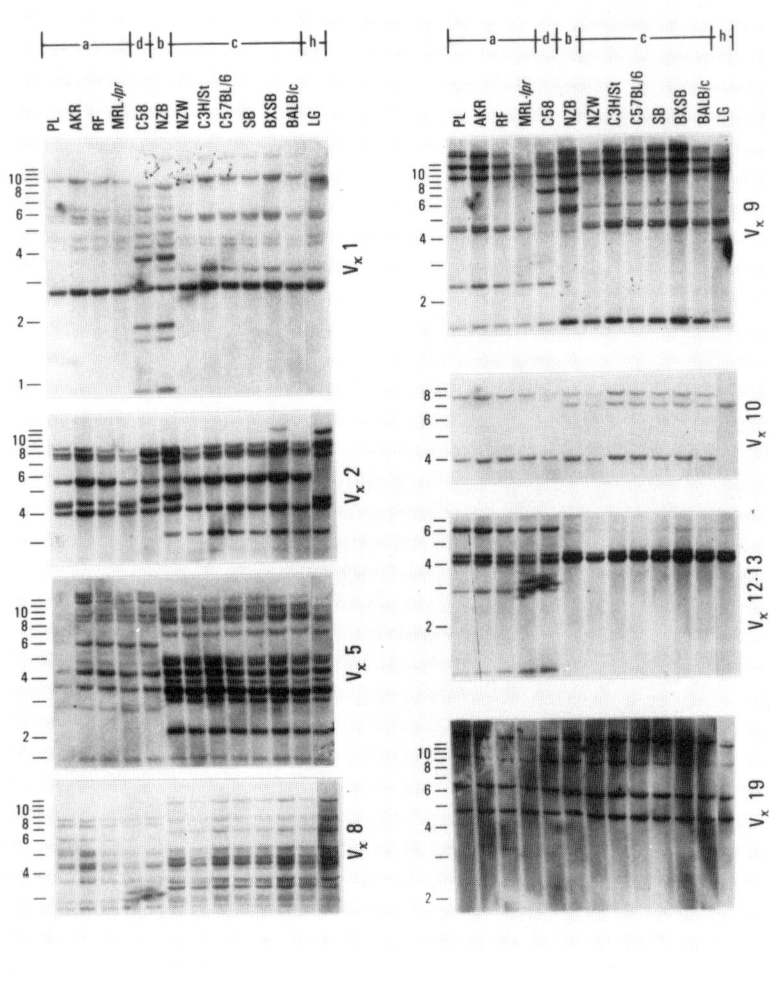

Fig. 1A. *Autoradiographs of restriction enzyme-digested, size-separated liver DNA from several lupus and other inbred strains of mice probed with ^{32}P-labeled DNA probes corresponding to several V_k gene families. Lowercase letters above strain designations denote their* Igk *haplo-types (5). One kilobase pair (kb) size markers are given on the left, the V_k gene probe on the right of each blot. Shown are HindIII digests except for V_k10, V_k28 (both PstI), and V_k19 (BamHI). Corresponding results were obtained with additional restriction enzymes (EcoRI, HindIII, PstI, BamHI) and probes for V_k11, V_k14, V_k23, and V_kRF gene families.*

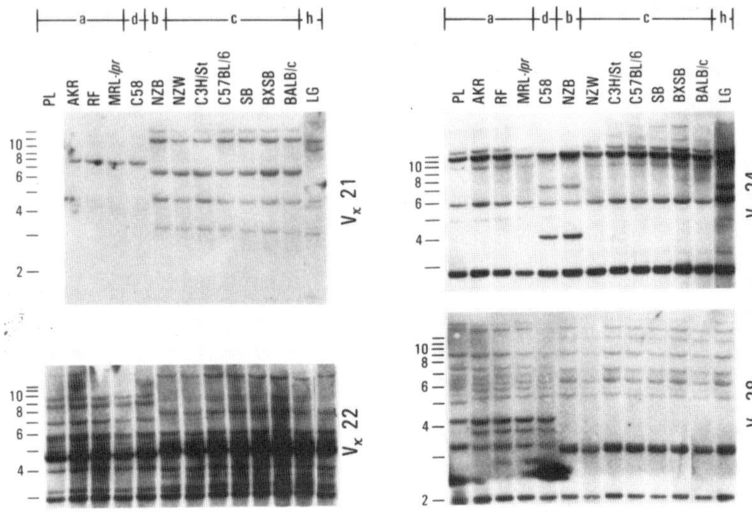

Fig. 1B. *(See Fig. 1A legend)*

28) as well as the J_k/C_k complex are indistinguishable from those of the "c" haplotype, whereas the remaining loci (V_k1, 2, 9, 11, 24, V_kRF) are very similar to, but not always identical with, the corresponding loci in C58 mice (haplotype "d"). The extent, if any, to which the NZB Igk haplotype contributes to disease etiology in this strain remains to be determined, since non-autoimmune strains such as LG and C58 also exhibited unique Igk haplotypes. Mice congenic for the *lpr*, *gld* (generalized lymphadenopathy), *me* (motheaten) and *tsk* (tight skin) genes, all of which induce autoimmune disease and/or autoantibody expression on various genetic backgrounds, and congenics for other genes of immunologic interest and various mutant strains were also tested using the entire probe panel and 3-4 different restriction enzymes. None of these mutations was associated with detectable alterations in the loci under scrutinity (exemplified in Figs. 2 and 3).

Our study contrasts with a similar analysis by Bona et al. (22), who found RFLPs between MRL and AKR, and between C57BL/6 and the congenic C57BL/6-*tsk* strains with V_k1, V_k10, and V_k19 DNA probes. These authors concluded that the V_k genes that are preferentially used by autoantibodies (see below), might derive from a set of germline genes present only in autoimmune-prone mouse strains. The reasons for the significant differences between our results and those of Dr. Bona are presently unexplained, although close scrutinity of fragment patterns obtained in the 2 laboratories shows 1 major additional fragment in the MRL and C57BL/6-*tsk* (as well as in non-autoimmune C3H and LG) lanes that is present at approximately the same molecular weight in 3 of their blots (V_k1, V_k10, and V_k19), but is absent from corresponding lanes on our blots. Although other explanations might exist, this divergence suggests that the unique fragments might be artifacts resulting from, for example, plasmid contaminations in the respective DNA preparations. Moreover, Dr. Bona's findings and the conclusions derived therefrom are not easily explained, particularly in the C57BL/6)-*tsk* strain. This strain is maintained by continuous backcrossing to C57BL/6-*pa* and selection against homozygosity at the *pa* (pallid) locus, thereby maintaining chromosome 2 (which harbors the *tsk* and *pa* mutations) in a heterozygous state (*pa*/-, -/*tsk*). Since C57BL/6-*pa* have normal Igk loci, the abnormal V_k genes specifically detected in the C57BL/6-*tsk* strain would have to reside on chromosome 2, which is surprising since the murine Igk gene complex is located on chromosome 6.

Our results on Ig heavy and kappa light chain gene loci in autoimmune mice agree with previous classical genetic analyses (23, 24) and the observation that lupus-like symptoms and/or autoantibodies can be induced in normal background mice by a variety of means (25-27). They strongly suggest that: a) defects within the Ig heavy and kappa light chain loci are not likely to be primary causes for murine SLE, and b) that there are no simple associations of Igh-V and Igk haplotypes with murine lupus.

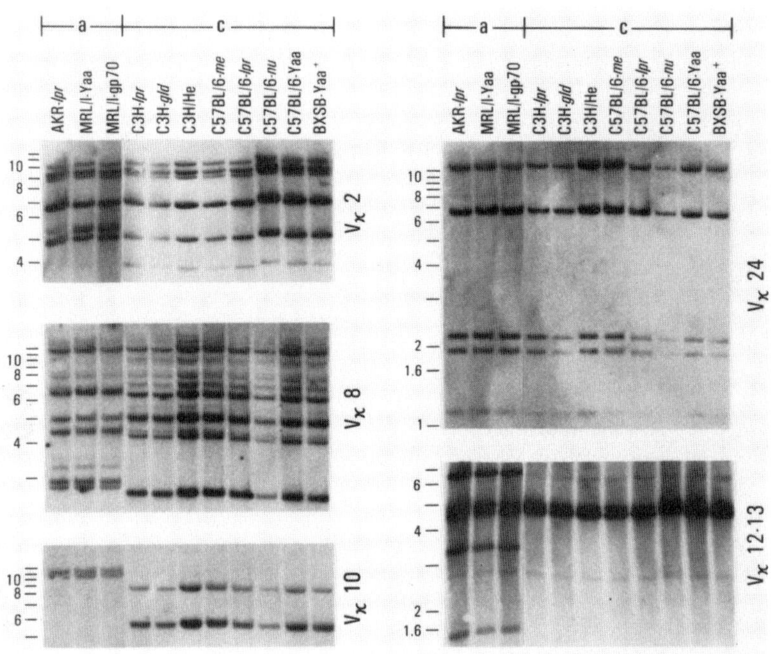

Fig. 2. *Autoradiographs of restriction enzyme-digested, size-separated DNA from mutant strains of mice probed with ^{32}P-labeled DNA corresponding to 5 V_k gene families. Lower-case letters above strain designations denote their Igk haplotypes (5). One kb size markers are given on the left, the V_k gene probe on the right of each blot. Shown are HindIII (V_k2 and V_k12-13) and BamHI (V_k8, 10, 24) digests. Corresponding results were obtained with additional restriction enzymes (EcoRI, PstI) and the remaining probes from our panel. Yaa, autoimmune accelerator, denotes strains consomic for the BXSB Y-chromosome; BXSB-Yaa+ is a BXSB substrain carrying the C57BL/6 Y-chromosome; MRL/l-gp70 is an MRL/MpScr-lpr/lpr congenic with low retroviral gp70 expression (35).*

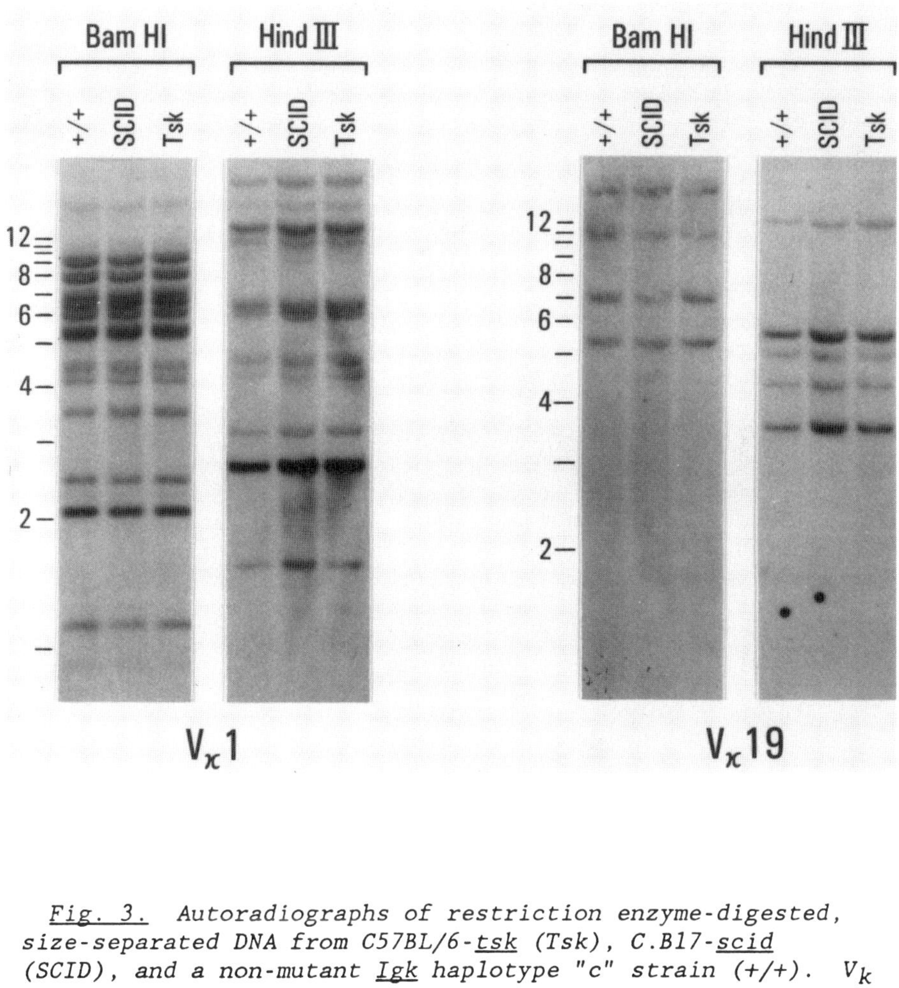

Fig. 3. Autoradiographs of restriction enzyme-digested, size-separated DNA from C57BL/6-tsk (Tsk), C.B17-scid (SCID), and a non-mutant Igk haplotype "c" strain (+/+). V_k gene probes are indicated below, restriction enzymes above, and 1 kb size markers on the left of each blot. Corresponding results were obtained with additional restriction enzymes (EcoRI, PstI) and the remaining probes from our panel.

III. IG GENE SEGMENTS ENCODING AUTOANTIBODIES

A. Autoantibody-Specific Genetic Elements

Although the above evidence suggests normal Ig germline genes in lupus mice, autoantibodies may still be encoded by unique V or D (diversity) gene segments that are not rearranged or used in response to exogenous antigens. To investigate such a possibility, which might suggest a defect in the control of V-(D)-J rearrangement in lupus disease, we cloned and sequenced mRNAs encoding heavy and light chains from 11 monoclonal autoantibodies (5,12,28,29). Table II summarizes the characteristics of these monoclonals and the structural genetic elements (V,D,J gene segments) encoding them. The respective nucleic acid and deduced amino acid sequences are depicted in Figures 4A and 4B. While J and C gene segments ($C\mu$ and C_k were sequenced from a representative autoantibody, 30) were identical or almost identical to those of BALB/c mice, some D segments could not be classified. However, novel D segments are frequently seen in antibodies to exogenous antigens and can be ascribed to alterations occuring during V/D/J joining, additional uncharacterized D families in the murine genome, allotypic differences, and a novel mechanism for D segment inversion reported by J.D. Capra at this meeting. Of interest, all

Table II. Genetic Elements Encoding Murine Lupus-Associated Autoantibodies

Monoclonal Ab Code	Specificity	Isotype	Heavy Chain			Light Chain	
			VH[a]	D	JH	Vk[b]	Jk
BXW-DNA7	ssDNA	IgM	J558	DFL16.1	JH1	n.d.	n.d.
BXW-DNA14	ssDNA	IgM	J558	DFL16.1	JH2	Vk2	Jk1
BXW-DNA16	ssDNA	IgM	J558	DFL16.1	JH2	Vk9	Jk2
MRL-DNA10	ssDNA	IgM	J558	n.a.	JH3	Vk1	Jk4
MRL-DNA4	ssDNA	IgG2a	VH10	n.a.	JH3	Vk1	Jk2
MRL-DNA22	ssDNA,dsDNA	IgM	J558	n.a.	JH4	Vk5	Jk4
MRL-RF7	IgG2b,ssDNA	IgM	J558	n.a.	JH1	n.d.	n.d.
MRL-RF14/9	IgG2a	IgM	J558	n.a.	JH4	Vk28	Jk1
MRL-RF24	IgG1,2a,3	IgM	J558	Q52	JH4	VkRF	Jk1
MRL-RF28	IgG2a,b	IgM	n.d.	n.d.	n.d.	Vk28	Jk1
MRL-Histone7	Histones	IgG3	Sm7	SP2	JH4	Vk5	Jk5

[a] V_H gene family designations according to refs. 4 and 9. Sm7 is a potential new V_H gene family formerly included in the large J558 family.
[b] V_k groups according to ref. 21. The MRL-RF24 Vk sequence could not be assigned to any known V_k group and represents the prototype of a new, single-member V_k gene family, termed V_kRF (5).
n.d., not determined;
n.a., not assigned.

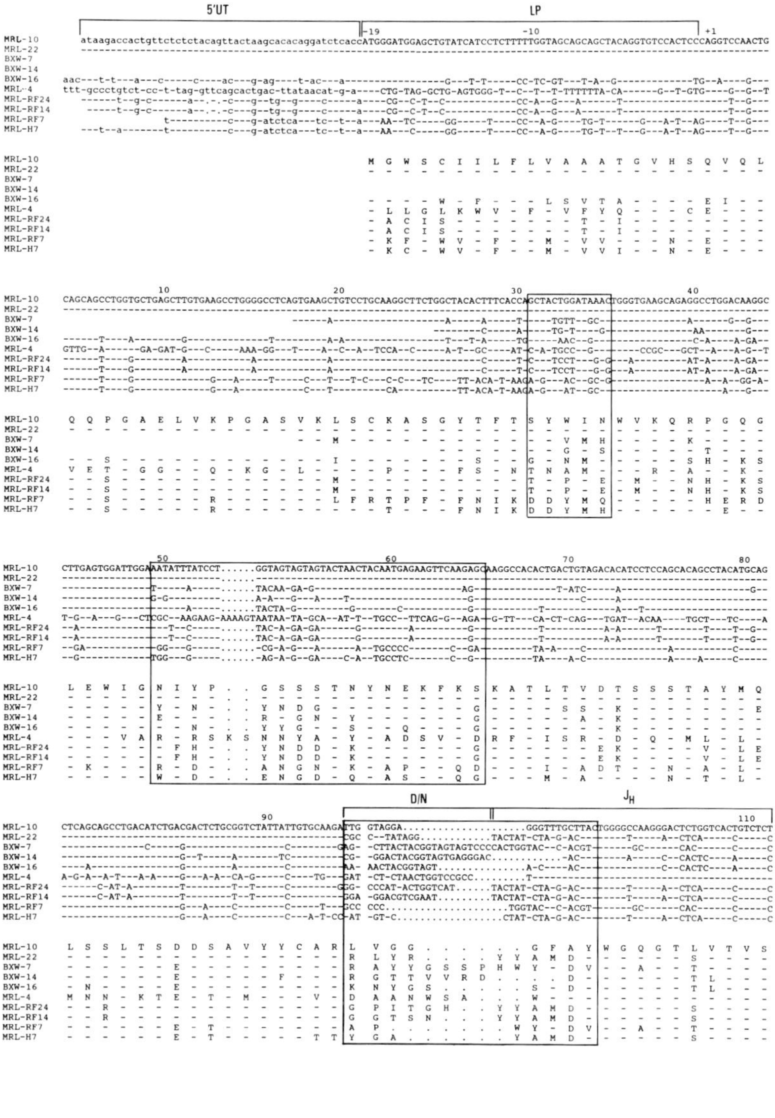

Fig. 4A. *Nucleic acid and deduced amino acid sequences of autoantibody heavy (A) and light (B) chain V regions. Dashes in sequence indicate identity to the MRL-DNA10 sequence at the top; dots indicate gaps introduced for proper alignment. Complementarity-determining regions are boxed; amino acid numbering is according to Kabat et al. (36). 5'UT, 5' untranslated region; LP, leader peptide.*

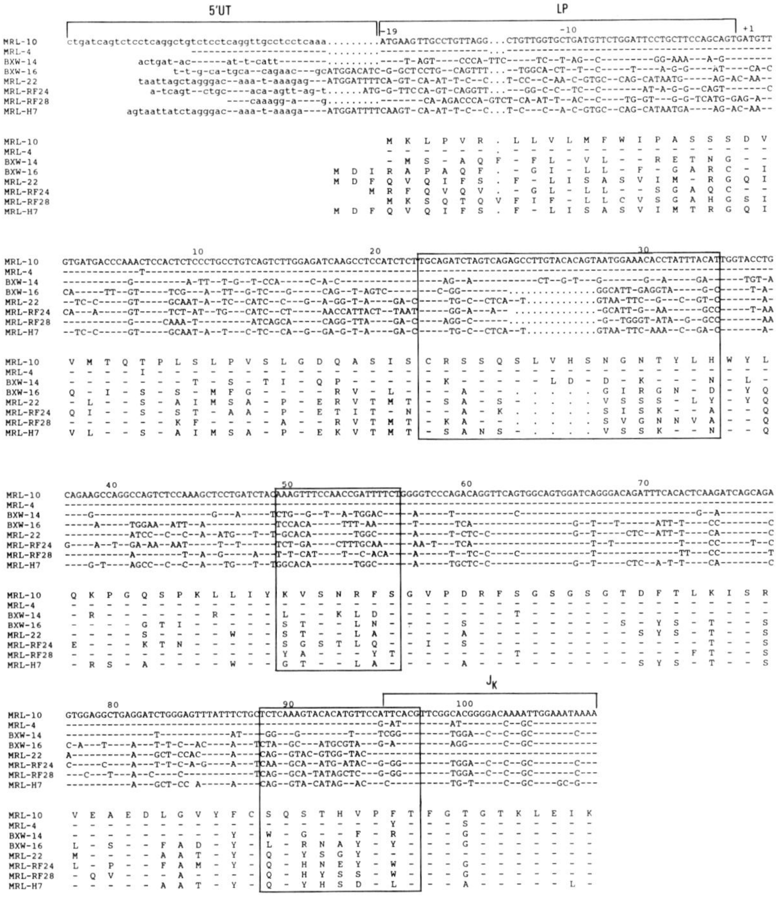

Fig. 4B. (See Fig. 4A legend)

unassigned D segments were clearly different, and the 3 FL16.1 D segments shared by $(BXW)F_1$ anti-DNAs were used in 2 reading frames and in context with different N-region sequences, resulting in quite different primary structures of the third complementarity-determining region (CDR). Furthermore, CDR-3 length, which is considered important for antigen and anti-idiotype recognition, was not conserved among these autoantibodies with different specificities. Almost all V genes investigated could be unambiguously assigned to existing V gene families. The only exceptions were the MRL-DNA4 V_H gene and the MRL-RF24 V_k gene, which define new V_H and V_k families, termed V_H10 (9) and, V_kRF (5), respectively. However, the organization of corresponding germline genes in lupus and normal mice of the same haplotype are indistinguishable by RFLP analysis (12, and this report), and V_H10 genes are also expressed in hybridomas from LPS-stimulated splenocytes of non-autoimmune mice (R. Dildrop, personal communication). The evidence available at present, therefore, strongly suggests that autoantibodies do not employ unique Ig gene segments, but are encoded by the same (or at least an overlapping) germline gene repertoire used by antibodies to exogenous antigens. This conclusion is in full agreement with a major postulate for generation of antibody diversity, *i.e.*, that an individual V gene participates in the generation of different specificities.

B. Genetic Restriction Among Autoantibodies

Common structural genetic elements among autoantibodies with different specificities might point towards common inducing agents, provide a structural explanation for how these molecules circumvent anti-idiotypic or other forms of immunologic regulation, and establish a basis for specific therapeutic interventions using anti-idiotypes. Preferential usage of V_H genes by autoantibodies with different specificities has indeed been suggested, particularly of those of the 7183 V_H gene family (31), and it was concluded that autoimmune disease may be related to a defective control of V_H gene expression (32). However, none of our sequenced autoantibodies derived from 3′ V_H gene families (Table II) and additional autoantibodies analyzed by us and others using nucleic acid hybridization and other techniques were encoded by representatives from all known V_H gene families (reviewed in 1). The proposed 7183 V_H gene overrepresentation appeared minimal, if existent, particularly if autoantibodies from spontaneously autoimmune mice were analyzed. More recently, preferential use of V_k gene families (V_k1, V_k10, V_k19) by autoantibodies has been suggested (22). However, the 9 V_k genes identified in our panel of autoantibodies derived from 6 different V_k gene families, and additional V_k gene families have been found to encode autoantibodies (1). Furthermore, one of the proposed autoantibody-restricting gene families (V_k1) also encodes exogenous responses at an unexpected high frequency (33). In this context, it is worth mentioning that an apparently non-random representation of V_H and V_k gene families in collections of hybridoma autoantibodies should be interpreted with caution, since neither the precise V germline gene number nor their expression frequency are known. Moreover, skewed representation might be due to small sample size, non-random representation of autoantibody specificities and, if RNA hybridization analyses (RNA-dot blotting, Northerns) are being used, technical reasons, as discussed elsewhere (1). The majority of current data suggests that the overall murine lupus-associated anti-self response shows little, if any, genetic restriction.

Of course, this does not exclude genetic restriction among autoantibodies of a given specificity, although this kind of restriction is more likely related to the structural requirements for generation of a particular binding site than to possible defects in V gene usage. Genetic restriction is common among antibodies against defined haptens and epitopes on complex exogenous antigens (34), and examples for anti-self specificities have been reported at this meeting.

VI. CONCLUSIONS

In this study, we have attempted to define the molecular and clonotypic origin of autoantibodies that typify systemic autoimmune diseases such as lupus and rheumatoid arthritis. Ig germline gene organization analysis in autoimmune strains of mice suggested that the disease can develop in different Ig heavy and light chain haplotypes, and that the Ig germline genes in lupus mice are probably normal. Analyses of the Ig gene segments expressed in monoclonal autoantibodies from autoimmune mice revealed that similar, and in some instances even identical, gene segments are expressed in autoantibodies and in antibodies to exogenous antigens, and that anti-self and anti-foreign responses are encoded by the same, or at least an overlapping, germline gene repertoire. A large variety of V, D, and J gene segments can encode autoantibodies with different specificities arguing against genetic restriction of the overall disease-associated anti-self response. These findings, in concert with additional data from our and other laboratories (reviewed in 1,7,29), suggest that gross abnormalities in the genes and mechanisms generating antibody diversity might not contribute to the etiology of generalized autoimmune diseases.

ACKNOWLEDGEMENTS

We thank Drs. J.D. Capra, N. Hozumi, P. Leder, R.P. Perry, and S.C. Riley for providing V_k probes, Drs. M.T. Aguado, M.A. Duchosal, R. Strohal, and P.A. Singer, for stimulating discussions, M.E. Johnson, S.T. Hogan, and C. Amundsen for excellent technical assistance, and M.K. Occhipinti for editing and preparing the manuscript.

References

1. Kofler, R., F.J. Dixon, and A.N. Theofilopoulos. (1987) Immunol. Today 8:374.
2. Tonegawa, S. (1983) Nature 302:575.
3. Alt, F.W., K. Blackwell, R.A. DePinho, M.G. Reth, and G.D. Yancopoulos. (1986) Immunol. Rev. 89:5.
4. Brodeur, P.H., and R. Riblet. (1984) Eur. J. Immunol. 14:922.
5. Kofler, R., M.A. Duchosal, and F.J. Dixon. (1989) Immunogenetics (in press).
6. D'Hoostelaere, L.A., K. Huppi, B. Mock, C. Mallett, and M. Potter. (1988) J. Immunol. 141:652.
7. Kofler, R., M.A. Duchosal, M.E. Johnson, M.T. Aguado, R. Strohal, G. Kroemer, and R. Faessler. (1987) Immunol. Lett. 16:265.
8. Winter, E., A. Radbruch, and U. Krawinkel. (1985) EMBO J. 4:2861.
9. Kofler, R. (1988) A new murine Ig VH gene family. J. Immunol. 140:4031.
10. Livant, D., C. Blatt, and L. Hood. (1986) Cell 47:461.
11. Kofler, R., R.M. Perlmutter, D.J. Noonan, F.J. Dixon, and A.N. Theofilopoulos. (1985) J. Exp. Med. 162:346.
12. Kofler, R., R. Strohal, R.S. Balderas, M.E. Johnson, D.J. Noonan, M.A. Duchosal, F.J. Dixon, and A.N. Theofilopoulos. (1988) J. Clin. Invest. 82:852.
13. Trepicchio, W.Jr., and K.J. Barrett. (1985) J. Immunol. 134:2734.

14. Painter, C., M. Monestier, B. Bonin, and C.A. Bona. (1986) Immunol. Rev. 94:75.
15. Theofilopoulos, A.N., and F.J. Dixon. (1985) Adv. Immunol. 37:269.
16. Theofilopoulos, A.N., R. Kofler, D. Noonan, P. Singer, and F.J. Dixon. (1986) Springer Semin. Immunopathol. 9:121.
17. Prud'homme, G.J., C.L. Park, T.M. Fieser, R. Kofler, F.J. Dixon, and A.N. Theofilopoulos. (1983) J. Exp. Med. 157:730.
18. Prud'homme, G.J., R.S. Balderas, F.J. Dixon, and A.N. Theofilopoulos. (1983) J. Exp. Med. 157:1815.
19. Augereau, P., and P. Chambon. (1986) EMBO J. 5:1791.
20. Sen, R., and D. Baltimore. (1986). Cell 46:705.
21. Potter, M., J.B. Newell, S. Rudikoff, and E. Haber. (1982) Mol. Immunol. 19:1619.
22. Bona, C. (1988). Ann. Rev. Immunol. 6:327.
23. Gavalchin, J., J.A. Nicklas, J.W. Eastcott, M.P. Madaio, B.D. Stollar, R.S. Schwartz, and S.K. Datta. (1985). J. Immunol. 134:885.
24. Bocchieri, M.H., A. Cooke, J.B. Smith, M. Weigert, and R.J. Riblet. (1982) Eur. J. Immunol. 12:349.
25. Onodera, T., A. Toniolo, U.R. Ray, A.B. Jenson, R.A. Knazek, and A.L. Notkins. (1981) J. Exp. Med. 153:1457.
26. Hang, LM., T.M. Aguado, F.J. Dixon, and A.N. Theofilopoulos. (1985) J. Exp. Med. 161:423.
27. Gleichmann, E., E.H. Van Elven, and J.P.W. Van Der Veen. (1982) Eur. J. Immunol. 12:152.
28. Kofler, R., D.J. Noonan, R. Strohal, R.S. Balderas, N.P.H. Moller, F.J. Dixon, and A.N. Theofilopoulos. (1987) Eur. J. Immunol. 17:91.
29. Kofler, R., F.J. Dixon, and A.N. Theofilopoulos. (1989) In: B Cells and B Cell Products. P. Del Guercio, editor. Karger Press, Basel, Switzerland (In Press).
30. Kofler, R., D.J. Noonan, D.E. Levy, M.C. Wilson, N.P.H. Moller, F.J. Dixon, and A.N. Theofilopoulos. (1985) J. Exp. Med. 161:805.
31. Monestier, M., A. Manheimer-Lori, B. Bellon, C. Painter, H. Dang, N. Talal, M. Zanetti, R. Schwartz, D. Pisetsky, R. Kuppers, N. Rose, J. Brochier, L. Klareskog, R. Holmdahl, B. Erlanger, F. Alt, and C. Bona. (1986) J. Clin. Invest. 78:753.
32. Stevenson, F.K. (1986) Immunol. Today 7:287.
33. Schiff, C., S. Corbet, and M. Fougereau. (1988) Immunol. Today 9:10.

34. Caton, A.J., G.G. Brownlee, L.M. Staudt, and W. Gerhard (1986) EMBO J. 5:1577.
35. Andrews, J., L.M. Hang, A.N. Theofilopoulos, and F.J. Dixon. (1986) J. Exp. Med. 163:458.
36. Kabat, E.A., T.T. Wu, M. Reid-Miller, H.M. Perry, and K.S. Gottesman. (1987) In: Sequences of proteins of immunological interest. 4th edition. U.S.Dept.Health & Human Services (PHS, NIH).

ESTABLISHMENT OF V-GENE REPERTOIRES IN NORMAL MICE

Dan Holmberg
Antonio Freitas

Unit of Applied Cell and Molecular Biology, Univeristy of Umeå, Sweden
Unité d´Immunobiologie, Départment d´Immunologie, Institut Pasteur, 75724 Paris Cedex 15, France

V-region compentarities mediating selection of actual B-cell repertoires

Differentiation from pluripotent stem cells in the bone marrow, through immunocompetent, resting B cells and to the effector stage of antibody-producing plasma cells, has classically been divided into two stages, the first independent of external antigen and the second driven by environmental stimuli into immune responses. It is well established that during the former stage an ongoing process of stimulation and selection of B cell repertoire occurs, leading to the establishment of what can be regarded as different compartments of the system. Addressing the question of antibody diversity we can thus define the following different levels (1-4).

1. The potential repertoire, including the total number of possible V-domains, that can be generated from the germline
2. The emergent repertoire, including the "cohort" of V-domains expressed by pre-B and B cells produced daily in the bone marrow
3. The available repertoire, constituted by the different V-domains that are currently expressed and which is therefore limited to the pool of immunocompetent B-cell clones
4. The actual repertoire which comprises the V-domains that are actually being utilized by antibody-producing effector cells

Observation of the characteristics of lymphocyte population dynamics, together with calculations of turnover rates of B-cells within these compartments, has led to the conclusions that the immune system only uses a minor fraction of its potential diversity and that selective mechanisms must act during these processes. Such an internal selection has been suggested to be based on V-region complementarities engaging both B-cells and antibodies, as well as T-B-cell interactions (5-7). If selection occurs based on interactions between the specificity receptors of lymphocytes, then the specificity repertoires of the different B-cell compartments would be unique.

To address this question, we have, a few years ago, initiated a project aimed at describing the composition of specificity repertoires of naturally activated B-cells. One of the approaches taken has been to establish large collections of B-cell hybridomas derived from normal non-immunized, neonatal or adult mice. The serological characterization of these hybridomas revealed the existence of a high frequency of V-region complementarities (8) with higher degrees of relative connectivity occurring in the neonatal compartment than in the adult (9). The sequence analysis of a dozen or so of these B-cell hybridomas also established the germline origin of these specificities. Thus, several of the hybridomas sequenced were found to express V_H- and V_L-regions identical to previously known germline genes and no indications of somatic mutations have so far been observed in this set of hybridomas (10). Taken together these data suggested to us that mechanisms acting at the stage of selecting cells for the actual B-cell repertoire involves interactions mediated by V-region complementarities. Moreover, as these interactions appear to be germline-encoded and occur with higher frequencies in early ontogeny we hypothesize that these mechanisms have been selected evolutionarily.

Recent progress in our understanding of the structure and organisation of the IgH-cluster has provided new possibilities to approach the characterization of V_H-gene repertoires. Based on nucleotide sequence homologies the V_H segments can be classified into families organized in overlapping clusters with variable degree of interspersion (11). Size estimates of each homology family varies from a few to hundreds of members. Relating to these V_H-families, data has been presented over the last few years that suggests developmentally controlled utilization of the most D-proximal V_H-gene segments (12,13). In line with these studies we have recently performed analysis of V_H-family utilization in the emergent, available and actual repertoires of neonatal and adult mice (14,15). For this purpose we have used an <u>in situ</u> hybridization technique that allows the detection of V_H-gene expression at the single cell level. From these data it is clear that the V_H-gene expression in neonatal mice is determined by nonrandom, position dependent processes which favour the utilization of the most D-proximal V_H-families. A similar position-dependent, preferential usage of D-proximal V_H-genes at early stages of maturation of B-cell development in the adult individual is also observed. The lack of such bias within the peripheral, immunocompetent cell pool of adults demonstrates the existence of selection mechanisms operating at the level of the emergent repertoire and the level of export of newly- formed B-cells into the periphery. Furthermore, local environmental factors can further modulate the V_H-gene expression within the peripheral, immunocompetent cell pool.

During establishment of different B-cell compartments

It is clear to us that during the process of developing a coherent immune system, mutual interactions between the T- and B-cell compartments must occur. Recently several examples of shaping of the T-cell repertoire by the B-cell compartment have been reported (6). We have also recently studied the possible role of T-lymphocytes in the selection of antibody repertoires by comparing V_H-family utilization in different B-cell compartments of normal and athymic mice (16). Using the technique of *in situ* hybridization as discussed above we could show decreased utilization of the V_HJ558-family within the effector compartment of the spleen and within the small B-cells of the lymph node of nude mice as compared to normal-aged matched controls. Furthermore, the transfer of mature T-cells from syngeneic donors into the athymic mice, increased the expression of the V_HJ558 in these two B-cell compartments. Taken together these data indicate that T-lymphocytes may play a fundamental role in the selection of antibody repertoires in normal, non-immunized mice.

Summary

Together the data outlined above represent examples of stages of the development and maintenance of B-cell repertoires at which selection of specificity repertoires occurs. On the basis of the described differences in serological properties and/or V_H utilization we hypothesize that the immune system may start as a highly connected, germline-encoded, idiotypic network. Further establishment of the mature system appears to included internally- driven selecting mechanisms based on interactions involving V-region complementarities.

This work was supported by the DRET and MFR.

References

1. Jerne, N.K. (1971) In Ciba Foundation Symposium: Ontogeny of acquired immunity. Elsevier, Amsterdam. p. 1.
2. Opselten, D. and Osmond, D.G. (1983) J. Immuol. 131, 2635.
3. Burnet, F.M. (1979) "The clonal selection theory of acquired immunity", Cambridge University Press, London, England.
4. Freitas, A.A.F., Rocha, B. and Coutinho, A. (1986) Immunol. Rev. 91, 5.
5. Coutinho, A., Forni, L., Holmberg, D., Ivars, F. and Vaz, N. (1984) Immunol. Rev. 79, 151.
6. Martinez-A., C., Pereira, P., Torbino, M.L., Marcos, M.A.R., Bandeira, A., De la Hera, A., Marquez, C., Cazenave, P.-A. and Coutinho, A. (1988) Immunol. Rev. 101.
7. Kearney, J. and Vakil, M. (1986) Immunol. Rev. 94, 39.
8. Holmberg, D., Forsgren, S., Ivars, F. and Coutinho, A. (1984) Eur. J. Immunol. 14, 435.
9. Holmberg, D., Wennerström, G., Andrade, L. and Coutinho, A. (1986) Eur. J. Immunol. 16, 82.
10. Carlsson, L., Andersson, Å. and Holmberg, D. (submitted for publication).
11. Brodeur, P.H. and Riblet, R. (1984) Eur. J. Immunol. 14, 992.
12. Yanacopoulos, G.D., Desiderio, S.V., Paskind, M., Kearney, J.F., Baltimore, D. and Alt, F.W. 81984) Nature 311, 727.
13. Perlmutter, R.M., Kearney, J.F., Chang, S.P. and Hood, L.E. Science 227, 1597.
14. Freitas, A.A., Lembezat, M.-P. and Coutinho, A. (submitted for publication).
15. Freitas, A.A., Andrade, L., Lembezat, M.-P. and Coutinho, A. (submitted for publication).
16. Freitas, A.A., Lembezat, M.-P. and Rocha, B. (submitted for publication).

CHARACTERIZATION OF A REGULATORY IDIOTOPE BY ANTIBODY ENGINEERING[1]

Maurizio Sollazzo
Daniele Castiglia
Rosario Billetta
Maurizio Zanetti

Department of Medicine
University of California, San Diego
San Diego, California 92103

I. INTRODUCTION

It is established that the response to conventional self antigens can be triggered or down regulated by modifying the equilibrium of the autoimmune network, a dynamic state based on idiotypic complementarity between receptors on B and T cells (Zanetti, 1986). Whereas it appears that only certain idiotypes (Id) are regulatory (Paul and Bona, 1982; Bottomly, 1984), their molecular basis is still poorly understood. We have addressed this issue using as a model system a putative regulatory idiotype (ReI), Id62, borne on murine autoantibodies to thyroglobulin (Tg). Id62 is recurrent, non-dominant component (<2%) of the autoantibody response to Tg in BALB/c mice, and is an autoimmunogen for B and T cells (Zanetti *et al.*, 1986). We found Id62$^+$ antibodies among hybridoma from unmanipulated neonatal BALB/c spleen cells, *i.e.*, at a developmental stage when ontogenic pressures by external antigen are minimal if any

[1]This work was supported by grants NSF DCB 850201, NIHAI23871 and Council for Tobacco Research, U.S.A. Inc., No. 2124.

(Glotz and Zanetti, 1986). Thus, Rel may be borne on variable (V) regions that are constitutive elements of the preimmune B cell repertoire. More recently, we focused on the molecular basis of Rel. In this communication we present data on: a) the molecular cloning of Id62$^+$ V regions; and b) the mapping of Id62 by site-directed mutagenesis.

II. PRIMARY SEQUENCE DATA

We determined the nucleotide sequence of two V_H regions expressing Id62, derived in one case from splenocytes of an adult hyperimmunized mouse (hybridoma 62), in the other from unimmunized and unstimulated neonatal (<24 hrs from birth) spleen cells (hybridoma B10H2) (Sollazzo *et al.*, submitted). Both monoclonal antibodies (mAb) bind to autologous Tg. As shown in Figure 1 the VDJ sequences of antibodies 62 and B10H2 are identical including the VD and DJ joints.

Since the two hybridoma were prepared from animals of different developmental stages, and the sequences are 100% identical, it is concluded that both parental cells utilized the same V_H, D, and J_H gene segments, and that somatic mutation had not occurred in the hybridoma isolated from the adult hyperimmunized mouse.

The V_H62 nucleotide sequence is most similar with the V_H of two rheumatoid factors (B13 and A26) reported by Shlomchick *et al.*, 1987. The identity is 98.5% in the V region, with only one amino acid difference in CDR1 at position 31, suggesting that the same V_H gene is utilized. However, the D regions are different (Fig 2). The similarity with other members of the V_H7183 gene family ranges between 94% and 88% amino acid identity. The J segment utilized is J_{H4} and is identical in sequence to germline J_{H4}. Interestingly, the D segment is only 50% similar to any murine D segments reported in the literature. While this D region could have resulted from several mechanisms including D to D fusion, gene conversion, D region inversion, TdT addition, on random insertion, it cannot be excluded that there are more D segments yet to be found in the murine germline.

Because of the striking identity between the two mAb the question arises about their possible germline origin. Identical amino acid sequences among antibodies generated from

GACGTGAAGCTGGTGGAGTCTGGGGGAGGATTAGTGAAGCTTGGAGGGTCCCTGAAACTCTCCTGTGCAGCCTCTGGGTT

CACTTTCAGT**AGGTATTACATGTCT**TGGGTTCGCCAGACTCCAGAGAAGAGGCTGGAGTTGGTCGCAGCC**ATTAAT**

AGTAATGGTGGTAGCACCTACTATCCAGACACTGTGAAGGGCCGATTCACCATCTCCAGAGACAATGCCAAAA

ACACCCTGTACCTGCAAATGAGCAGTCTGAAGTCTGAGGACACAGCCTTGTATTACTGTGCAAGAA**AGGCCTACTCTC**

ATGGTATGGACTACTGGGGTCAAGGAACCTCA

FIG.1. *The nucleotide sequence of V_H62 is shown (top line) compared to the V_HB10H2 (dotted line). In bold are denoted the hypervariable regions. The V_H62 belongs to the V_H7183 gene family.*

separate fusions have been documented in murine anti-idiotypes to the random terpolymer glu-ala-tyr (GAT) (Ollier *et al.*, 1985), and between an anti-GAT and an anti-[(4-hydroxy-3-nytrophenyl) acetyl] (NP) (Rocca-Serra *et al.*, 1983). In these cases the utilization of identical V_H, D, and J_H gene segments was interpreted as evidence for the germline origin of identical antibodies.

III. INDEPENDENT EXPRESSION OF Id62 ON THE H CHAIN

Previous studies based on immunochemical techniques had shown that Id62 is independently expressed on the H and light (L) polypeptide chains (Zanetti *et al.*, 1985; Zanetti and Rogers, 1986). Recently we have expanded the original information confirming that the L chain is not required for the expression of this Id by the H chain.

To determine the role played by the L chain in Id expression (as well as antigen specificity) we also cloned the genomic DNA rearrangement encoding the L chain variable (V) region from the unrelated MOPC21 myeloma cell, so that H and L chain expression vectors could be constructed and used in transfection experiments to produce immunoglobulins (Ig) with different L chain combinations. The H chain plasmid vector pN$\gamma_1$62 was electroporated (Sollazzo *et al.*, 1988) in one instance into J558L myeloma cells, that express a lambda1 L chain (Morrison, 1985), and in the other into P3X3 Ag8 hybridoma cells together with the L chain vector pSVCkVkM21 to express the Vk MOPC21 L chain. Following transfection and expression the recombinant Ig were tested for the presence of Id62 and binding to antigen (Tg).

Table I indicates that while in both instances the expression of Id62 is maintained, none of the chimeric Ig binds the original antigen (Tg).

TABLE I: DETECTION OF Id62 AND Tg BINDING ON RECOMBINANT LIGHT CHAIN Ab MOLECULES

Antibody	Id 62 expression*	Tg binding**
V_H62 /V_L*Lambda-1*	+	-
V_H62 /V_LMOPC21	+	-
mAb 62 (IgG1, k)	+	+

**Expression detected as % of inhibition of the canonical Id-anti-Id ELISA binding using 0.5 µg/ml antibody solution.*
***Binding to Tg measured by ELISA on rat Tg - coated polyvinyl microtiter wells using 5 µg/ml antibody solution.*

Thus, these results clearly suggest that Id62 is expressed on the H chain independently from the association with the L chain. Furthermore, this finding implies that in spite of the heterologous junction between a murine V_H and a human C_H1, efficient folding of the V_H region had occurred. It appears that the expression of the antigen binding site, unlike for the Id, requires the association between the parental V_H62 and V_L62 polypeptide chains.

IV. IDIOTOPE MAPPING BY SITE-DIRECTED MUTAGENESIS

To investigate the structural correlate for Id62, V_H62 variants were generated by site-directed mutagenesis according to Zoller and Smith (1983). Recombinant V_H62 chains were transfected by electroporation into J558L cells and expressed. The rationale for designing the mutations was provided by the comparative analysis of several Id62⁻ antibodies whose V_H share identical framework residues with V_H62 but show marked differences clustered in the complementarity determining regions (CDR) (Figure 2).

```
                                                         CDR1
                                                       30
62       DVKLVESGGGLVKLGGSLKLSCAASGFTFSRYYMSWVRQTPEKRLELVAA
A26      _____________________________S ___________________
B13      _____________________________S ___________________
MOPC21   __Q_________QP______R________SFG_H___A___G____W_Y
66E-3    E_M________V_MEP_____________A _______________W T

             CDR2
                60                                    90
62       INSNGGSTYYPDTVKGRFTISRDNAKNTLYLQMSSLKSEDTALYYCAR
A26      ________________________________________________
B13      ________________________________________________
MPOC21   _S_GSSTLH_A_____________P____F___T__R______M______
66E-3    _S_G_S_HLPSRQCE_____________________R______M______

     CDR3

62       KAYSHG        MDYWGQGTS
A26      HELTGTALFA     _______LV
B13      QALLSIHYFA    ________TL
MOPC21   WGNPYYA       _________
66E-3    PPLSLLDAYA    _________
```

FIG.2 *The amino acid sequences of mAb A26, and B13 (Shlomchick* et al., *1987), MOPC21 (Milstein, 1974) and 66E-3 (Cabilly* et al., *1984), are compared with the sequence of* V_H *62.*

Briefly, mutants were constructed according to Kunkel *et al.* (1987) using synthetic oligonucleotides carrying the desired mutation. That mutations were correctly introduced was determined by sequence analysis using a V_H62 specific primer. Mutated V_H genes were then subcloned into the pNy1 expression vector and electroporated into J558L host cells. The genetically-engineered Ig were purified from stable transfectoma cell lines by Protein A-Sepharose 4B chromatography and tested for Id62 expression by ELISA. The results are shown in Table II.

TABLE II: Id62 EXPRESSION ON RECOMBINANT V_H62 MUTANT ANTIBODIES

Transfectoma	Site Mutation	Type Mutation	aa Change	Position	Id62*
γ_1 wt	none	-	-	-	+
γ1 Δ133/34	CDR1	deletion	two aa	33-34	-
γ1 33S	CDR1	substitution	Y → S	33	+
γ1 34K	CDR1	substitution	M → K	34	-
γ1 52bI	CDR2	substitution	N → I	52b	+
γ1 56D	CDR2	substitution	Y → D	56	+
γ1 94VP	CDR3	subst/insert	A → V/P	94 /95	-
γ1 95N	CDR3	substitution	Y → N	95	-

* Expression of Id62 in fluid supernatant or purified protein based on competitive inhibition of Id62 binding in ELISA.

A. *Point mutations in CDR1 and CDR3 abrogate Id expression*

The CDR1 deletion mutant (Δ1) in which amino acid residues Tyr 33 and Met 34 were deleted no longer expresses Id62. The amino acid substitution 33 Tyr→Ser is neutral, while substitution Met 34→Lys abrogates Id expression. CDR3 mutant 94 Ala→Val/+ Pro lost Id expression. Mutant 95N, in which a single Tyr→Asn substitution was introduced, also lost Id expression. Thus, amino acid residues Met 34 and Tyr 95 in CDR1 and CDR3, respectively, contribute to the stabilization of the Id-anti-Id complex. Moreover, this indirectly suggests that both CDRs are exposed on the surface of the Ig molecule and are accessible to anti-Id antibodies.

B. *Mutations in CDR2 do not affect Id expression*

Two amino acid substitutions in the second CDR, namely 52b Asn→Ile and 56 Tyr→Asp, did not affect Id62 expression. This result is supported by the observation that rabbit antibodies raised against a synthetic peptide with the CDR2 sequence recognize in Western blot, under reducing and non-reducing conditions, all Ig expressing Id62. However, these antibodies do not behave as conventional anti-Id as they do not inhibit the canonical Id-anti-Id binding (M. Zanetti, unpublished work). Additionally, molar excess of free CDR2 peptide fails to inhibit the Id binding. Taking all these facts into consideration, it appears that amino acid residues in CDR2 do not directly contribute to the expression of Id62.

V. DISCUSSION

In this communication we present the molecular characterization of an autoantibody V region carrying a putative Rel. It was previously demonstrated that this V region is a naturally occurring element in the preimmune repertoire and modulates quantitatively the *in vivo* autoimmune response of normal BALB/c mice - involving in this process both B and T cells. Here we show that Id62 is encoded by at least two elements in germline configuration (V_H and J_H) and its expression is affected by amino acid substitution in CDR1 and CDR3, but not in CDR2. Amino acid Met 34 and Tyr 95 play an essential role in the stabilization of Id anti-Id complex.

Our results are in agreement with previously reported data (for review see Davie *et al.*,1986) suggesting that the structural correlate for idiotypy is preferentially located in the CDR regions and that among them CDR3 is the most often involved one. Possibly, the third CDR is a privileged site for exposure to solvents and consequently for contact with complementary residues of anti-Id antibodies. Indeed, X-ray crystallographic analyses suggest that the D region is constituted by an external loop lying at the ß bend between the eighth and ninth ß-plated sheet exposed to solvents (Navia *et al.*,1979) with intrinsic mobility and immunogenicity (Tainer *et al.*,1985; Westhof *et al.*,1984).

Interestingly, recombination experiments suggest that the L chain plays little if any role in the expression of Id62 by the H chain. However, since the CDR of both V_H and V_L are topographically proximal and likely interact with each other in the native molecule (Alzari *et al.*, 1988), the L chain seems to provide the proper positioning to the H polypeptide chain.

Id-anti-Id interactions obey to the same rules that govern the interaction between two protein molecules. In protein-protein interactions, contacting residues play a critical role in the formation of a stable complex. Our strategy for Id mapping clearly can not unambiguously distinguish between amino acids physically contributing to Id expression from those whose substitution yields distant conformational adjustments that can, *per se*, influence Id expression. However, several examples exist where new information on antibody structure-function has been obtained by site-directed mutagenesis (Radbruch *et al.*, 1985; Sharon *et al.*,1986; Sharon, 1988; Roberts and Rees,1986).

The available crystallographic studies suggest that in general structural perturbations accompanying conservative mutation are rare (Grutter *et al.*,1979; Perutz *et al.*,1984; Villafranca *et al.*, 1986). Therefore, our biochemical approach remains useful in current efforts to better understand the structural correlate for Rel and the molecular basis of regulatory events involving both B and T cells.

ACKNOWLEDGEMENTS

M.S. is on leave from Instituto di Biologia dello Sviluppo (CNR), Palermo, Italy. M.Z. is a scholar of the Leukemia Society of America, Inc.

REFERENCES

Alzari, P.M., Lascombe, M.B. and Poljak, R.J. (1988) *Ann. Rev. Immunol.* ***6***:555 580.

Bottomly, K. (1984) *Immunol. Reviews* ***79***:45.

Cabilly, S., Riggs A.D., Pande H., Shively J.E., Holmes W.E., Rey M., Perry L.J., Wetzel R. and Heyneker H.L. (1984) *Proc. Natl. Acad. Sci. USA* ***81***:3273.

Davie, J.M., Seiden, M.V., Greenspan, N.S., Lutz, C.T., Bartholow, T.L. and Clevinger, B.L. (1986) *Ann. Rev. Immunol.* ***4***:147.

Glotz, D. and Zanetti, M. (1986) *J. Immunol.* ***137***:223.

Grutter, M., Hawkes, R. and Matthews, B. (1979) *Nature* ***277***:667.

Milstein, C., Adetugbo, K., Cowan, N.J. and Secherr, D.S. (1974) *Prog. Immunol.* ***2***:157.

Kunkel, T.A., Roberts, J.D. and Zakour, R.A. (1987) *Methods Enzymol* ***154***:367.

Morrison, S.L. (1985) *Science* ***229***:1202.
Navia, M.A., Segal, D.M., Padlan, E.A., Davies, D.R., Rao, D.N., Rudikoff, S. and Potter, M. (1979) *Proc. Natl. Acad. Sci. USA* ***76***:4971.
Ollier, P., Rocca-Serra, J., Somme, G., Theze, J. and Fougereau, M. (1985) *EMBO J.* ***4***:3681.
Paul, W.E. and Bona, C.A. (1982) *Immunol Today* ***3***:230.
Perutz, M.F., Fermi, G. and Shih, T.B. (1984) *Proc. Natl. Acad. Sci. USA* ***81***:4781.
Rocca-Serra, J., Tonnelle, C. and Fougerau, M. (1983) *Nature* ***304***:353.
Radbruch, A., Zaiss, S., Kappen, C., Bruggemann, M., Beyreuther, K.and Rajewsky, K. (1985) *Nature* ***315***:506.
Roberts, S. and Rees, A.R. (1986) *Protein Engineering* ***1***:59.
Sharon, J., Gefter, M.L., Manser, T. and Ptashne, M. (1986) *Proc. Natl. Acad. Sci. USA* ***83***:2628.
Sharon, J. (1988) *J. Immunol.* ***140***:2666-2669.
Shlomchick, M., Nemazee, D., Van Snick, J. and Weigert, M. (1987) *J. Exp. Med.* ***165***:970.
Sollazzo, M., Hasemann, C.A., Meek, K.D, Glotz, D., Capra, J.D. and Zanetti, M. (1989), *Eur. J. Immunol*, in press.
Sollazzo, M., Zanetti, M. and Judd, S. (1988) *Focus* ***10***:64.
Tainer, J.A., Getzoff, E.D., Paterson, Y., Olson, A.J. and Lerner, R.A. (1985) *Ann. Rev. Immunol.* ***3***:305.
Villafranca, J.E., Howell, E.E., Oatley, S.J., Warren, M.S. and Kraut, J. (1986) *Phil. Trans. R. Soc. Lond.* ***A317***:405.
Westhof, E., Altschuh, D., Moras, D., Bloomer, A.C., Mondragon, A., Klug, A. and Van Regenmortel, M.H. (1984) *Nature* ***311***:123.
Zanetti, M., Liu, F.-T., Rogers, J., and Katz, D.H. (1985) *J. Immunol.* ***135***:1245.
Zanetti, M., Glotz, D. and Rogers, J. (1986) *J. Immunol.* ***137***:3140.
Zanetti, M. (1986) *C.R.C. Crit . Rev. Immunol.* ***6***:151.
Zanetti, M. and Rogers, J. (1986) *J. Immunol.* ***137***:3140.
Zoller, M. and Smith, M. (1983) *Methods Enzymol.* ***100***:468.

EPIBODIES IN THE IMMUNE RESPONSE TO THE ACETYLCHOLINE RECEPTOR

Donard S. Dwyer[1]
Joachim Bartels

Neuropsychiatry Research Program
University of Alabama at Birmingham
Birmingham, Alabama

I. INTRODUCTION

According to the idiotypic network hypothesis of Jerne, the variable regions of immunoglobulin molecules interact with each other establishing functional networks and providing regulation of immune responses (1). In this view, every antibody may be considered an autoantibody because they react with self antigens, namely autologous idiotopes (Ids). More typically, autoantibodies are defined as antibodies directed against non-immunoglobulin self antigens, such as thyroglobulin, the acetylcholine receptor (AChR), or DNA. In this chapter, a special class of autoantibody will be considered- the epibody. Epibodies were first described by Bona et al. and are defined as anti-idiotypic antibodies that bind not only to the Id but also to the same antigen recognized by the Id-bearing antibody (2). Recently, a more restricted set of epibodies has been described that exhibits self-binding via idiotypic interactions. These self-reactive epibodies, known as autobodies, have been obtained from the immune responses to phosphorylcholine (3) and type II collagen (4). In most of the cases reported so far, the epibodies have been autoreactive, binding to the Fc portion of IgG (i.e. rheumatoid factors [RFs]) or to the AChR (5). Therefore, epibodies appear to define a special subset of anti-Ids that are true autoantibodies.

---

[1]Dr. Dwyer is supported by a grant from the NIH (NS-23532).

The topic of this chapter will be epibodies from the immune response to the AChR. In the human autoimmune disease, myasthenia gravis (MG), 90% of the patients produce detectable levels of serum antibodies against AChR (6,7). It has been demonstrated that these autoantibodies cause impairment in neuromuscular function through complement fixation and increased turnover of membrane AChR (8). Experimental models of MG can be produced by immunizing animals with purified AChR (9) or by transferring monoclonal antibodies (Mabs) against the AChR to mice (10) or rats (11,12), and represent a faithful counterpart to the human disease. Because autoantibody is the key pathogenic factor in MG, it will be important to know how epibodies reactive with the AChR contribute to the autoimmune process.

The role of epibodies in normal immune function is not known. It is possible that they are simply autoantibodies that have the unusual property of reacting with Ids of other autoantibodies with similar specificity. Alternatively, epibodies may participate in the regulation of autoimmune responses. An initial step towards understanding the function of these antibodies would be the characterization of epibody binding. This chapter will examine the molecular basis for epibody-antigen recognition and discuss the functional consequences of this interaction. As outlined below, epibody binding is considered as another example of protein interactions mediated by regions of similarity between the interacting proteins.

II. CHARACTERISTICS OF EPIBODIES FROM THE IMMUNE RESPONSE TO THE AChR

As mentioned above, the first epibodies described were produced against human IgM antibodies that exhibited RF activity, i.e. they reacted with the Fc portion of human IgG. Some of the anti-Ids that were obtained from A/J mice also bound specifically to the Fc region of IgG, prompting the classification of these antibodies as epibodies (2). In this instance, the epibody and corresponding Id were not syngeneic; the epibodies were derived from mice, whereas the RF was of human origin. In contrast, the epibodies described here all react with syngeneic Ids, suggesting a more fundamental role for these unusual antibodies. Table I shows the origination and specificty of the various epibodies that will be discussed in this chapter.

Several points should be emphasized here. First, the epibodies were derived in a variety of ways; two were obtained after repeated boosting with the relevant antigen (JMC 2 and Sh 264), whereas AH 9 was obtained from mice treated with anti-Ids and challenged once with muscle AChR, and another (BA 6) was produced spontaneously by spleen cells of a two-day old mouse. Second, the epibodies do not utilize a single heavy or light chain isotype, reflecting at least a certain degree of heterogeneity among these antibodies. Finally, as will be seen later, the epibodies do not recognize a single Id or even the same epitope on the AChR, again suggesting structural diversity.

Table I. Origins and Specificities of Epibodies[a]

	Isotype	Origin	Specificity
JMC 2	IgM, λ	challenge with BGT	BGT, AChR, ACR 24, EB3-7, Sh 174
AH 9	IgM, κ	anti-Id treated mice, challenged with AChR	AChR, ACR 24, EB3-7, Sh 174
BA 6	IgM, κ	spleen fusion, 2-day old mice	AChR, ACR 24, EB3-7, Sh 174
Sh 264	IgG1, κ	challenge with AChR	AChR, Sh 14, BC 18

[a]These Mabs were produced and assayed for specificity as described previously (10). BA 6 was a gift from Dr. John Kearney (University of Alabama at Birmingham). BGT denotes α bungarotoxin.

Why do these antibodies qualify as epibodies? The binding specificity of three of the epibodies is shown in Table II. BA 6 is virtually identical to AH 9 (although the two antibodies can be differentiated by anti-idiotypic reagents) and will only be mentioned sporadically in this chapter. As reported elsewhere, JMC 2 binds to both α bungarotoxin (BGT) and the AChR (13) and to certain anti-AChR antibodies like ACR 24, Sh 174 and Sh 14, but not to other antibodies (BC 18) or even other anti-AChR antibodies (EBG 4). In addition, JMC 2 recognizes Ids associated with EB3-7 (an anti-J558 antibody from the dextran immune response) and GB 4-10 (an anti-Id from the phosphorylcholine response). AH 9 is less cross-reactive than JMC 2 and binds to AChR, the anti AChR antibodies- ACR 24 and Sh 174, and to EB3-7. In contrast, Sh 264 does not recognize the purified fish AChR used for this assay, but reacts strongly with rodent muscle AChR (see Table III). Furthermore, Sh 264 binds to Sh 14, and BC 18 (which reacts with the P2 protein). These Mabs have been tested against a larger panel of antibodies than that represented here and were negative for the most part, although occasional positive reactions were observed (e.g. Sh 264 binds to the anti-Ia Mab, MKD6). Thus, JMC 2, AH 9 and Sh 264 may be considered epibodies because they react with both the AChR and with certain anti-AChR antibodies, such as Sh 174 or ACR 24. Interestingly, JMC 2 binds to both members of another ligand-receptor pair, namely BGT and the AChR. Therefore, an epibody should probably be defined more broadly as an antibody that reacts with both members of a complementary pair of interacting molecules.

Table II. Binding of epibodies to various proteins and antibodies[a]

	Isotype	JMC 2	AH 9	Sh 264
Narcine AChR		++	++	-
ovalbumin		-	-	-
cytochrome c		-	-	-
BGT		++	-	-
ACR 24	IgG 1, κ	+++	++	nt
Sh 14	IgG 2a, κ	+++	-	+++
Sh 174	IgG 2b, κ	++	+	+
S 3.7	IgG 1, κ	-	-	nt
EB3-7	IgG 1, κ	++	+	nt
BC 18	IgG 2a, κ	-	-	++
EBG 4	IgG 2a, κ	-	-	-
GB4-10	IgG 1, κ	+++	-	nt

[a]The epibodies were tested against a panel of antigens with an ELISA that has been described before (10). The plates were read after 30 min. of reaction with substrate. The values here correspond to absorbance readings of 0.000-0.150 (-), 0.200-0.400 (+), 0.400-0.800 (++), and >0.800 (+++). nt- not tested.

The binding data obtained with the epibodies suggested that the fine specificity of these antibodies differed. For instance, AH 9 reacted with ACR 24 and Sh 174, but not with Sh 14, whereas Sh 264 bound to Sh 14 and weakly to Sh 174, and JMC 2 recognized all three anti-AChR Mabs. In addition, the antibodies could be distinguished by their reactivity with muscle or fish AChR. These data are presented in Table III. As can be seen, AH 9 reacts equally well with AChR purified from either electric organ of Narcine or muscle tissue; JMC 2 also reacts with both kinds of AChR but favors interaction with fish receptor. On the other hand, Sh 264 is very specific recognizing only rodent muscle AChR. These findings suggest that the epibodies either react with several distinct epitopes of the AChR or else the Mabs are binding to nearly the same site, however, subtle differences in the AChR from different species alter the affinity of the antibody interaction to differing degrees. In addition, the results obtained with BGT are shown here. Only JMC 2 precipitates labeled BGT, independently confirming the ELISA data in Table II.

Table III. Immunoprecipitation of AChR and BGT by epibodies[a]

	Narcine AChR	muscle AChR (cpm)	BGT
AH 9	471	412	12
JMC 2	1203	153	480
Sh 264	38	2665	0

[a]An immunoprecipitation assay was used to determine binding to the AChR and BGT. The AChR was prepared from either Narcine electric organ or denervated rat muscle tissue. Non-specific background precipitation with control Mabs was measured and has already been subtracted from the values shown here.

To analyze in more detail the specificity of the epibodies, competitive binding assays were performed. A limitation to these studies was discovered in preliminary experiments. As shown in previous studies, AH 9 (and JMC 2) does not bind very well to soluble Id, if at all, preferring instead the Id bound to the ELISA plate (5). In this same paper, we discussed the apparent directional binding of certain anti-Ids (particularly those belonging to the IgM class) that serve as important regulatory antibodies. Thus, the inability to bind soluble Id does not correlate with a lack of functional behavior. Sh 264 differed from JMC 2 and AH 9 in binding to the soluble Id (Sh 14). The results of inhibition assays are shown in Table IV. First, it is clear that soluble Sh 14 inhibits binding of Sh 264 to the Sh 14-coated plates. A second inhibitor used for these studies is the Mab, N 4.3. N 4.3 is a highly specific, syngeneic anti-Id that was raised by immunizing mice with purified Sh 14. The data here demonstrate that N 4.3 competes effectively with Sh 264 for binding to Sh 14 suggesting that Sh 264 and N 4.3 recognize Ids that are in close proximity. As mentioned above, Sh 264 also binds to the Mab, BC 18, which reacts with P2 protein. BC 18 can also compete with Sh 14 for binding to Sh 264 indicating idiotypic similarities between these antibodies.

Data are presented in the lower part of Table IV that were obtained by inhibiting the binding of AH 9 to Sh 174 with AChR. Sh 174 is the only anti-AChR Mab that can be used for these studies because it does not bind fish AChR very well, whereas ACR 24 and Sh 14 both interact with this type of receptor complicating interpretation of the experiment. AH 9 can easily bind to soluble AChR, therefore this protein might be expected to compete with the immobilized Id for binding to the epibody. It is clear that the addition of AChR to the assay inhibits binding of AH 9 to Sh 174 suggesting that the Id and the antigen resemble each other in some respect. Further discussion of this possibility is reserved for the section on the molecular basis of recognition.

Table IV. Competitive binding assays with the epibodies[a]

		Inhibitor added (μg/ml)			
		10	20	40	80
Sh 264-Sh 14	+ control Mab	0.860	1.011	0.973	0.997
	+ N4.3	0.412	0.351	0.298	0.261
	+ Sh 14	0.191	0.169	0.168	0.177
		6.67	20		47
AH 9-Sh174	+ PBS	0.566	0.498		0.511
	+ AChR	0.262	0.223		0.174

[a]Polyvinyl plates were coated with either Sh 14 or Sh 174 and competitor was added at the concentrations shown. For comparison, the interaction of Sh 264 or AH 9 with these substances was also measured in the presence of contol Mab or PBS. The values refer to the A_{405} reading after 30 min. of reaction with substrate.

III. POSSIBLE INVOLVEMENT OF EPIBODIES IN THE IMMUNE RESPONSE

The function of epibodies is still a mystery. Several possibilities will be discussed in this section, however, additional studies will be necessary to substantiate any of these ideas. A sheme is depicted in Figure 1 which integrates the epibodies into the immune response to the AChR and to certain foreign antigens. The dashed lines represent indirect connections to the antigens via anti-Ids (i.e. AH 9 and JMC 2 do not directly bind to DEX, but react with EB3-7 which is an anti-Id in the DEX response). By the orientation of this scheme, the role of epibodies may be viewed in several different ways.

1) The epibodies may primarily be rather low affinity (cross-reactive) autoantibodies against AChR that arise early in this autoimmune response, but which are later replaced by high affinity antibodies. Because the epibodies also bind to the Ids of some of the higher affinity antibodies, immune complexes may be formed locally that stimulate further production of autoantibody. In this view, the epibodies would have a potentiating effect on the autoimmune response.

2) Alternatively, the anti-idiotypic properties of the epibodies may be their most significant feature. According to this notion, the epibodies would behave like classical anti-Ids and specifically regulate the immune response to the AChR, possibly by suppressing the production of the corresponding Id. Binding of AChR by the epibodies would merely be a

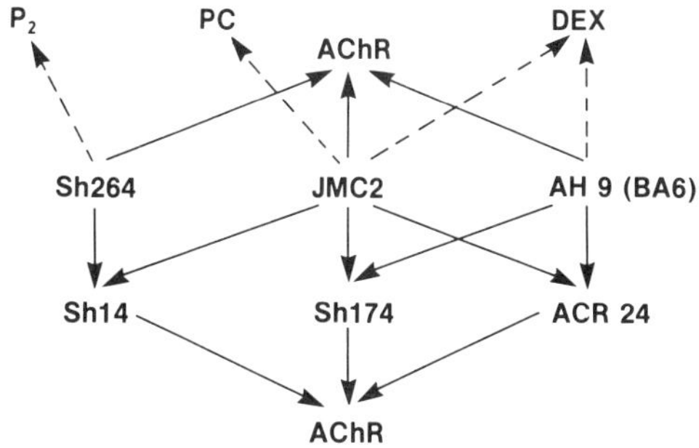

Fig. 1. Idiotypic connections of epibodies from the immune response to the AChR. DEX and PC refer to the immune responses to α 1,3 dextran and phosphorylcholine, respectively.

fortuitous cross-reaction between Id and AChR. On the other hand, the epibody could reduce the activity of autoantibodies against the AChR not only by down-regulating production of these antibodies via idiotypic connections, but also by competing for binding to the AChR with the more harmful autoantibodies. Thus, epibodies may have a protective influence on the development of autoimmunity.

3) Finally, the epibodies may belong to a special subset of antibodies termed 'superorganizers' that are important for cross-regulation of immune responses. Superorganizers are typically IgM class antibodies that are somewhat cross-reactive and recognize a variety of Ids and anti-Ids involved in a number of different immune responses (14). For example, JMC 2 could potentially participate in the immune responses to the AChR, DEX and PC, providing key regulatory signals in each of these systems. The unusual recognition pattern of epibodies (i.e. binding to Id and antigen) would be viewed simply as a manifestation of their cross-reactivity and would have no further meaning. This last issue will be discussed in more detail in the next section.

IV. MOLECULAR BASIS OF EPIBODY RECOGNITION

Epibody binding is puzzling and appears to be contradictory according to prevailing notions that ligand-receptor interactions are lock and key arrangements. Because antibody-antigen binding is often viewed in this way, it is difficult to imagine how the epibody can bind to both the lock and the key at the same time. However, as will be discussed in this section, epibody recognition may resemble dimer formation more than it does classical ligand-receptor interactions.

```
        ______________FR1_____________|*CDR1*|______FR2____|*******CDR2********|____
        --------10--------20--------30-----AB---40--------50--ABC------60--------70
        .........|.........|.........|...........|.........|............|.........|
Sh 174         GGGLVKPGGSPKLSCAASGFTFSSYAMoooooooooooooooooooooooooooooooooVKGRFIIS
Sh 264                 GSLKLSCAASGFTFSSYGMS  WVRQTPDKRLEWVoTISS  GGVYTYYooooooooooo
ACR 24                GGSLKLSCAASGFTFSSYGMS  WVvds dKRLEWVATISq yvvSYTYYPDtsKoooooo

        ____________FR3___________|*******CDR3********|___FR4____
        --------80--ABC------90-------100ABCDEFGHIJK-------110---
        .........|.............|.........|....................|...
Sh 174  RDNAKNTLFLQMRSLRSEDTAMYYCASRISTVGG              FGYWGQGTLVTLSA
Sh 264  oooooooooLQMSSLKSEDTAMYYCARRGVWPH              AMDYWGQGToVTVSS
ACR 24  oooooooooooooooooooooLYYCASRGGIGP            QMAMDYWGSRTDAoVSS
```

Fig. 2. Amino acid sequences of V_H segments of the anti-AChR antibodies. cDNA was prepared using reverse transcriptase, and in some cases, was amplified by the polymerase chain reaction, PCR (19). cDNA was either sequenced directly according to Maxam and Gilbert (20), or after PCR amplification by the chain terminator method (21,22). The amino acids specified by the codons are shown here using the single letter code. The corresponding amino acids are grouped below according to relatedness as determined by Dayhoff (23): S (serine), T (threonine), P (proline), A (alanine), and G (glycine); N (asparagine), D (aspartic acid), E (glutamic acid), and Q (glutamine); H (histidine), R (arginine), and K (lysine); M (methionine), I (isoleucine), L (leucine), and V (valine); F (phenylalanine), Y (tyrosine), and W (tryptophan); C (cysteine). The gaps in sequence were inserted to maintain alignment, whereas the 'o' symbols represent regions where the sequence is not available. Small letters indicate uncertainty about the identity of the residue.

A. Amino Acid Sequences of Immunoglobulin Heavy and Light Chains

Already, limited information is available concerning the molecular basis for epibody binding. Chen et al. were able to produce epibodies in rabbits by immunizing the animals with a synthetic peptide corresponding to the first complementarity-determining region (CDR) of the light chain of an IgM RF (15). The epibodies reacted with an Id shared by several RFs and also bound to the Fc portion of human IgG. The structure of the immunizing peptide and analysis of the amino acid sequence of the various antigens bound by the epibodies led these investigators to suggest that the sequence ser-ser-ser constituted the common epitope shared by the RF light chains and the Fc portion of IgG.

Using a different approach, Kang et al. have identified segments of the variable region of the heavy chain that appear to be involved in autobody recognition (16). Interesting regions of the heavy chain were selected for further study by the analytical methods of Blalock and Smith that examine the hydropathic complementarity of amino acids specified by the coding and noncoding strands of DNA (17). A synthetic peptide based on this analysis (derived from the CDR2) was found to inhibit the self-recognition and antigen binding of the autobody, implying that this portion of the heavy chain was involved in the specific interactions.

The immune response to the AChR is ideally suited for similar studies of the molecular basis of epibody recognition. Monoclonal versions of the anti-AChR antibodies and epibodies are available and the amino acid sequence of the AChR from a number of species is known. As a first step in attempting to identify a common epitope recognized by the epibodies, we have begun sequencing the variable regions of the antibodies depicted in Figure 1. mRNA was isolated from the hybridomas of interest and cDNA prepared by the primer extension method described by Caton et al. (18). The results obtained by sequencing the variable regions are presented in Figures 2 (heavy chains) and 3 (light chains). Although the data are incomplete, certain trends may already be evident. For the three heavy chains shown here, the sequences are fairly similar to each other, even in the CDRs to some extent. It appears that all three heavy chains belong to the same family (subgroup IIID according to Kabat et al. (24), which is a subset of the J558 family), although complete sequences will be necessary to make definitive assignments. For instance, Sh 174 is also similar to the MOPC 21 heavy chain of the 7183 family. In any event, the data suggest there may be somewhat restricted expression of V_H genes by autoantibodies against the AChR, at least in BALB/c mice. Of course, the antibodies examined in these studies were selected not only for binding to the AChR, but also because of their idiotypic similarities, therefore the apparent restricted V_H gene usage observed here may be a consequence of the selection process. Other anti-AChR Mabs that do not share the Id recognized by JMC 2 and AH 9 may utilize a much broader array of V_H genes. Additional sequence information will be required to address this issue.

```
         |__________FR1_________|*******CDR1******|_____FR2_____|**CDR2*|____________
         |--------10--------20-------ABCDEF-30--------40--------50--------60---------
_________|...................................................................
Sh 174   |          LAVTAGEKVTMTCKFSQSLLNSGNQKNYLTWYQQKPGQPPKLLIYWASTRESGVPDRFTGSGSVT
Sh 264   |                                                                   FSGSGQGQ
ACR 24   |                  VTITCRASE     NISGYLAWYQQKQGKSPQLLVYNAKTLAEGVPSRFSGSGSGT
Sh14.4   |                                                     IYYTSRLHSGVPSRFSGSGSGA
EB 3     |
```

```
         |_______FR3________|******CDR3*****|___FR4___|__
         |70-------80--------90-----ABCDEF--100------A---
_________|...............................................
Sh 174   |DFTLTISSVRAEDLAVYYCQNDYSYP      LTFWDRAGARRP
Sh 264   |fqlsvsnSVEPEDVGVYYCQNGHSFP      WTFGGGTK
ACR 24   |QFSLKINSLQPEDFGSYSCQHHYGPP      WTFGGGTKLDI
Sh14.4   |DYSLTISNLEQEDIATYFCQQGYTLP      YTFGGGTKLEI KRA
EB 3     |                YHCGQGYSYP      YTFGGGT
```

Fig. 3. Amino acid sequences of the V regions of the light chains. The methods for obtaining these sequences are described in the legend to Figure 2.

In examining the light chain sequences in Figure 3, it would appear that the V_L genes used by these autoantibodies are more diverse. The light chain used by Sh 174 is quite similar to that of the myeloma protein MCPC 603 which is a member of the Vκ8 family (23). On the other hand, the ACR 24 light chain is similar to that of A31.9 and MOPC149 of the Vκ12,13 family (25). The sequence information from the other three light chains is not sufficient for assignment to a family. In the next section, the similarities between V regions will be discussed in relation to strategies for identifying counterparts in the AChR.

B. V Region Similarities with the AChR

To localize regions of the AChR that are recognized by the epibodies, we have adopted the following stategy. Amino acid sequences of the CDRs of the antibodies bearing the cross-reactive Ids will be compared with the sequence of the AChR. If areas of similarity are observed, synthetic peptides based on the homologous regions will be prepared to confirm the involvement of that particular sequence in epibody recognition. Preliminary analysis of the partial sequences already obtained has revealed one area of potential interest. The epibody, JMC 2, binds to all of the the anti-AChR antibodies listed in Figure 1. The CDR3s of the corresponding light chains are somewhat similar to each other and to portions of the AChR as seen in Figure 4. For instance, ACR 24 and a segment from the α chain of the AChR have the consensus sequence: basic amino acid-x-gly-x-small polar-trp-thr-aromatic amino acid. A second region of the AChR (γ chain) also shows the pattern of alternating small hydrophilic and aromatic amino acids which is characteristic of the CDR3 segments of these antibodies. Once the complete V region sequences are available, it may be possible to identify other portions of the AChR which bear even greater similarity to a sequence commonly observed in another CDR.

Why should the antibodies that bind to AChR resemble the AChR in anyway? First, it would explain how the epibody can react with both the Id and the AChR (i.e. via the common amino acid sequence and resulting structure). Second, as will be discussed in more detail below, amino acid sequence similarities between ligands and their receptors may be a more general phenomenon relevant to the molecular recognition of many proteins.

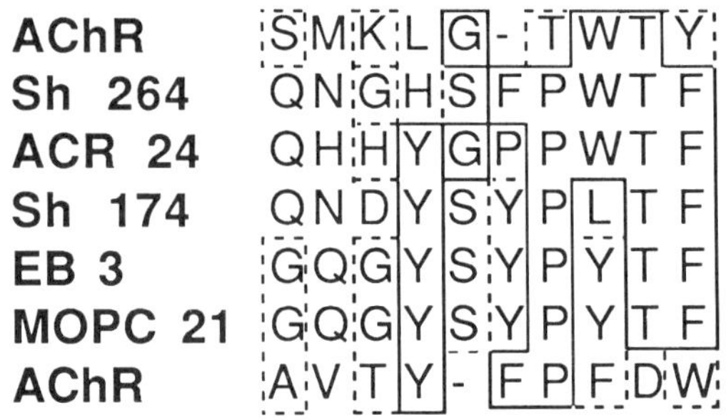

Fig. 4. Amino acid sequence similarities between the AChR and the CDR3 of light chains from anti-AChR antibodies. The single letter amino acid code is again used to represent the residues. The AChR sequences have been previously reported by Noda et al. (26), top (residues 143-151), and Claudio et al. (27), bottom (131-139). Solid lines represent identical amino acids, whereas dashed lines denote conservative changes.

C. Protein-Protein Interactions Mediated by Regions of Homology

In general, ligand-receptor interactions have been likened to a key fitting a lock. Antibody-antigen binding is also viewed in this way, in part, due to crystallographic evidence demonstrating that the antibody binding site can form a pocket or groove (28). However, more recent X-ray diffraction data indicate that the antibody-antigen interface can also be a rather flat surface (29,30). These findings suggest that complementarity of shape is not a prerequisite for the interaction of antibody with antigen, and as will be suggested here, chemical complementarity between the amino acid residues themselves may not be necessary either.

In contrast to the lock-and-key paradigm for receptor interactions, we have recently proposed that there may actually be limited areas of homology between a ligand and its receptor, and further, that these regions of similarity define the interaction sites (13). To illustrate this point, one example from our original paper will be discussed here, namely amino acid sequence homology between BGT and the AChR. BGT binds nearly irreversibly to the AChR and is often used as a specific label for the receptor. As mentioned above, JMC 2 reacts with both the AChR and BGT. To discover the possible basis for this cross-reaction, the amino acid sequences of these two proteins were examined for any regions of homology. Several small homologous segments were identified and the most interesting of these is shown in Figure 5. Stretches of 12 amino acids from BGT and from the AChR of either Torpedo electric organ or mouse muscle tissue have been aligned. The overall amino acid composition of these sequences is very similar with 10 of 12 residues from BGT also

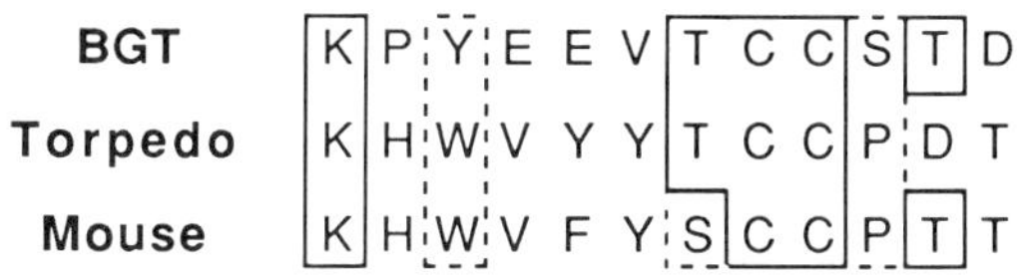
BGT K P Y E E V T C C S T D
Torpedo K H W V Y Y T C C P D T
Mouse K H W V F Y S C C P T T

Fig. 5. Identification of amino acid sequence similarities between BGT and the AChR. The AChR sequences were reported by Boulter et al. (31) and the BGT sequence was published by Mebs et al. (32). The AChR sequence encompasses residues 185 to 196 of the α subunit, and the BGT segment represents amino acids 52 to 63.

present in the AChR. In addition, 5 of 12 amino acids from BGT are identical to residues in the receptor, and two others (tyrosine and serine) are conservative changes from the AChR sequence.

Interestingly, a synthetic peptide based on the Torpedo sequence depicted here bound BGT, indicating that this region of the AChR defines the ligand binding site (33). Because BGT forms dimers, it seemed possible that the portion of BGT represented in Figure 5 could behave like the AChR and serve as an acceptor site for toxin, thus explaining the self association. In addition to BGT and the AChR, several other examples of amino acid sequence homology between ligand-receptor pairs (e.g. interleukin 2 and its receptor) were reported (13). A general principle was formulated for locating protein interaction sites by first identifying regions of amino acid sequence similarity between the two interacting proteins.

The initial observation that an antibody (epibody) could bind to both Id and the corresponding antigen was surprising and unexpected. However, the paradoxical epibody specificity is easily explained as illustrated in Figure 6. A region of amino acid sequence similarity has been represented with three ridges on the AChR and the anti-AChR antibody (labelled Id). The protein interaction between antibody and antigen is accomplished via this homologous segment. Anti-Ids would fall into two categories: (i) those that bind to the homologous protein interaction site would be epibodies because they bind to both Id and antigen, and (ii) those that bind to Ids outside this region would be conventional anti-Ids. Furthermore, antibodies similar to the Id portrayed in Figure 6 could conceivably bind themselves in the same manner, thus explaining autobody recognition.

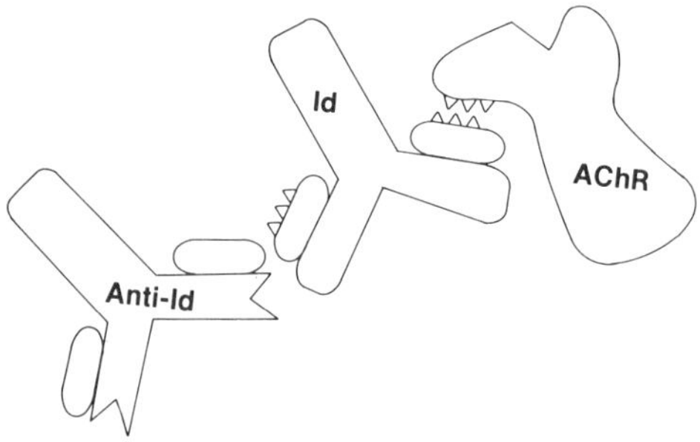

Fig. 6. Schematic representation of epibody recognition.

Is this type of antibody interaction, via regions of similarity, consistent with the kinds of binding interaction that have already been analyzed by X-ray crystallography? High affinity antibodies can bind to antigen using a relatively flat surface, with the juxtaposition of complementary charges increasing the affinity of the reaction (29,30). The lower affinity binding observed here may instead be accomplished by amino acids that are similar to each other, for instance, hydrophobic or amphipathic residues, particularly those capable of hydrogen bonding. In this way, epibody recognition would resemble dimer formation in proteins where identical polypeptide chains associate, much like the autobodies that have recently been described (3,4). Thus, the lock-and-key, ridge-and-cleft type of binding characteristic of high affinity ligand-receptor or antibody-antigen interactions may not be adequate for modelling molecular recognition by epibodies. Future studies will be aimed at discovering precisely how an epibody recognizes both Id and antigen.

V. SUMMARY AND PERSPECTIVES

In this chapter, a number of epibodies from the immune response to the AChR have been described. Unlike the first epibodies that were characterized, these are syngeneic with the Id-bearing antibodies. Moreover, they arose from a variety of circumstances: following deliberate immunization with antigen, after treatment with anti-Ids, or spontaneously in newborn mice. Based on these observations, we conclude that epibody production is not an isolated event, and further, that epibodies may be involved in normal regulation of immune responses. In examining the molecular basis of epibody recognition, nucleotide sequencing of key antibodies has revealed certain similarities among the V regions used by these antibodies. According to the view of ligand-receptor interactions presented here, limited areas of homology between the Ids and antigen (AChR) would be expected to occur. In the future, it may be possible to design synthetic idiotypic peptides based on these regions of similarity for in vivo studies of regulation of autoimmunity.

The existence of epibodies potentially offers clues about the origins of autoantibodies in MG. Because epibodies react with both antigen and Id, the chances of activating the corresponding B cells would be increased. Thus, epibodies may be the earliest manifestation of autoreactivity arising as a consequence of inadvertent activation via idiotypic networks. The dual specificity for antigen and Id may enable the epibody to enhance T cell activation or antibody production in response to autoantigen. Amplification of the autoimmune response would soon dilute the concentration of epibodies, leading to their eventual replacement by the more specific, higher affinity autoantibodies characteristic of the full-blown disease. On the other hand, epibodies may be drawn from a special pool of so-called 'natural' antibodies that are very cross-reactive (often autoreactive) and which appear to play an important regulatory role in the internal activation of the immune system. If so, epibodies may provide important regulatory signals throughout the autoimmune response. Functional involvement of these antibodies in autoimmunity would demonstrate that the epibody is not merely an oddity of idiotypic networks, but is also a full-fledged partner in the regulation of immune responsiveness.

REFERENCES

1. Jerne, N.K. (1974). Ann. Immunol. (Paris) 125C, 373.
2. Bona, C.A., Finley, S., Waters, S., and Kunkel, H.G. (1982). J. Exp. Med. 156, 986.
3. Kang, C.-Y., and Kohler, H. (1986). J. Exp. Med. 163, 787.
4. Punjabi, C.J., Wood, D.D., and Wooley, P.H. (1988). J. Immunol. 141, 3819.
5. Dwyer, D.S. (1988). In "Biological Applications of Anti-Idiotypes " (C. Bona, ed.), Vol. II, p. 55. CRC Press, Inc., Boca Raton, FL.
6. Lindstrom, J. (1977). Clin. Immunol. Immunopathol. 7, 36.
7. Monnier, V.M., and Fulpius, B.W. (1977). Clin. Exp. Immunol. 29, 16.
8. Drachman, D. (1981). Annu. Rev. Neurosci. 4, 195.
9. Patrick, J., and Lindstrom, J. (1973). Science 180, 871.
10. Dwyer, D.S., Kearney, J.F., Bradley, R.J., Kemp, G.E., and Oh, S.J. (1981). Ann. N.Y. Acad. Sci. 377, 143.
11. Lennon, V.A., and Lambert, E.H. (1980). Nature 285, 238.
12. Richman, D.P., Gomez, C.M., Berman, P.W., Burres, S.A., Fitch, F.W., and Arnason, B.G. (1980). Nature 286, 738.
13. Dwyer, D.S. (1988). submitted for publication.
14. Dwyer, D.S., Vakil, M., and Kearney, J.F. (1986). J. Exp. Med. 164, 1310.
15. Chen, P.P., Fong, S., Houghten, R.A., and Carson, D.A. (1985). J. Exp. Med. 161, 323.

16. Kang, C.-Y., Brunck, T.K., Kieber-Emmons, T., Blalock, J.E., and Kohler, H. (1988). Science 240, 1034.
17. Blalock, J.E., and Smith, E.M. (1984). Biochem. Biophys. Res. Comm. 121, 203.
18. Caton, A.J., Brownlee, G.G., Staudt, L.M., and Gerhard, W. (1986). EMBO J. 5, 1577.
19. Saiki, R.K., Gelfand, D. H., Stoffel, S., Scharf, S.J., Higuchi, R., Horn, G.T., Mullis, K.B., and Erlich, H.A. (1988). Science 239, 487.
20. Maxam, A.M., and Gilbert, W. (1980). Methods Enzymol. 65, 499.
21. Sanger, F., Nicklen, S., and Coulson, A.R. (1977). Proc. Natl. Acad. Sci. (USA) 74, 5463.
22. Wong, C., Dowling, C.E., Saiki, R.K., Higuchi, R.G., Erlich, H.A., and Kazazian, H.H. (1987). Nature 330, 384.
23. Dayhoff, M.O. (1972). In "Atlas of Protein Sequence and Structure" Vol. 5, National Biomedical Research Foundation, Washington, DC.
24. Kabat, E.A., Wu, T.T., Reid-Miller, M., Perry, H.M., and Gottesman, K.S. (1987) In "Sequences of Proteins of Immunological Interest" U.S. Department of Health and Human Services, Public Health Service, National Institutes of Health.
25. Potter, M., Newell, J.B., Rudikoff, S., and Haber, E. (1982). Molec. Immunol. 19, 1619.
26. Noda, M., Takahashi, H., Tanabe, T., Toyosato, M., Furutani, Y., Hirose, T., Asai, M., Inayama, S., Miyata, T., and Numa, S. (1982). Nature 299, 793.
27. Claudio, T., Ballivet, M., Patrick, J., and Heinemann, S. (1983). Proc. Natl. Acad. Sci. (USA) 80, 1111.
28. Amzel, L.M., Poljak, R.J., Saul, F., Varga, J.M., and Richards, F.F. (1974). Proc. Natl. Acad. Sci. (USA) 71, 1427.
29. Amit, A.G., Mariuzza, R.A., Phillips, S.E.V., and Poljak, R.J. (1986). Science 233, 747.
30. Sheriff, S., Silverton, E.W., Padlan, E.A., Cohen, G.H., Smith-Gill, S.J., Finzel, B.C., and Davies, D.R. (1987). Proc. Natl. Acad. Sci. (USA) 84, 8075.
31. Boulter, J., Luyten, W., Evans, K., Mason, P., Ballivet, M., Goldman, D., Stengelin, S., Martin, G., Heinemann, S., and Patrick, J. (1985). J. Neurosci. 9, 2545.
32. Mebs, D., Narita, K., and Lee, C.Y. (1971). Biochem. Biophys. Res. Comm. 44, 711.
33. Neumann, D., Barchan, D., Safran, A., Gershoni, J.M., and Fuchs, S. (1986). Proc. Natl. Acad. Sci. (USA) 83, 3008.

INTERSPECIES IDIOTYPES ON ANTI-Sm ANTIBODIES[1]

Howard Dang
Masami Takei[2]
Norman Talal

Clinical Immunology Section
Audie L. Murphy Memorial Veterans Hospital, and the
Department of Medicine
The University of Texas Health Science Center
San Antonio, Texas

I. INTRODUCTION

Systemic lupus erythematosus (SLE) is a generalized autoimmune disease characterized by serum antibodies to various self constituents (1). In the past we have been interested in antibodies directed against an acidic nonhistone nucleoprotein designated Sm. These autoantibodies are present in approximately 30% of SLE patients and are helpful in making a diagnosis of the disease (2,3). Interestingly, anti-Sm antibodies are also spontaneously present in 30% of MRL mice (4), a murine model of SLE (5). Although not directly shown, immunoglobulin heavy chain analysis of the anti-Sm antibody response in both MRL mice and lupus patients suggests T cell involvement (6,7).

Migliorini et al (8) showed that some anti-Sm antibodies from MRL mice may have anti-idiotype (anti-Id) specificities suggesting that such antibodies are involved in an Id network. According to Jerne's network hypothesis of immune interactions (9), anti-Id/Id interactions are important in maintaining the preimmune repertoire. Taken altogether anti-Sm antibodies and the Id that it expresses may be important in normal immune regulation in the mouse.

[1] Supported by USPHS Grant AM30487.
[2] Present address: Nihon University, First Department of Medicine, Tokyo, Japan.

Furthermore, such antibodies and their Id may be conserved throughout nature.

A. Interspecies Id Expression in SLE

We have focused on an Id expressed on a monoclonal anti-Sm antibody designated Y2 which was derived from an MRL mouse (10). Using a rabbit anti-Y2 Id antiserum, we studied Id expression in SLE sera by solid-phase radioimmunoassay (11). Twenty-five of 51 patients (49%) positive for anti-Sm antibodies had elevated levels of the Y2 Id compared to a normal control group. Moreover, 9 of 28 patients (32%) negative for anti-Sm antibodies also showed increased Y2 Id expression. Appropriate controls ruled out rheumatoid factor-like activity as an explanation for the finding. Furthermore, anti-Y2 Id serum inhibited the ability of 12 of the 25 anti-Sm positive lupus sera to bind Sm. These data suggest that the Y2 Id is highly conserved and partially related to anti-Sm binding activity. Similar observations concerning the expression of the Y2 Id have been made in the MRL mouse strain (12).

In extension of these studies (13), sera from 29 SLE patients and 81 first-degree healthy family members were tested for quantitative expression of the Y2 Id. Forty-one percent of SLE patients and 27% of all relatives showed increased serum levels of the Y2 Id compared to 6% in a normal, unrelated control group. In addition, female relatives of SLE patients showed slightly increased levels of anti-Sm antibodies compared to male relatives (15% vs 3%). In one of the 28 families and three unrelated SLE patients studied, there was a significant correlation between Y2 Id expression and expression of another Id present on anti-DNA antibodies (134Id). Affinity column absorption studies showed that these two Ids were present on different antibody molecules.

To further understand the significance of this Id, B cell hybridomas were made from the fusion of pokeweed mitogen stimulated peripheral blood lymphocytes from an SLE patient (M.C.) and GM4672, a lymphoblastoid cell line (14). Of the seven successful hybrids, two produced monoclonal antibodies (designated 4B4 and 3C3) against the Sm antigen as detected by ELISA. Both monoclonal antibodies are comprised of IgM, K chains. Antigen inhibition studies showed that anti-Sm binding was only inhibited by Sm and not by nDNA, dDNA, poly(rA), keyhole limpet hemacyanin or ovalbumin. In addition, 4B4 did not show any rheumatoid factor activity. The rabbit anti-Id serum made against the murine monoclonal anti-Sm antibody Y2 also reacted with the two human monoclonal antibodies. The rabbit anti-Id binds to the μ heavy chain of 4B4 and to both IgM and IgG in the serum of patient M.C. Competitive inhibition studies showed that the Id expressed on the human monoclonal antibody 4B4 is similar but not identical to the Y2 Id.

Furthermore, rabbit anti-Id antibodies were made against the 4B4 Id and were used to look for the expression of this Id in sera previously studied for Y2 Id expression. We find that approximately 48% of 76 SLE patients showed elevated levels of the 4B4 Id compared to sera from 26 normal healthy individuals. In addition, there was a linear correlation between Y2 and 4B4 Id expression in the SLE sera studied suggesting that these two Ids may be on the same molecule.

Recent collaboration with Dr. Donald Capra's laboratory (Dallas, TX) has allowed us to study the V_H region sequences of our human monoclonal antibody 4B4 (15). A cDNA library was made from our hybridoma and screened with a μ chain and a V_H family DNA probe. Subsequently, full length cDNAs were subcloned into M13 mp18 vectors and sequenced using the dideoxy chain termination method. The resulting V_H sequence was studied using the GENEBANK computer program. Dramatically, the V segment is totally identical to a unique human V region sequence found in a fetal cDNA library designated 20P1 (16). Further analysis suggests that 4B4 utilizes a small subfamily (2-3 members) of the V_H III_b gene family which has not been seen in the adult repertoire.

The D segment is 29 nucleotides in length and cannot be ascribed to any of the reported germline D region genes. Furthermore, it does not show any significant homology to any of the published D segments. On the other hand, the J segment is identical to the J_H4 germline gene except for a single silent mutation.

II. DISCUSSION

Interspecies Id have been described in several antigen/antibody systems. These include antibodies to both foreign (17-19) and self (20-23) antigens. We have focused our attention on an Id related to anti-Sm antibodies. This Id is shared between a mouse and human monoclonal anti-Sm antibody as well as Ig in lupus sera.

Since this Id is conserved in nature one may predict that the genes encoding these Id^+ antibodies would also be conserved. Indeed, we find that the V_H and J_H segments of 4B4 are encoded by germline genes. It must be noted, however, that it is not clear what selective advantages such Id have in order to be retained in the germline.

We have used antibodies to synthetic peptides to determine the nature of this interspecies cross-reactivity. Our preliminary studies using antibodies made against a peptide corresponding to the V_H CDR2 region of 4B4 suggests that the basis of the cross-reactivity lies near or at that region of the Ig molecule. Comparison between the V_H sequences of Y2 and 4B4 indicate that it does not appear that the interspecies Id is defined solely by a primary sequence but may include secondary structures. Nevertheless, antibodies to synthetic Id peptide will help elucidate the molecular basis of this conserved Id.

The use of peptide specific antibodies which recognizes Ig Id can be used to study Id inheritance. We have evidence that the expression of the Y2/4B4 interspecies Id requires a genetic predisposition (13). However, it is difficult to interpret the inheritance of this Id without sequence analysis. To circumvent this problem, anti-synthetic Id peptide antibodies can be employed.

In summary, we have proceeded from defining the Y2/4B4 interspecies Id in sera to identifying a germline gene. Further studies with anti-synthetic Id peptide antibodies should provide insight into the nature of this cross-reactivity and its regulation in autoimmune diseases.

REFERENCES

1. Sharp, G.L., Irwin, W.S., LaRogue, R.L., Velez, C., Kaiser, A.D., and Holman, H.R. (1971). J. Clin. Invest. 50, 350.
2. Munves, E.E., and Shur, P.H. (1983). Arthritis Rheum. 26, 848.
3. Field, M., Williams, D.G., Charles R., and Maini, R.N. (1988). Ann. Rheum. Dis. 47, 820.
4. Eisenberg, R.A., Tan, E.M., and Dixon, F.J. (1978). J. Exp. Med. 147, 582.

5. Andrews, B.S., Eisenberg, R.A., Theofilopoulos, A.N., Izui, S., Wilson, C.B., McConahey, P.J., Murphy, E.D., Roths, J.B., and Dixon, F.J. (1978). J. Exp. Med. 148, 1198.
6. Eisenberg, R.A., Winfield, J.B., and Cohen, P.L. (1982). J. Immunol. 129, 2146.
7. Eisenberg, R.A., Dyer, K., Craven, S.Y., Fuller, C.R., and Yount, W.J. (1985). J. Clin. Invest. 75, 1270.
8. Migliorini, P., Ardman, B.. Kaburaki, J., and Schwartz, R.A. (1987). J. Exp. Med. 165, 483.
9. Jerne, N.K. (1974). Ann. Immunol. (Paris). 125C, 373.
10. Lerner, E.A., Lerner, M.R., Janeway, C.A., Jr., and Steitz, J.A. (1981). Proc. Natl. Acad. Sci. (USA). 78, 2737.
11. Takei, M., Dang, H., and Talal, N. (1987). Clin. Exp. Immunol. 70, 546.
12. Pisetsky, D.S., Semper, K.F., and Eisenberg, R.A. (1984). J. Immunol. 133, 2085.
13. Dang, H., Takei, M., Isenberg, D.A., Shoenfeld, Y. Blachimer, R., Rauch, J., and Talal, N. (1988). Clin. Exp. Immunol. 71, 445.
14. Takei, M., Dang, H., Wang, R.J., and Talal, N. (1988). J. Immunol. 140, 3108.
15. Sanz, I., Dang, H., Takei, M., Talal, N., and Capra, J.D. (1989). J. Immunol. (January, in press).
16. Schroeder, H.W., Hillson, J.L., and Perlmutter, R.M. (1987). Science 238, 791.
17. Ju, S.T., Benacerraf, B., and Dorf, M.E. (1978). Proc. Natl. Acad. Sci. USA 75, 6192.
18. Butler, J.D., Cambier, J.C., and Klobasa, F. (1985). Mol. Immunol. 22, 1159.
19. Sigal, N.H., Chan, M., Reale, M.A., Moran, T., Berlin, Y., Schulman, J.L., and Bona, C. (1987). J. Immunol. 139, 1985.
20. Eilat, D., Fishel, R., and Zlotnick, A. (1985). Eur. J. Immunol. 15, 368.
21. Morgan, A., Isenberg, D.A., Naparstek, Y., Rauch, J., Duggan, D., Khiroya, R., Staines, N.A., and Schattner, A. (1985). Immunology 55, 393.
22. Ruiz-Arguelles, A. (1988). J. Clin. Invest. 82, 958.

SPECIFICITIES AND IDIOTYPY OF ANTI-HISTONE H1 AUTOANTIBODIES

Marc Monestier
Institute of Molecular Immunology
Center for Molecular Medicine and Immunology
University of Medicine and Dentistry of New Jersey
Newark, NJ 07103

Thomas M. Fasy
Department of Pathology
Mount Sinai School of Medicine
of the City University of New York
New York, NY 10029

I. INTRODUCTION

The production of autoantibodies to a variety of nuclear antigens is one of the hallmarks of systemic autoimmune syndromes (1). Histones are the major protein components of the nucleus and they are frequent targets of such autoreactivity. Histones are small DNA-binding proteins rich in basic amino acids and found in the nuclei of eukaryotic cells. The 5 major classes of histones (H1, H2A, H2B, H3, H4) were originally defined according to their respective contents in lysine and arginine amino acids. The 4 smaller histones (11 to 14 kd) are present in the form of an octameric core complex which contains 2 molecules each of H2A, H2B, H3 and H4. 167 bp of DNA lie on the surface of each oligomeric core where they are wound in 2 superhelical turns. The resulting discrete particles are called nucleosomes and are connected by linker DNA to form nucleosome chains. The very lysine-rich histone H1 plays a double role in the packaging of DNA: (i) located external to the nucleosome, it binds to the DNA and locks together the 2 coils at the point where they enter and leave the nucleosome; (ii) H1 is required for the formation of the higher-order structures and aggregates of chromatin fibers, and of the compact chromatin fibers, even though few details are known about these interactions (2). The histone H1 molecule is composed of about 210 amino acid residues and consists of 3 structural domains: N, a short (about 35 residues) NH2-terminal segment, consisting of alanine, proline, serine and clusters of basic residues; G, a central, hydrophobic globular domain of about 80 conserved amino acid residues; C, a long (about 100 residues) and basic COOH-terminal segment (figure 1). The G domain is compact and contains all of the secondary and tertiary structure of the H1 molecule, whereas N and C are randomly coiled chains. The utilization of histone H1 fragments corresponding to 1 or 2 of these domains has shown that certain functions of the H1 molecules can be mapped to a particular domain. For instance, the central G domain alone is able to close 2 full turns of nucleosomal DNA, while C is involved in chromatin condensation (3).

In contrast to the core histones which have been remarkably conserved during evolution, histone H1 molecules exhibit a great variability. The number of variants and their amount differ from one tissue to another, and for a given organ, differ from one species to another. The heterogeneity of H1 variants is due not only to differences in the sequence and the length of the primary structure, particularly in the carboxy-terminal half of the molecule, but also to post-translational modifications: methylation, acetylation, ADP-ribosylation and phosphorylation. The physiological role of these modifications is still controversial, but certain correlations between functional phases of interphase chromatin and histone modifications have been observed. Two particularly interesting variants are $H1^{o}$, found mainly in non-dividing cells, and H5, found in amphibian and avian erythrocyte nuclei. Both are very similar in their globular domains, but they differ significantly from H1 in the same domain,which is usually conserved among the other variants (4).

Anti-histone autoantibodies can be detected in the sera of up to 70% of patients afflicted with systemic lupus erythematosus (1) and they are also found, albeit at a lower frequency, in other spontaneous autoimmune diseases, such as rheumatoid arthritis (1). Nevertheless, their incidence is highest (95%) in drug-induced lupus (5). For instance, IgG antibodies to the histone complex H2A-H2B are particularly characteristic of patients with clinically active procainamide-induced lupus (5). Even though significant discrepancies are found in the results of various laboratories (1), anti-H1 appear to be the most commonly found population of anti-histone antibodies in systemic lupus erythematosus (6). Mice belonging to strains prone to develop spontaneous lupus-like syndromes, such as MRL lpr/lpr or NZBxNZW/F1, also produce significant amounts of anti-histone autoantibodies (7). These mice represent valuable models to study the specificities of anti-histone autoantibodies and the immunological abnormalities leading to their production.

II. SPECIFICITIES OF ANTI-HISTONE H1 AUTOANTIBODIES

The incidence of anti-histone antibodies is very high among autoimmune mice, particularly among MRL lpr/lpr, NZB and NZBxNZW/F1 animals where virtually every single animal has elevated antibody titers (figure 1). Antibodies to H1 represent a significant fraction of these anti-histone autoantibodies (not shown).

Further studies on the specificities of anti-histone autoantibodies were conducted using proteolytic fragments encompassing 1 or 2 domains of the H1 molecule (8). These studies showed that, in MRL lpr/lpr and NZB mice, the main reactivities were directed against GC-H1 (33-210), a fragment encompassing both the central globular and the basic COOH-terminal domains. Interestingly, only limited reactions were observed against the individual fragments G-H1 (33-122) and C-H1 (123-210). When binding to these fragments was assayed using isotype-specific reagents, IgG antibodies reacted mostly with the GC-H1 fragment, suggesting that these antibodies recognize either a determinant at the G-C junction or a conformational determinant requiring the integrity and the native linkage of the G and C domains. On the other hand, IgM antibodies showed equal binding to both GC-H1 and C-H1 fragments, indicating that IgM anti-H1 antibodies react mainly with determinants located in the C domain of the molecule.

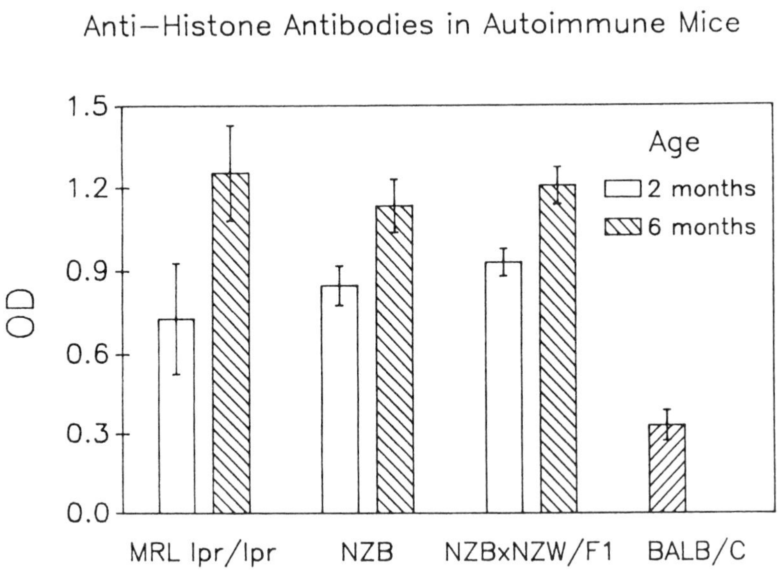

Fig. 1. Anti-histone antibodies in autoimmune mice. Antibodies were detected by ELISA on microtitration plates coated with 10 μg/ml of purified calf thymus histones. Mouse sera were assayed at a 1/500 dilution. In comparison with normal BALB/c mice, all animals have significant levels of anti-histone antibodies, even at the age of 2 months, when clinical symptoms are not yet apparent.

When murine autoimmune sera were studied with respect to the development of the disease (from the ages of 6 weeks to 6 months), IgM antibodies were detected early in life and persisted at constant levels, whereas IgG anti-GC-H1 antibodies increased with age. These results were further assessed by evaluating the binding of the same autoimmune murine sera to cleaved H1 molecules. The cleavage of H1 with N-bromosuccinimide at position 72 (a tyrosine residue located within the G domain) alters the secondary structure of the H1 molecule (the N-bromosuccinimide cleavage site is indicated in figure 1). Following N-bromosuccinimide cleavage, the binding to H1 of IgM antibodies was not affected, as expected since IgM antibodies recognize a determinant in the C domain. However, the binding of IgG antibodies to cleaved H1 was significantly reduced in comparison with intact H1. Since N-bromosuccinimide cleavage takes place at about 50 amino acid residues from the G-C junction, these data are not compatible with the recognition of a segmental epitope at this location. Therefore, most IgG anti-Hl antibodies recognize a conformational determinant resulting from the contiguity of the intact G and C domains. Moreover, since some residual binding to cleaved Hl was detected with IgG antibodies, it is also likely that some IgG antibodies bind segmental determinants located probably in the C domain. Nevertheless, this anti-Hl antibody profile is not found in all autoimmune murine strains: in NZBxNZW/F1 mice, most of the reactivity (IgM or IgG) is directed to the C domain whereas almost no binding to the GC-Hl fragment is detected. The data obtained with murine sera were confirmed by studying spontaneous monoclonal anti-Hl antibodies obtained from animals belonging to these autoimmune strains. All IgM monoclonal antibodies bound determinants located in the C domain and their binding was not affected by cleavage of histone Hl with N-bromosuccinimide. Of 8 IgG monoclonal antibodies tested, 2 exhibited a binding pattern identical to the one observed with monoclonal IgM antibodies, whereas the other 6 IgG antibodies were specific for the GC-Hl fragment and had their binding greatly reduced after N-bromosuccinimide cleavage, in a pattern similar to the data obtained with serum IgG. To ensure that N-bromosuccinimide did not cleave within a sequential determinant, monoclonal antibodies were also assayed against histone Hl that had been subjected to limited chymotrypsin digestion, resulting in cleavage at position 106 (a phenylalanine residue). The results were similar to those obtained following N-bromosuccinimide cleavage: IgM antibody binding was not affected, whereas 6 of 8 IgG antibodies had their binding to histone Hl greatly decreased by the chymotrypsin digestion. Since the N-bromosuccinimide and chymotrypsin cleavage sites are 34 amino acid residues apart, these results rule out the possibility that IgG antibodies recognize a sequential determinant on the Hl molecule and strongly suggest the existence of a conformational determinant requiring the integrity of the G domain and at least part of the C domain.

As in mice, anti-histone Hl antibodies can be detected in a significant number of patients with systemic lupus erythematosus. In studies where histone Hl was cleaved at position 106 with chymotrypsin and the fragments tested for reactivity after electrophoretic separation, most sera reacted with determinants located in the carboxy-terminal half of the molecule but showed limited binding to the

NH2-terminal moiety, suggesting that, as in autoimmune mice, the C and possibly G domains are the main targets for autoimmune recognition (9, 10). However, in a more detailed study where the binding of human lupus sera to purified polypeptides encompassing 1 or 2 domains of the H1 molecule was assayed by immunoblotting and ELISA, most of the reactivity (of both IgM and IgG antibodies) was directed to the C domain without any requirement for the presence of the G domain (11). Therefore, contrary to what is observed in autoimmune mice, it does not appear that the G domain plays an important role in the autoantibody recognition of the histone H1 molecule, nor does there exist any difference in regional specificity with respect to antibody isotype.

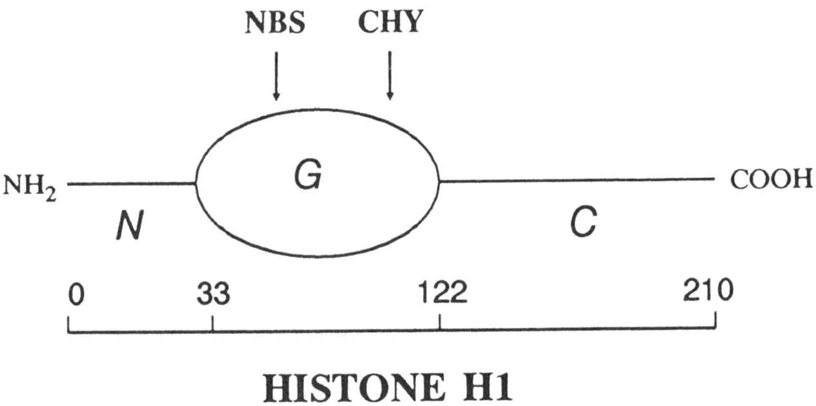

Fig. 2. Schematic representation of the histone H1 molecule. N is the NH2-terminal domain, G the globular domain and C the COOH-terminal domain. The cleavage sites of N-bromosuccinimide (NBS) at position 72 and of chymotrypsin (CHY) at position 106 are indicated.

As mentioned above, significant amino acid sequence differences exist between H1 molecules from various species. When sera from MRL lpr/lpr mice were tested against mouse, bovine, duck, trout and sea urchin sperm H1 molecules or chicken erythrocyte H5, IgM antibodies reacted with a similar intensity to all these H1 variants. On the other hand, IgG antibodies from these mice reacted less with H1 molecules from duck and trout. If the activation of autoreactive clones is indeed driven by the autoantigen itself, this result is logical since both these molecules are phylogenetically distant from mammalian histone H1.

Surprisingly, a strong IgG reactivity against sea urchin sperm H1 and chicken erythrocyte H5 was observed, but it is unlikely that the activity against these variants was due to direct stimulation Interestingly, these two H1 variants possess strong sequence homologies to $H1^{o}$, a variant found mostly in non-dividing tissues (12). Indeed, $H1^{o}$ seems to be more closely related to H5 than to H1, since it was shown that antibodies to H5 cross-react with $H1^{o}$ but not with H1 (13). Therefore, it is likely that the binding to sea urchin sperm H1 and chicken H5 is due to the cross-reactivities of anti-$H1^{o}$ antibodies present in the sera of these MRL lpr/lpr mice. One could envision that, following the death of non-dividing cells (such as neutrophils), nuclei containing significant amounts of $H1^{o}$ are released which might exert direct stimulatory effects on the proliferation of autoreactive clones.

Multispecificity, namely the ability of one antibody to bind several antigens, is a property common among autoantibodies (14, 15), including anti-histone autoantibodies. Indeed, anti-histone antibodies present in the sera of human autoimmune patients have been shown to cross-react with other autoantigens, such as plasma membrane or centromere (16, 17). Rheumatoid factors are known for their extensive polyreactivities and 10% of the rheumatoid factors found in rheumatoid arthritis patients have anti-histone activity (18). A human monoclonal rheumatoid factor from a patient with mixed cryoglobulinemia also reacted with histones H1 and H3 and it was shown by competitive inhibition experiments that 2 different sites were involved in the binding to the Fc region of IgG and histones (19). In a study of 2 monoclonal anti-histone antibodies isolated from MRL lpr/lpr mice, both antibodies reacted with several (but not all) of the core histones and various cationic antigens: one antibody reacted with H2A, H2B, H3 and poly-L-lysine while the other bound H2A, H3, H4, poly-L-arginine and protamine sulfate (20).

III. IDIOTYPES OF ANTI-HISTONE H1 AUTOANTIBODIES

Little is known about the mechanisms triggering the production of anti-nuclear autoantibodies or about their pathogenic importance. The controversy of polyclonal B cell stimulation versus autoantigen-driven activation of autoreactive cells is still unresolved (21) and the pathogenic role of these antinuclear autoantibodies remains hypothetical since most nuclear structures are not directly accessible to circulating antibodies. Among several hypothesis, it has been proposed that anti-nucleic acid antibodies are themselves anti-idiotype antibodies against another population of antibodies. Indeed, Reeves and Chiorazzi (22) have observed, in the sera of some systemic lupus erythematosus patients, the coexistence of anti-DNA antibodies and antibodies directed against p70/p80, a cellular DNA-binding complex. These two populations of antibodies were shown to interact in an idiotypic manner in patient's cryoglobulins. Therefore, one can imagine that certain anti-DNA antibodies are internal images of p70/p80 and that, reciprocally, anti-p70/p80 antibodies possess structural similarities to epitopes found on nucleic acids. The existence of idiotypic interactions between different populations of anti-nuclear antibodies is specially important: certain nuclear antigens, such as nucleic acids or histones are weak immunogens, therefore unlikely to elicit by themselves the expansion of autoreactive clones. A possible origin of such autoantibodies is through an idiotype-anti-idiotype networking mechanism. For instance, it was proposed that antibodies to Ul RNA are elicited as anti-idiotype antibodies to certain autoantibodies directed against the Ul RNA binding domain of a ribonucleoprotein (23). Following immunization with RNA polymerase I, rabbits developed antibodies against the immunogen and also against nucleic acids (24). Even though this hypothesis was not envisioned by the authors, it is conceivable that these anti-nucleic acids antibodies arose as anti-idiotypes to anti-RNA polymerase I antibodies. Passive transfer of KSm2, a monoclonal MRL lpr/lpr antibody to the 16 kD polypeptide of Sm, was able to induce anti-DNA antibodies and antibodies directed against the other major immunoreactive polypeptides of Sm (25). Similarly, after immunization with 16/6, a human anti-DNA idiotype, C3H.SW mice develop a systemic lupus erythematosus-like syndrome with anti-16/6 and anti-anti-16/6 antibodies (26), both studies evoking the triggering of an idiotype cascade by the original immunogen. We have obtained several anti-H1 histone monoclonal IgG autoantibodies from MRL lpr/lpr mice binding to conformational epitopes involving the globular domain and possibly a contiguous segment of the C domain. This same region of the H1 molecule has been reported to contain the major binding sites for DNA. Therefore, it is conceivable that some anti-DNA autoantibodies might in fact be anti-anti-histone H1 antibodies whose binding sites mimic DNA contact domains on the H1 molecule (figure 3).

This hypothesis is further supported by the observations that histone H1 and anti-DNA antibodies share several ligand binding properties. Like H1 (27, 28), anti-DNA antibodies can bind both to single stranded and double stranded DNA (29, 30), and like H1 (31), some anti-DNA antibodies bind to certain phospholipid molecules (29, 32).

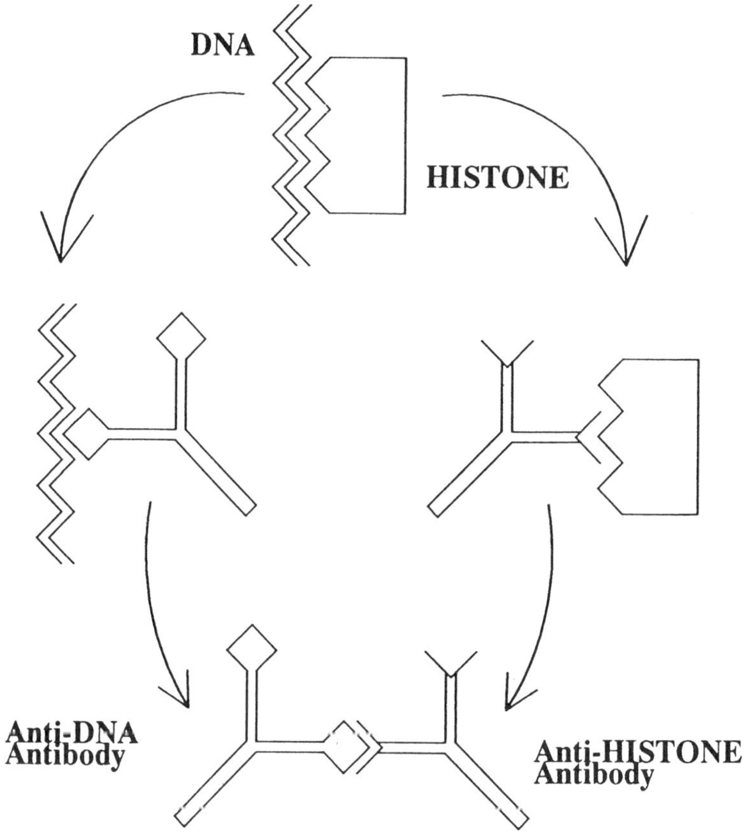

Fig. 3. Anti-histone H1 and anti-DNA antibodies are internal images of epitopes on nuclear autoantigens.

Murine polyclonal antibodies against MRA12, an IgG_{2a} antibody specific for a conformational epitope on histone H1, were shown to be idiotypically specific (figure 4). Interestingly, these anti-MRA12 antibodies were shown to express a significant anti-single stranded DNA activity, suggesting that a portion of these anti-idiotype antibodies recognized a determinant on MRA12 presenting structural homologies to DNA epitopes (figure 4).

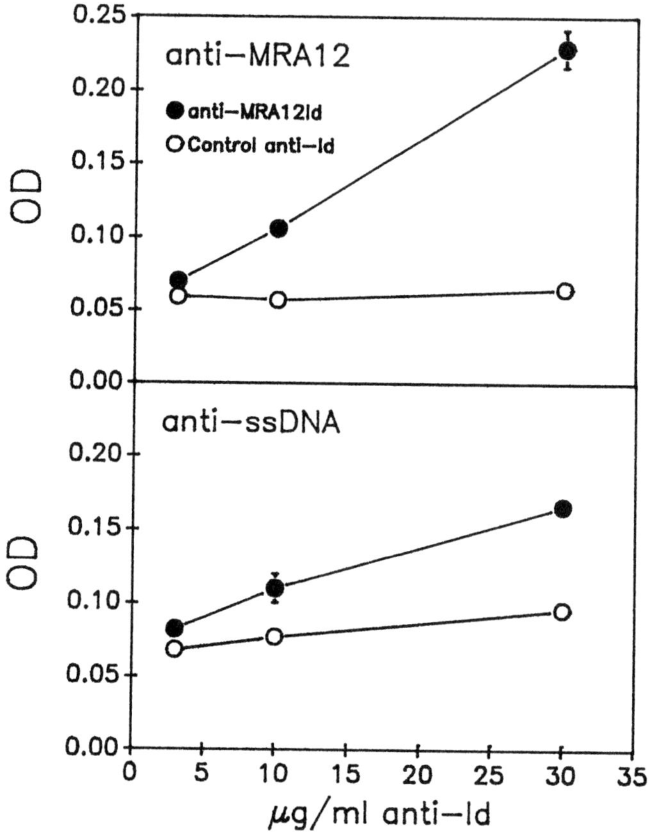

Fig. 4. Top: Specificity of the binding of anti-idiotype antibodies to MRA12, a monoclonal anti-histone H1 IgG_{2a}; no binding was observed with control anti-idiotype antibodies against NP-4, a monoclonal antibody to carcinoembryonic antigen. Bottom: Anti-MRA12 idiotype antibodies show binding to single stranded DNA whereas no significant binding is observed with the control anti-idiotype antibodies.

Another important consequence of idiotypic interactions among anti-nuclear antibodies could be the formation of potentially pathogenic immune complexes. Indeed, idiotype-anti-idiotype immune complexes deposits are found in the renal glomeruli of BALB/c mice following polyclonal B cell activation with LPS (33). Similarly, idiotypic interactions have been reported between the IgM and IgG fractions of human cryoglobulins (34). Since they recognize various nuclear components that can be complementary to each other, anti-nuclear antibodies might very well interact idiotypically and participate in the formation of pathogenic immune complexes.

ACKNOWLEDGEMENTS

The work of the authors was supported by grants from the National Institutes of Health (AI26665), the SLE Foundation and the Lupus Foundation of America.

REFERENCES

1. Rubin, R.L., and Waga, S. (1987) J. Rheumatol. 14 (suppl. 13), 118.

2. Pederson, D. S., Thoma, F., and Simpson, R.T. (1986) Ann. Rev. Cell. Biol. 2, 117.

3. Bohm, L., and Crane-Robinson, C. (1984) Bioscience Rep. 4, 365.

4. Cole, R.D. (1987) Int. J. Peptide Protein Res. 30, 433.

5. Totoritis, M.C., Tan, E.M., Mc Nally, E., and Rubin, R.L. (1988) N. Engl. J. Med. 318, 1431.

6. Costa, O., and Monier, J.-C. (1986) J. Rheumatol. 13, 722.

7. Costa, O., and Monier, J.-C. (1986) Clin. Immunol. Immunopathol. 40, 276.

8. Monestier, M., Fasy, T. M., and Bohm, L. (1989) (submitted).

9. Hardin, J.A., and Thomas, J. O. (1983) Proc. Natl. Acad. Sci. USA 80, 7410.

10. Costa, O., Tchouatcha-Tchouassom, J.-C., Roux, B., and Monier, J.-C. (1985) Clin. Exp. Immunol. 63, 608.

11. Gohill, J., and Fritzler, M.J. (1987) Mol. Immunol. 24, 275.

12. Panyim, S., and Chalkley, R. (1969) Biochem. Biophys. Res. Com. 37, 1042.

13. Yasuda, H., Logan, K.L., and Bradbury, E.M. (1984) FEBS Letters 166, 263.

14. Monestier, M., and Bona., C. (1988) Int. Rev. Immunol. 3, 59.

15. Monestier, M., Bonin, B., Migliorini, P., Dang, H., Datta, S., Kuppers, R., Rose, N., Maurer, P., Talal, N., and Bona, C. (1987) J. Exp. Med. 166, 1109.

16. Rekvig, O.P., Muller, S., Miand, J.P., Skogen, B., and van Regenmortel, M.H.V. (1987) Immunol. Invest. 16, 535.

17. Ayer, L.M., and Fritzler, M.J. (1984) Mol. Immunol. 21, 761.

18. Francoeur, A. (1985) Scand. J. Rheumatol. Suppl.56, 46.

19. Pasquali, J.L., Azerad, G., Martin, T., and Muller, S. (1988) Eur. J. Immunol. 18, 1127.

20. Kotzin, B.L., Lafferty, J.A., Portanova, J.P., Rubin, R.L., and Tan, E.M. (1984) J. Immunol. 133, 2554.

21. Klinman, D.M., and Steinberg, A.D. (1987) J. Exp. Med. 165, 1755.

22. Reeves, W.H., and Chiorazzi, N. (1986) J. Exp. Med. 164, 1029.

23. Deutscher, S.L., and Keene, J.D. (1988) Proc. Natl. Acad. Sci. USA 85: 3299.

24. Stetler, D.A., and Jacob, S.T. (1985) Proc. Natl. Acad. Sci. USA 82, 6797.

25. Stocks, M.R., Williams, D.G., and Maini, R.N. (1987) Clin. Exp. Immunol. 67, 492.

26. Mendlovic, S., Brocke, S., Shoenfeld, Y., Ben-Bassat, M., Meshorer, A., Bakimer, R., and Mozes, E. (1988) Proc. Natl. Acad. Sci. USA 85, 2260.

27. Umanskii, S.R., Korol, B.A., Piker, E.G., Runova, Y.N. (1975) Mol. Biol. 8, 393.

28. Fisher, S.G., and Laemmli, U.K. (1980) Biochem. 19, 2240.

29. Schwartz, R.S., and Stollar, B.D. (1985) J. Clin. Invest. 75, 321.

30. Pollard, K.M., Jones, J.E., Tan, E.M., Theofilopoulos, A.E., Dixon, F.J., and Rubin, R.L. (1986) Clin. Immunol. Immunopathol. 40, 197.

31. Capitani, S., Cocco, L., Matteuci, A., Caramelli, E., Papa, S., and Manzoli, F.A. (1984) Cell. Biol. Intern. Rep. 8, 289.

32. Lafer, E.M., Rauch, J., Andrzejewski, C., Mudd, D., Furie, B., Furie, B., Schwartz, R.S., and Stollar, B.D. (1981) J. Exp. Med. 153, 897.

33. Goldman, M., Rose, L.M., Hochmann, A., and Lambert, P.H. (1982) J. Exp. Med. 155, 1385.

34. Renversez, J.C., Roussel, S., Vallee, M.J., Brighouse, G., and Lambert, P.H. (1984) Blood Transfusion Immunohaematol. 27, 737.

EXPERIMENTAL MODELS OF T CELL TOLERANCE

Lorise C. Gahring
William O. Weigle

Department of Immunology
Research Institute of Scripps Clinic
La Jolla, California

INTRODUCTION

One view of the generation of autoimmunity is that tolerance to a self-antigen is lost. Loss of tolerance, followed by the induction of autoreactivity, ultimately results in the elimination of the antigen and cells bearing the antigen. While this is an oversimplified view of autoimmunity, it serves to stress the importance of understanding the mechanisms regulating the induction and maintenance of tolerance. Several mechanisms have been proposed to explain the induction of specific immunologic tolerance. These include deletion, anergy or active suppression of self reactive lymphocytes. The induction of tolerance to self molecules of the major histocompatibility complex (MHC) results from the deletion of self reactive T cell clones in the thymus of neonatal mice (1-3). The mechanisms of tolerance induction to many other self antigens including those which are not cell associated have yet to be determined. This laboratory and others have employed models of tolerance to antigens which are non cell-associated, non-MHC proteins (4-6). One such antigen, human gamma globulin (HGG), induces an antigen specific tolerance in adult mice. Tolerance to HGG is unique in that one form of the antigen

This work was supported in part by a U.S. Public Health Service Grant no. AI07007 and Biomedical Research Grant no. RR05514. L.C.G. was supported by American Cancer Society Postdoctoral Fellowship no. PF3074.

(deaggregated HGG) is tolerogenic in adult mice and other forms (aggregated HGG) are immunogenic. For most antigens, a tolerogenic form does not exist. Such is the case for thyroglobulin which is another non cell-associated antigen. Autoreactive T cell clones to thyroglobulin can induce a form of autoimmune thyroiditis known as Hashimoto's thyroiditis. In this report, we will summarize recent results obtained from the study of tolerance to human gamma globulin (HGG) and thyroglobulin (Tg).

TABLE I
Tolerance to Human Gamma Globulin *In Vivo*

Group #	DHGG[a]	Challenge[a]	ELISA[b] units/ml
1	-	400 μg AHGG	121 + 27
2	+	400 μg AHGG	7 + 5
3	-	200 μg HGG in CFA	252 + 46
4	+	200 μg HGG in CFA	5 + 1

[a] Groups of 5 mice were treated with 1 mg of DHGG i.p. 10 days following DHGG treatment mice were challenged with either 400 μg of AHGG (intravenously) or 200 μg of HGG emulsified in complete Freund's adjuvant (CFA) by footpad injection.

[b] Mice were bled 10 days after challenge with AHGG or 7 days after challenge with HGG in CFA. Anti-HGG titers were determined for individual serum samples obtained from normal and DHGG treated mice.

The Induction of Tolerance to HGG. The induction of tolerance to HGG is dependent on the form of the antigen administered (4-7). The results presented in Table 1 demonstrate that when monomeric or deaggregated HGG (DHGG) is injected into adult mice and these animals are then challenged with aggregated HGG (AHGG) or HGG emulsified in complete Freunds adjuvant (CFA) they fail to respond to the immunogenic form of HGG. This induced tolerance to HGG is antigen specific and long lasting (greater than 180 days for T cells and approximately 60 days for B cells).

The induction of tolerance to HGG can be inhibited by modulation of the normal processes required for the generation of an immunologic response. In order to elicit an immune response, antigen must be ingested by antigen presenting cells (APC), processed by these cells and presented to the appropriate T lymphocyte. Interleukin-1 (IL-1), an accessory molecule produced by APC such as macrophages, is thought to play a role in antigen presentation to T cells. AHGG, upon incubation with macrophages induces the release of IL-1 into culture supernates (8,9). However, DHGG does not stimulate detectable levels of IL-1 in supernates upon culture with macrophages _in vitro_ (8,9). Therefore, we have examined the possibility that the lack of IL-1 production during antigen presentation of DHGG may play a role in the generation of tolerance to HGG. The results of several experiments suggest that IL-1 is indeed involved in the mechanisms of tolerance induction to HGG. First, injection of exogenous inducers of IL-1, such as bacterial lipopolysaccharide (LPS), 2 hours after the injection of tolerogen (DHGG) inhibits the induction of tolerance (10,11). However, animals which are first desensitized to LPS (by daily injection of this substance) such that they fail to respond to LPS by producing IL-1, then the administration of LPS 2 hours after injection of tolerogen does not interfere with the induction of tolerance to HGG (12). More direct evidence that IL-1 inhibits the generation of tolerance was obtained by injection of IL-1 shortly after DHGG treatment. Such injection of IL-1 results in the inhibition of tolerance induction. Therefore, the failure of IL-1 production following administration of DHGG appears to play a pivotal role in the generation of tolerance to HGG _in vivo_.

T Cell Tolerance to HGG. T cell unresponsiveness to HGG was initially observed as the inability to provide T cell help in HGG plaque assays (13). More recently, we have taken a direct approach to the question of HGG-induced T cell unresponsiveness by determining the proliferative responsiveness of T cells from HGG tolerant mice to HGG _in vitro_. T cells were obtained from mice which were first tolerized by injection of 1 mg of DHGG and then challenged with HGG emulsified in complete Freund's adjuvant (CFA). Age matched naive mice received only a challenge dose of HGG in CFA. Results shown in Table 2 demonstrate that T cells from tolerized mice do not proliferate upon incubation with HGG _in vitro_. However, T cells from tolerized mice respond as well as normal mice to the mycobacterial antigen purified protein derivative (PPD) and to the mitogen concanavalin A (Con A). These results demonstrate the antigen specific tolerance of T cells from DHGG treated mice.

TABLE II
Proliferation of Lymph Node T Cells From Normal and HGG Tolerized Mice *In Vitro* [c]

Mice[a]	Antibody[b] (EU/ml)	^{3}H-Thymidine Incorporation[d] (ΔCPM) HGG	PPD	Con A
Normal	512±37	15,419±414	20,289±521	168,294±3965
Tolerized	9± 5	1,579±386	23,180±636	156,276±4398

[a] Normal or tolerized CBA/CaJ mice were challenged with 200 μg of HGG emulsified in CFA by footpad injection. Eight days following challenge, animals were bled, lymphocytes were isolated and T cell enriched by passage over nylon wool columns.
[b] Anti-HGG antibody titers (ELISA units/ml, EU/ml) were determined for individual serum samples obtained from normal and DHGG treated mice. All mice were challenged with HGG-CFA. Results are expressed as mean ± S.E.M.
[c] APC were obtained from the spleens of naive CBA/CaJ mice. These APC were irradiated prior to addition to lymphocytes.
[d] Cells were incubated in the presence of either 400 μg HGG, 25 μg PPD or 2.5 μg/ml Con A. Con A stimulated cultures were pulsed with 0.5 μCi of ^{3}H-thymidine for the final 6 hrs of the 48 hrs assay period. PPD and HGG stimulated cultures were pulsed with 0.5 μCi of ^{3}H-Thymidine at 72 hrs and then harvested at 96 hrs. Results are expressed as CPM +/- SEM.

HGG tolerant mice that were challenged either 5, 10, or 21 days after the administration of tolerogen fail to proliferate in response to HGG *in vitro* (Table 3). Therefore, tolerance is induced as early as 5 days following tolerogen injection and is maintained for at least 21 days. These results coincide with the previous studies which have shown that tolerance at the T cell level can be induced as early as 2 days following tolerogen administration and persists for prolonged periods in the animal (greater than 180 days) (7). The role of suppressor T cells in the induction and maintenance of tolerance to HGG has been difficult to

TABLE III
Kinetics of HGG-Induced Unresponsiveness in CBA/CaJ mice and the Involvement of T-Suppressor Lymphocytes

Day of Challenge[a]	Mice[b]	Serum Antibody[b] (EU/ml)	^{3}H-Thymidine Incorporation[c] (ΔCPM) Untreated	Anti-lyt-2 treated
5	Normal	445±57	31,717± 353	38,029±1,633
	Tolerized	10±2	2,581± 101	4,690± 126
10	Normal	336±22	33,066±2,906	40,408±2,703
	Tolerized	5±3	2,036± 141	1,714± 355
21	Normal	333±22	10,918±1,135	17,123±1,064
	Tolerized	1±05	519± 56	1,159± 149

[a] Groups of 5 CBA/CaJ mice were tolerized to HGG by injection of 1 mg DHGG on day 0. Normal or tolerized mice were challenged with 200 μg HGG in CFA on either day 5, day 10 or day 20.
[b] Mice were bled 8 days post challenge and serum samples from individual mice titered for anti-HGG antibody. Results are expressed as the mean ± SEM.
[c] T lymphocyte enriched lymph node cells were incubated with 400 μg of HGG per well *in vitro.* Prior to culture cells were either incubated with anti-Lyt-2.1 plus complement (anti-Lyt 2 treated) or with complement alone (untreated). Cells were pulsed with 0.5 μCi ^{3}H-Thymidine at 72 hrs and harvested at 96 hrs. Results are expressed as ΔCPM (^{3}H-Thymidine incorporation of T cells, APC and HGG minus incorporation of T cells plus HGG).

determine. Several reports suggest that T suppressor cells (Ts) are induced following administration of DHGG and that these cells are responsible for the induction and maintenance of this tolerance (14). However, it has also been observed that tolerance to HGG can be induced in the absence of any detectable suppressor cell activity (15). In an attempt to clarify the role of suppressor cells in HGG-induced T cell tolerance, the role of Ts in the proliferative responsiveness of T cells from HGG tolerized and normal mice was determined. Results shown in Table 2 demonstrate that removal of Ts by treatment of lymph node T cells with anti-Lyt 2.1 plus complement did not alter the proliferative response of cells obtained from normal mice or mice tolerized with HGG. This result was found to be true for T cells from animals challenged either 5, 10, or 21 days after tolerization. Further, addition of T cells obtained from tolerized mice to T cells from normal mice did not inhibit the normal cells proliferative response to HGG *in vitro* (Table 4).

TABLE IV
T Cells From HGG Tolerized CBA/CaJ Mice Do Not Suppress the Proliferative Response of Lymphocytes From HGG-Immune Mice

Day of challenge[a]	Lymphocytes[b] (cells/wells)		^{3}H-Thymidine Incorporation[c]
	Normal	Tolerant	(ΔCPM)
5	1 x 10^5	none	10,407 ± 500
	none	1 x 10^5	1,461 ± 172
	1 x 10^5	1 x 10^5	15,729 ± 1,000
10	1 x 10^5	none	7,334 ± 1,060
	none	1 x 10^5	569 ± 147
	1 x 10^5	1 x 10^5	9,433 ± 406
21	1 x 10^5	none	5,105 ± 400
	none	1 x 10^5	464 ± 113
	1 x 10^5	1 x 10^5	5,229 ± 391

[a] CBA/CaJ mice were tolerized with 1 mg DHGG on Day 0. These animals as well as normal CBA/CaJ mice were challenged with 200 μg of HGG in CFA on either day 5, day 10 or day 21.
[b] T lymphocytes from normal or tolerant mice were obtained as previously described. These cells were added to wells along with gamma irradiated APC from naive CBA/CaJ mice and 400 μg of HGG.
[c] Cultures were pulsed at 72 hrs with 0.5 μCi ^{3}H-Thymidine and harvested 24 hrs later. Results are expressed as ΔCPM.

The A/J strain of mouse has been most commonly used in this laboratory for the study of HGG tolerance. Therefore, the involvement of suppressor cells in the maintenance of HGG induced tolerance of A/J mice was tested and compared to the tolerance induced in CBA/CaJ mice. Results in Table 5 demonstrate that suppressor cell independent non-responsiveness of T cells from tolerant mice was observed for both the A/J and CBA/CaJ strains of mice. Thus, it can be concluded that lymph node T cells from DHGG tolerized mice fail to proliferate in response to HGG *in vitro* and this lack of responsiveness is not due to the presence of suppressor cell activity at any of the time points tested.

TABLE V
Comparison of Tolerance Induction in CBA/CaJ Mice With A/J Mice

Lymphocytes[a]	Anti-Lyt 2[b] plus C'	^{3}H-Thymidine Incorporation (ΔCPM) A/J	CBA/CaJ
Normal	-	2,236 ± 64	9,324 ± 99
Normal	+	3,862 ± 246	25,102 ± 210
Tolerant	-	332 ± 69	448 ± 67
Tolerant	+	316 ± 149	594 ± 95

[a] CBA/CaJ mice and A/J mice were tolerized with 1 mg DHGG i.p. on day 0. Both normal and tolerized mice were challenged with 200 μg HGG in CFA. Lymph node cells were harvested 8 days after challenge and enriched for T cells.
[b] Nylon wool enriched T cells were treated with either anti-Lyt 2.1 (CBA/CaJ cells) or anti-Lyt 2.2 (A/J cells). Both antibody treated and untreated cells were then incubated with complement.

The Role of the Thymus in HGG Induced Tolerance. To determine if the induced tolerance to HGG *in vivo* was one of central unresponsiveness which required the presence of a functional thymus, mice were thymectomized prior to tolerization. Adult thymectomized mice were injected with a tolerizing dose of DHGG and then challenged with HGG in CFA either 10 or 30 days following tolerization. Mice were bled 8 days after challenge. The level of serum anti-HGG antibody in normal verses thymectomized mice is shown in Table 6. Thymectomized mice which were injected with DHGG fail to elicit an antibody response to the challenge dose of HGG. Further, results in Table 6 demonstrate that T lymphocytes from thymectomized mice do not proliferate to any appreciable extent upon incubation with HGG *in vitro*.

TABLE VI
Induction of Tolerance to HGG in Normal and Adult Thymectomized CBA/CaJ Mice.

CBA/CaJ Mice[a]	Tolerized[b] (1mg DHGG)	Day of Challenge	Serum Antibody[c] (EU/ml)	^{3}H-Thymidine Incorporation[e] (ΔCPM)
	-	10	1,569±191	26,462± 15.25
	+	10	36± 7(98)[d]	2,398± 239 (91)
Normal	-	30	3,080±195	15,712± 341
	+	30	521± 78(83)	2,996± 386 (81)
	-	10	2,393±510	50,381±2187
Thymec-tomized	+	10	41± 11(98)	6,032± 812 (88)
	-	30	3,086±320	46,813±1,337
	+	30	379±121(88)	9,479±1,267(80)

[a] Groups of 5 normal or 5 thymectomized CBA/CaJ mice were used.
[b] Normal and thymectomized mice were challenged either 10 or 30 days after injection of 1 mg DHGG i.p.
[c] All animals were bled eight days after challenge and individual serum samples were tested for the presence of anti-HGG antibody.
[d] Numbers in parentheses refer to the percent suppression.
[e] Lymphocytes were harvested from animals eight days after challenge, enriched for T cells, and incubated with naive CBA/CaJ APC and 400 μg HGG/well. Cultures were pulsed at 72 hrs with ^{3}H-thymidine and harvested 24 hrs later.

TABLE VII
Transfer of Thyroid Lesions with Cloned T Cells

T Cell Clone injected[a]	Recipient[b]	Day 7 Thyroid Lesions					Presence of Polymorpho-nuclear Cells
		Negative	1+	2+	3+	4+	
A7	Normal	5	0	0	0	0	
A7	Irradiated	2	2	2	4	0	0/8
B7	Normal	5	0	0	0	0	
B7	Irradiated	2	0	0	5	3	8/8
Irradiated B7	Irradiated	5	0	0	0	0	
D2	Normal	5	0	0	0	0	
D2	Irradiated	5	0	0	0	0	

[a] 2×10^6 T cells injected i.v. 3 days after activation with 50 µg/ml of Tg. Cells that were irradiated received 3000 rad.

[b] CBA/CaJ female mice. Irradiated recipients received 475 rad.

Thus, thymectomized mice can be tolerized to HGG as easy as normal animals which suggests that this type of tolerance involves the induction of unresponsiveness in mature peripheral T cells of adult animals.

Tolerance in HGG Specific T Cell Clones. The induction of T cell tolerance to HGG has also been investigated through the use of T cell clones and lines which are specific to HGG. It was found that exposure of these T cell clones to DHGG *in vitro* resulted in the induction of tolerance to HGG. Tolerance was determined by the inability of DHGG treated clones to reconstitute the plaque forming response of HGG-primed B cells (13). It has also been determined that HGG specific T cell clones which are incubated with DHGG in the presence of IL-1 fail to become tolerant (13). This result further substantiates the role of IL-1 in the induction of tolerance to HGG. More recent studies are revealing possible mechanisms of T cell tolerance induction by establishing which types of T cells are tolerizable (Th^1 type clones verses Th^2 type clones), the lymphokines that are secreted by tolerized verses nontolerized clones, and at what stage in their cell cycle the clones can be tolerized to HGG (16).

Molecular Mechanisms of T cell Unresponsiveness.

The activation of T cell clones results in a cascade of

cellular events that are rapidly being elucidated. Occupation of the T cell receptor induces cleavage of phosphatidyl inositol-4,5-biphosphate to 1,4,5,-inositol triphosphate (ITP) and diacylglycerol. ITP then induces an increase in intracellular calcium levels which subsequently stimulates transcription of the IL-2 gene (17-19). Jenkins et al have induced T cell unresponiveness to an antigenic peptide of pigeon cytochrome C by incubation of T cell clones with macrophages which have been fixed with carbodiimide. The T cell tolerance induced by carbodiimide treated macrophages could be mimicked by treatment of these clones with the calcium ionophore, ionomycin (17). These results suggest that calcium influx was required for the induction of tolerance in this system. However, the influx of Ca^{++} was not accompanied by phosphatidyl inositol metabolism. Therefore, it has been suggested that inactivation of antigen specific T cells results from the dissociation of signals required for T cell activation.

Autoreactive T Cell Clones.

It has been previously demonstrated by others (20) and ourselves (21) that autoreactive T cell lines or clones generated to mouse thyroglobulin (Tg) are capable of transferring severe experimental autoimmune thyroiditis (EAT) to syngeneic mice. $CD4^+$ ($L3T4^+$) clones have been generated which proliferate to mouse Tg and when transferred to irradiated (475R) syngeneic mice causes the development of either monocytic or a combination of monocytic and polymorphonucleacytic infiltration of their thyroid glands which is associated with T helper function of the clone (21). Another clone showing Tg-specific proliferation and T helper function, however, was incapable of transferring lesions (Table 7). It was previously shown by others that pretreatment of antigen-specific Th_1 clones with ionophore results in the inability of these clones to proliferate to antigen at a later time. Similarly, pretreatment of the Th_2 Tg-specific T cell clone with 1 μM ionomycin resulted in the inability of that clone to respond to Tg 24 hrs later (C.G. Romball, unpublished observations). Such unresponsiveness was transient and was not obvious 4 days later. On the other hand, the Tg-unresponsive ionomycin-treated clones responded equally as well to Concanavalin A and recombinant interleukin-2 (rIL-2) as did the non-treated clones. It is of interest that anti-CD3, which is reactive with the T cell receptor (TcR) complex, also failed to cause proliferation of the ionomycin-pretreated T cell clones, suggesting that activation of these clones through the TcR complex follows a proliferative pathway different than that induced by either Concanavalin A or the IL-2 receptor.

CONCLUSIONS

Monomeric HGG induces T cell tolerance in the peripheral lymph nodes of adult mice. This type of tolerance is a unique model of tolerance that is neither suppressor cell ($CD8^+$) nor thymus dependent. The results that support this conclusion are 1) T cells from tolerized mice do not proliferate in response to HGG *in vitro*, 2) elimination of $CD8^+$ cells from T cells obtained from HGG tolerant mice does not alter the unresponsiveness to HGG *in vitro*, 3) addition of T cells from tolerant mice to normal HGG-primed T cells does not inhibit the primed T cell response to HGG *in vitro*, and 4) thymectomized mice can be tolerized to HGG. Many questions concerning tolerance to HGG remain unanswered. For example, is tolerance to HGG the result of peripheral deletion of HGG responsive T cells or a result of clonal anergy? Evidence for clonal anergy of B cells has been demonstrated. Nossal and co-workers found that B cells tolerized (via the placental route) to hapten-conjugated HGG are capable of binding the hapten and are present in normal numbers in the tolerized animal yet they are incapable of responding to the hapten (22,23). Goodnow et al. have recently demonstrated B cell anergy in transgenic mice (24). Anergy of mature T cells to a non-self and non-MHC antigen has also been demonstrated (17-19). T cell clones can be rendered tolerant if the antigen is presented by "fixed" splenocytes *in vitro* (17-19). Further, T cell clones specifically reactive to HGG can be rendered anergic to HGG *in vitro* if monomeric HGG is incubated with the clones (8,13,16) or if HGG-pulsed, paraformaldehyde fixed splenic accessory cells are used as APC for the clones (16).

The induction of an immune response to Tg can result in the generation of the autoimmune disease thyroiditis. Transfer of T cell clones which are specified to Tg to irradiated syngeneic mice can result in lesions in the thyroid of the recipient animals. T cell clones can be tolerized *in vitro* to Tg by treatment with the ionophore ionomycin. These results suggest that uncoupling of the signals required to stimulate T cells may instead lead to the generation of specific immunologic tolerance.

Tolerance to either HGG or Tg represents tolerance of mature T cells. These experimental models of tolerance to non-MHC molecules should markedly enhance our understanding of the mechanisms required to maintain tolerance in the peripheral lymphoid organs of adult animals.

REFERENCES

1. Kappler, J.W., Roehm, N., and Marrack, P. (1987). Cell. 49:273.
2. Kappler, J.W., Staerze, U., White, J., and Marrack, P., (1988). Nature. 332:35.
3. MacDonald, H., Schneider, R., Lees, R.K., Howe, R.C., Ocha-Orbca, H., Festenstein, H., Zinkernagel, R.M., and Hengartner, H. (1988). Nature. 332:40.
4. Weigle, W.O. (1980) Adv. Immunol. 30:159.
5. Dressor, D.W. (1962). Immunology. 5:378.
6. Basten, A., Miller, J.A.F.P., Loblay, R., Johnson, P., Gamble, J., Chia, E., Pritchard-Briscoe, H., Callard, R., and McKenzie, I.F.C. (1978). Eur. J. Immunol. 8:360.
7. Chiller, J.M., Habict, G.S., and Weigle, W.O. (1971). Science. 171:813.
8. Levich, J.D., Signorella, A.P., Wittenberg, G., and Weigle, W.O. (1987). J. Immunol. 138:3675.
9. Weigle, W.O., Scheuer, W.V., Hobbs, M.V., Morgan, E.L., and Parks, P.E. (1987). J. Immunol. 138:2069.
10. Louis, J.A., Chiller, J.M., and Weigle, W.O. (1973). J. Exp. Med. 138:1481.
11. Parks, D.E., Walker, S.M., and Weigle, W.O. (1981). J. Immunol. 126:938.
12. Weigle, W.O., Gahring, L.C., Romball, C.G., and Goodman, M.G. (1989). J. Immunol. 142:1107.
13. Levich, J.D., Parks, D.E., and Weigle, W.O. (1985). J. Immunol. 135:873.
14. Loblay, R.H., Fazekas, B., St. Groth, D.E., Pritchard-Briscoe, H., and Basten, A. (1983). J. Exp. Med. 157:957.
15. Parks, D.E., Doyle, M.V., and Weigle, W.O. (1978). J. Exp. Med. 148:625.
16. Gilbert, K.M., Hoang, K.D., and Weigle, W.O. (1989). Federation Proc. (in press).
17. Jenkins, M.K., Pardoll, P.M., Mizuguchi, J., Chused, T.M., and Schwartz, R.H. (1987). Proc. Natl. Acad. Sci. 84:5409.
18. Jenkins, M.K., Pardoll, D.M., Mizuguchi, J., Quill, H., and Schwartz, R.H. (1987) Immun. Rev. 95:113.
19. Jenkins, M.K., and Schwartz, R.H. (1987). J. Exp. Med. 165:302.
20. Maron, R., Zerubauel, R., Friedman, A., and Cohen, I.R. (1983). J. Immunol. 131:2316.
21. Romball, C.G., and Weigle, W.O. (1987). J. Immunol. 138:1092.
22. Nossal, G.J.V., and Pike, B.L. (1980). Proc. Natl. Acad, Sci. USA 77: 1602.

23. Pike, B.L., Kay, T.W., and Nossal, G.J.V. (1982). Proc. Natl. Acad. Sci. USA 79: 2013.
24. Goodnow, C.C., Crosbie, J., Adelstein, S., Lavoie, T.B, Smith-Gill, S.J., Brink, R.A., Pritchard-Briscoe, H., Witherspoon, R.H., Loblay, R.H., Raphail, K., Trent, R.J., and Basten, A. (1988). Nature 334: 676.

GENOMIC AND EXPRESSED T CELL ANTIGEN RECEPTOR REPERTOIRE IN AUTOIMMUNE MURINE MODELS[1]

Argyrios N. Theofilopoulos
Paul A. Singer

Department of Immunology
Scripps Clinic and Research Foundation
La Jolla, California

I. INTRODUCTION

Several studies in animal models have clearly documented the primary role of T cells in the pathogenesis of systemic and organ-specific autoimmune diseases, either in the form of helper activities required for autoantibody production or self-reactive cytotoxic T cells. Thus, neonatally thymectomized MRL-*lpr/lpr* mice do not exhibit the lymphoid hyperplasia and early-life severe lupus seen in control animals (1,2), and (NZBxNZW)F_1 *nu/nu* mice do not develop autoimmune disease unless a syngeneic thymus is engrafted (3). The involvement of T cells in the induction of autoimmune syndromes has also been supported by cell transfer experiments (4-6) and by the inhibitory or ameliorating effects of administered anti-L3T4 (CD4) antibodies in spontaneous models of autoimmunity such as murine strains with lupus (7,8) and in the NOD mouse with insulin-dependent diabetes (9,10) as well as models of experimentally-induced autoimmune syndromes such as collagen arthritis (11), allergic thyroiditis (5), experimental allergic encephalomyelitis (EAE) (12) and myasthenia gravis (13). In fact, preliminary evidence has suggested that

[1]This is Publication Number 5740IMM from the Department of Immunology, Research Institute of Scripps Clinic, 10666 North Torrey Pines Road, La Jolla, CA 92037. The work reported herein was supported by NIH Grants AR33826, AR31203 and AR39555.

The Molecular Aspects of Autoimmunity

an allelic variant of the T cell antigen receptor (TCR) Vβ6 gene is necessary for the development of experimental collagen arthritis in mice (14). Moreover, a limited set of TCR Vα-Jα and Vβ-Jβ genes has been identified in T helper clones specific for the encephalitogenic portion of mouse myelin basic protein (MBP), and a monoclonal antibody recognizing the product of one of these genes was found to block T helper clone recognition of the specific encephalitogenic MBP peptide *in vitro* and to significantly reduce the susceptibility of appropriate mice to peptide-induced EAE (15-17).

For the reasons cited above, we and others believe that a detailed investigation into the genomic composition and expression of TCR genes in mice predisposed to autoimmunity will be paramount to our efforts to determine why tolerance to self is circumvented. Significant TCR genomic polymorphisms may be identified that could correlate with the autoimmune predisposition. Furthermore, aberrant TCR expression patterns might emerge that will indicate either selective activation of certain clones or abnormalities in thymic selection and maturation processes in these diseases. Below, we summarize the current understanding of TCR gene biology and describe our recent studies on the genomic composition and expressed repertoire of these genes in several autoimmune and normal mouse strains.

II. TCR GENE DIVERSITY AND T CELL MATURATION

The two types of murine TCR heterodimeric structures (α:β and γ:δ) and their corresponding genes have been well-defined (reviewed in 18-20), with the α:β structure found on the majority (≈98%) of mature peripheral helper ($CD4^+8^-$) and cytotoxic ($CD8^+4^-$) MHC class II- or class I-restricted T cells, respectively. The γ:δ is found on a small (≈2%), but distinct, population of peripheral T cells and on the majority of dendritic T cells in the skin; the function of the γ:δ-bearing cells remains unknown. Both heterodimers are independently expressed on the cell surface of these T cell populations in a non-covalent association with the multichain (5 chains; γ, δ, ε, ζ, η) invariant CD3 complex.

The mouse β-chain locus (chromosome 6) consists of an estimated 20-30 V genes, arranged in a minimum of 17 one-to-three member subfamilies, and two C-region genes, each with a single upstream D element and 6 functional J elements (Fig. 1). Strains of mice (SJL, SWR, C57L, C57BR) have been identified that have deleted a large fraction (≈50%) of

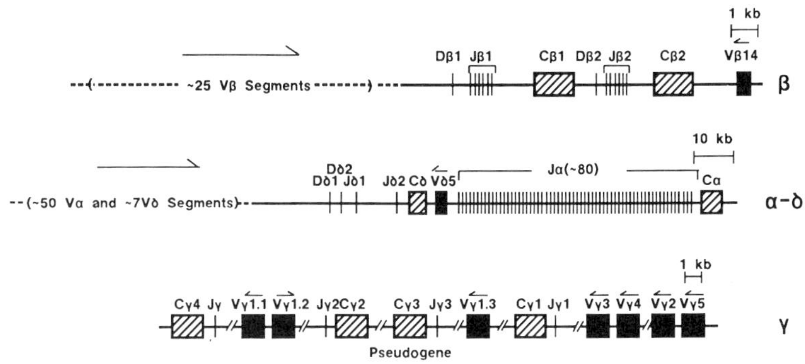

Fig. 1. Genomic organization of the T cell receptor loci in the mouse. Transcriptional orientations are indicated with arrows.

these Vβ segments, yet appear immunologically normal (21). The murine α-chain locus (chromosome 14) consists of perhaps 100-150 V genes, arranged in 15-20 subfamilies, each consisting of 1 to 10 members and a single C-region gene with a large number (≈50%) of upstream J elements (no Dα gene element has been identified). The δ locus (chromosome 14) is unique in that it is located between the V and J segments of the α gene and is deleted in α:β-bearing T cells. Although there is some overlap in V region usage, the V gene segments used for α and δ chains are largely distinct, with only ≈7 V segments identified for the δ chain. Finally, the TCR γ locus (chromosome 13) is less diverse, with three different functional Jγ-Cγ loci and ≈7 Vγ gene segments. TCRs appear to diversify primarily by recombination of their various genetic elements, but not by somatic hypermutation, which occurs for Ig genes.

Although there is no complete consensus among the prevailing views, it is reasonably established that the normal pathway of T cell differentiation involves the following steps (reviewed in 22-25; Fig. 2): a) emigration of precursor T cells ($CD4^-8^-$, TCR^-) from the bone marrow to the thymic cortex; b) transcription of the genes encoding the multichain CD3 complex; c) rearrangements of the γ and δ loci, initial rearrangements of the β locus, and acquisition of surface γ:δ dimeric structures together with CD3 in a few such cells; d) in the majority of $CD4^-8^-$ cells where

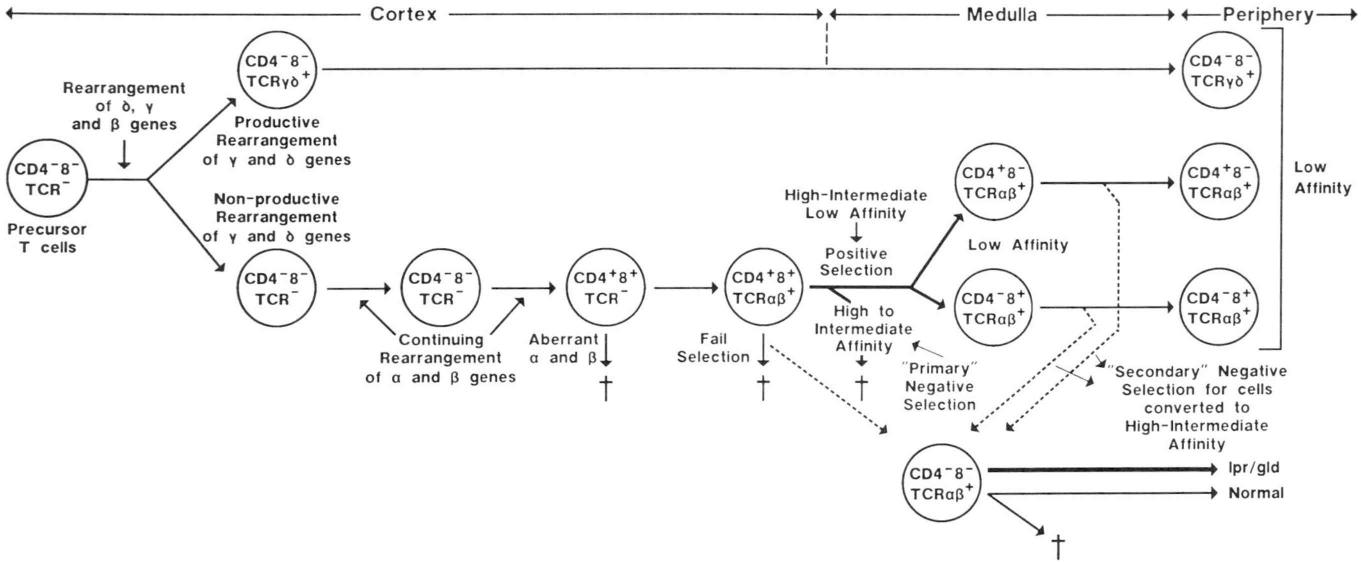

Fig. 2. Developmental pathways for murine T cells (see text).

γ, δ rearrangements are non-productive, continued maturation with further β-chain gene rearrangements and mRNA expression, followed by acquisition of CD4 and CD8 accessory molecules ($CD4^+8^+$ or double-positive cells), with CD8 appearing prior to CD4; e) the subsequent rearrangement of α-chain genes and the appearance of surface CD3 together with $\alpha:\beta$ dimeric structures on ≈50% of these cells; f) the so-called "positive" (26-28) and "negative" (29-33) selection processes, i.e., positive selection for cells having TCRs that will recognize antigen fragments only if presented by self-MHC, and negative selection against cells having TCRs that would confer autoreactivity in the mature T cells, and, finally g) the development of some of these cells into mature $CD4^+8^-$ (helper) or $CD8^+4^-$ (cytotoxic) thymocytes and their eventual exit to the periphery. It is generally thought that positive selection precedes negative selection, primarily because positive selection seems to involve an interaction between the TCR and MHC molecules expressed on thymic cortical epithelial cells (25,34), the thymic cortex being the site at which double-positive thymocytes are found. Similarly, negative selection requires the presence of cells derived from bone marrow (macrophages, dentritic cells) (25,35), which are believed to be found primarily in the thymic medulla, a site occupied by more mature thymocytes. It is far from clear, however, what the actual sequence of events is since several studies suggest, somewhat paradoxically, that both positive and negative selections begin at the double-positive stage (23,36,37). Janeway (23) has offered several plausible scenarios for these events, Sprent and Webb (25) have suggested that, to the contrary, negative selection of cells displaying TCRs with intermediate to high anti-self MHC affinity precedes positive selection of cells displaying TCRs with low anti-self MHC affinity, and Marrack and Kappler (24) suggested that these events are related to the different spectrum of self-peptides bound to thymic epithelial cells (positive selection) and self-peptides bound to bone marrow-derived cells (negative selection). Whichever model of thymic selection is correct, it is now clear that positive selection determines the CD4/CD8 phenotype of the developing thymocyte (26-28), this determination being based on whether the TCR has reactivity for self class I (CD8-selected) or class II (CD4-selected). Although the exact mechanism of this selection process has not been delineated, the end result is down-regulation of the unselected CD4 or CD8 accessory molecule, either as a result of a preprogrammed event or through an active negative signal, giving rise to single-positive $CD8^+4^-$ or $CD4^+8^-$ cells, with the $CD4^+8^-$ subset appearing first. A portion of these cells, selected for low anti-self

MHC reactivity, are then exported to the periphery, where they form the pool of self-MHC-restricted helper ($CD4^+8^-$) and cytotoxic ($CD8^+4^-$) T cells. Thus, out of the $>50x10^6$ T cells produced in the thymus per day, only $1\text{-}2x10^6$ per day are exported as mature functional T cells (24,25). The majority of T cells die intrathymically, presumably because a) their TCR gene rearrangements are not productive; b) their TCRs do not exhibit reactivity for self-MHC so as to be positively selected, or c) they are eliminated by negative selection.

In addition to the $CD4^+8^-$ and $CD8^+4^-$ TCR $\alpha:\beta^+$ cells, a small subset of $CD4^-8^-$ TCR $\alpha:\beta^+$ cells consisting ≈2-30% of $CD4^-8^-$ thymocytes (themselves representing ≈5% of the total thymocytes) has been identified (22,38-41), but its origin remains enigmatic. This subset appears relatively late in ontogeny (between birth and day 5 of life, increasing to ≈20-30% of double-negative thymocytes in 2-4 week-old mice) and thus is unlikely to be the precursor to the TCR $\alpha:\beta^+$ single-positive cells already present at birth. Furthermore, this double-negative TCR $\alpha:\beta^+$ subset cannot recolonize thymuses, nor give rise to medullary T cell types, further substantiating its late developmental stage (40). As postulated in a later section of this chapter, these cells, exhibiting many phenotypic characteristics similar to the abnormally expanded T cells of autoimmune mice homozygous for the *lpr* or *gld* mutations, may represent a heterogeneous population derived from: a) cells that never express CD4 and CD8; b) cells that have failed to be selected, and c) moderately self-reactive cells that have escaped clonal deletion, but have downregulated their accessory molecules.

From the foregoing, it becomes apparent that TCR genomic modifications (allelic variants, genomic deletions), alterations imposed during thymic positive and negative selection, and oligoclonal restrictions in autoaggressive T cells might be important in the pathogenesis of autoimmune disorders. Aspects of our investigations in these areas are outlined below.

III. GERMLINE TCR α AND β GENES IN AUTOIMMUNE STRAINS

At least two situations can be envisioned in which the germline TCR genes could contribute to autoimmunity: 1) autoimmune strains could exhibit alterations in TCR genomic organization (deletions of certain VDJC elements) which could lead to autoreactivity through immunoregulatory imbalances, and 2) autoimmune strains could have unique allelic variants of TCR V genes, including one or more V genes predisposing to the development of autoreactive T cells.

A. Cα and Cβ Genes

In an initial structural analysis of the TCR locus (42), we screened genomic DNAs of classical autoimmune strains along with additional ancestral strains for gross alterations in TCR Cα and Cβ genes. Hybridization of the α-chain C region probe to EcoRI-digested DNA identified genomic DNA fragments (4.4 and 6.8 kb) encoding the Cα gene, but revealed no polymorphisms among the strains tested (data not shown). Hybridization of BamHI-digested DNA with a TCR β-chain (CDJ) probe also disclosed nonpolymorphic DNA fragments (6 and 10 kb) in 16 of the 18 strains tested. The two exceptions were NZW mice, in which only one hybridization band (9kb) was detected, and (NZBxNZW)F_1, which had the expected composite NZB and NZW profiles (6, 9 and 10 kb; data not shown). Considering the published restriction map for the TCR β gene locus, additional digests and actual cDNA cloning and sequencing of the NZW DJC elements (42), we concluded that this profile was caused by an ≈8.8 kb deletion beginning at the first exon of Cβ1 and extending to the beginning of the first exon of Cβ2, thereby creating a Cβ locus lacking the Cβ1, Dβ2 and Jβ2 segments (Fig. 3).

A meiotic recombination event can be evoked to explain this deletion, with an unequal crossing over between the precisely aligned first exon of the Cβ1 gene on one chromatid and the Cβ2 gene on its homologue. Based on Southern blot analysis only, Kotzin et al. (43) independently derived similar conclusions. Due to this deletion, only Dβ1-Jβ1, and not Dβ2-Jβ2 or Dβ1-Jβ2, joinings are possible in NZW mice; thus, these mice may be able to generate considerably less TCR β-chain diversity than other strains. In spite of this seemingly dramatic impairment, the effects on T cell responses of these mice are not readily apparent. Furthermore, despite the contrary claims (44), our studies with (NZBxNZW)F_2 mice (45) and those of Kotzin and Palmer (46) with (NZBxNZW) backcrosses to NZB have not disclosed any primary role for this deletion in the development of autoimmune manifestations in these mice.

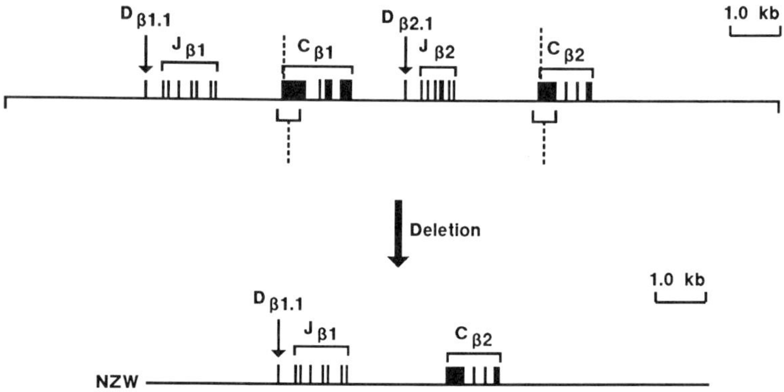

Fig. 3. A schematic representation of the TCR β-chain deletion identified in NZW mice. Hatched lines denote breakpoint regions as determined by previous sequence analysis.

B. Vβ Haplotypes

We first used a complete set of 17 Vβ subfamily probes (i.e., Vβ1-17, according to nomenclature in ref. 47) to analyze genomic blots containing DNA from a number of normal, autoimmune-susceptible or autoimmune-contributing murine strains not previously characterized in the literature, including autoimmune BXSB, MRL, NZB, NZW, NOD mice and their ancestors (when known) (48). Using EcoRI, HindIII and BamHI, we detected no new RFLPs beyond those previously described (21) defining the two Vβ haplotypes, i.e., $V\beta^a$ that includes the above-described Vβ-deleted strains (SWR, SJL, C57L, C57BR with deletions in Vβ5, 8, 9, 11, 12 and 13), and $V\beta^b$ haplotype that includes all other non-Vβ deleted strains (data not shown).

C. Vα Haplotypes

When genomic blots of various strains were hybridized with 9 Vα subfamily probes (Vα1,2,4,5,6,7,8,9,11), numerous RFLPs were detected (Fig. 4), identifying four distinct haplotypes, which we have designated $V\alpha^a$, $V\alpha^b$, $V\alpha^c$ and $V\alpha^d$ (48). Specific RFLPs were detected for each haplotype and for all of the Vα subfamilies analyzed, in most cases regardless of which restriction enzyme was used. In contrast to the situation in the murine Vβ locus, no Vα haplotypes were found in which one or more entire subfamilies had been

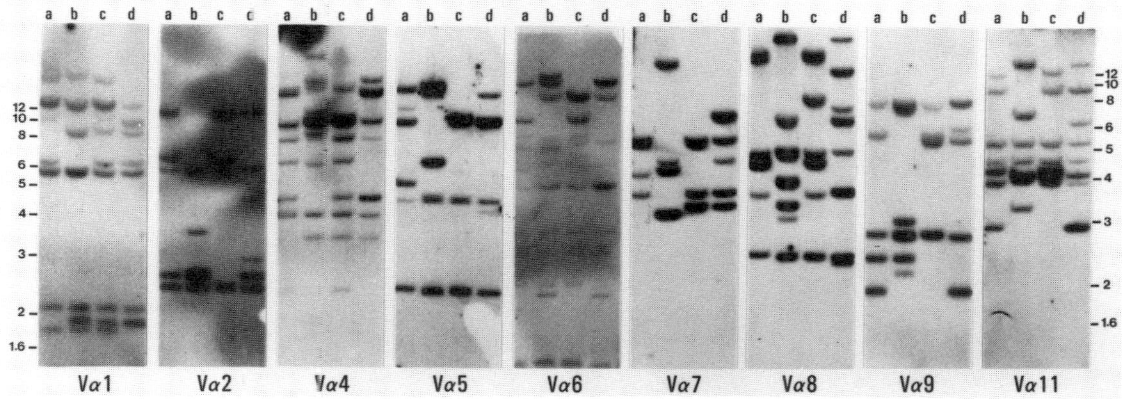

Fig. 4. *RFLPs distinguishing murine TCR Vα haplotypes. Lanes a-d correspond to Vα haplotypes $V\alpha^a$, $V\alpha^b$, $V\alpha^c$, and $V\alpha^d$. Genomic DNAs were obtained from strains BALB/c (lane a), BXSB (lane b), NZB (lane c), and NZW (lane d). Vα4 and 5 panels are BamHI digests; all others are HindIII digests. Size markers (in kilobases, Kb) are indicated (for blots Vα1, -2, -7, -8 and -9 at the left, and for blots Vα4, -5, -6 and -11 at right).*

deleted; however, deletions of some specific genes or gene sets within some subfamilies were detected (data not shown).

Table I lists the strain distribution among the four $V\alpha$ haplotypes. The larger group carries the $V\alpha^a$ haplotype, including a number of normal laboratory strains such as BALB/c, CBA, and A/J; the autoimmune MRL mouse and its major progenitor strains, LG, AKR and C3H and the autoimmunity-contributing strain SB/Le. The C57 strains carry the $V\alpha^b$ haplotype (or a subtype thereof), as does the autoimmune-prone BXSB mouse, which is a cross between the C57BL/6 and SB/Le parental strains. SJL and SWR, on the other hand, are $V\alpha^c$, as are NZB, PL/J and NOD mice. Finally, $V\alpha^d$ is carried only by NZW mice of all the strains tested. No apparent relationship of MHC with $V\alpha$ haplotype emerged from these studies.

TABLE I. Strain Distribution Among the Four $V\alpha$ Haplotypes

$V\alpha$ Haplotype	Strains
a	BALB/c, AKR, C3H, CBA, A/J, LG, SB/Le, MRL
b	C57BL/6, C57BL/10, BXSB C57L, C57BR (subtypes)
c	SJL, SWR, NZB, PL/J, NOD
d	NZW

Based on these findings, it can be stated that in murine models of systemic autoimmunity, correlations with $V\alpha$ haplotype were not clearly apparent. Thus, the prototypic lupus models were distributed in all four $V\alpha$ haplotypes. In addition, on the basis of the nine $V\alpha$ subfamilies analyzed in this study, autoimmune MRL and BXSB mice are shown to have $V\alpha$ and MHC haplotypes (i.e., $V\alpha^a$/ H-2^k and $V\alpha^b$/H-2^b, respectively) identical to at least one of their normal progenitor strains. It therefore seems unlikely that disease expression in these lupus models is caused by abnormalities encoded in a particular $V\alpha$ (or $V\beta$) haplotype *per se* or by novel combinations of $V\alpha$ haplotypes with MHC alleles. However, these examples do not preclude the possibility that, in particular cases, an otherwise normal Vα haplotype may nonetheless contribute to the unique constellation of factors allowing the autoimmune response to occur. Of interest in this regard, the $V\alpha^{c}$ haplotype was found to be common to a diverse group of autoimmune-prone or autoimmune-contributing strains, but this association may be fortuitous.

IV. EXPRESSED TCR Vβ REPERTOIRE IN AUTOIMMUNE MODELS

Following the genomic studies outlined above, we examined the expression patterns of TCR Vβ genes in primary lymphoid organs of autoimmune and other types of mice in an attempt to identify unique expression patterns or abnormalities in T cell maturation and selection phenomena, particularly in tolerance-related clonal deletions.

A. Multiprobe TCR Vβ RNAse Protection Assay

To define TCR gene expression characteristics of autoimmune and normal mice, we adapted and modified an RNAse protection assay (48,49) whereby the quantity and quality of an mRNA species in the total cellular RNA from any tissue source can be analyzed.

In this assay, diagrammatically depicted in Fig. 5, a single-stranded anti-sense radioactive RNA probe of defined length, complementary to the mRNA sequence to be quantitated, is hybridized in solution to the target mRNA under conditions of probe excess and high Rot value, such that essentially all target mRNA present becomes hybridized to the probe. After hybridization, the excess probe is removed by RNAse digestion, leaving the hybridized probe:mRNA duplex intact (i.e., "protected"). The protected probe is electrophoresed on polyacrylamide sequencing gels and identified as a specific band by autoradiography or other means (e.g., direct beta scanning). The strength of the radioactive signal in a given band is directly proportional to the quantity of protected probe corresponding to that band, and hence to the quantity of target mRNA present in the original RNA sample.

With a goal of having an accurate and rapid assay for determining the entire TCR V gene usage at the RNA level, we modified this basic assay into what can be described as a fingerprinting method, or multiprobe RNAse protection assay. Briefly, cDNA probes corresponding to all known Vβ genes (and several Vα genes) have been made through recombinant

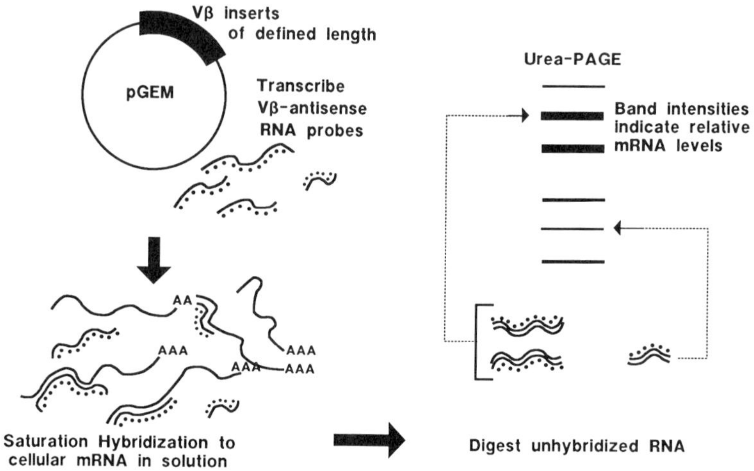

Fig. 5. A schematic representation of the multiprobe RNAse protection assay for the analysis of expressed TCR repertoires in lymphoid cells (see text).

DNA techniques into defined length fragments (from ≈40 to ≈360 bp long) and subcloned into pGEM, a riboprobe vector. Importantly, the probe design has been made in such a way that the size of a given protected band uniquely identifies a single Vβ (or Vα) gene. The fingerprinting or ladder RNAse protection assay for analyzing multiple genes simultaneously works as follows: Several radiolabeled individual antisense riboprobes (a probe set), each of defined length recognizing different Vβ (or Vα) mRNAs, together with an aliquot of the RNA preparation to be analyzed, are hybridized in a single tube, digested with RNAse A+T1, and run on a single lane of a polyacrylamide sequencing gel. In the final autoradiography, intensities of different bands correspond to the level of the TCR V gene mRNAs present, thus creating a V gene fingerprint for the relevant T cell population. The use of probe sets over individual probes increases the information that can be obtained from a given amount of RNA, and increases the accuracy of the results, since the relative levels of the individual probes within a probe set are internally controlled. Good band definition of Vβs can currently be performed with 6-8 probes/probe set. Vβ expression patterns, using the above-outlined approach on total mouse thymocytes and double-positive thymocyte RNAs are shown in Fig. 6, where the reference prototype template with 4 probe sets is also shown. As expected, the profiles of total thymocytes and

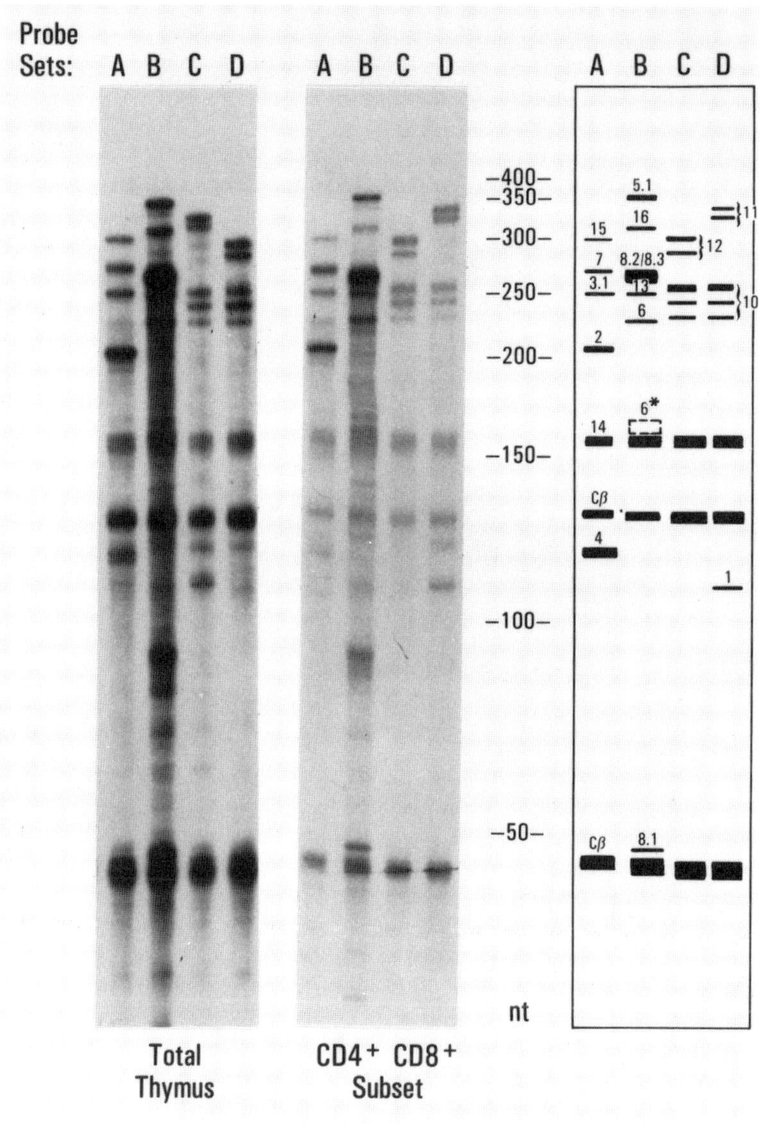

Fig. 6. Results obtained by the RNAse protection assay with unseparated total thymocytes and double-positive ($CD4^+8^+$) thymocytes, and the corresponding, diagrammatically depicted, prototypic template with four probe sets (A, B, C, D) encompassing most of the known murine Vβ genes. nt = nucleotide.

double-positive cells (consisting ≈80% of total thymocytes that, in their majority, have not yet undergone thymic selection, but highly transcribe Vβ genes) are identical.

B. Genomic Impositions on TCR Vβ Gene Expression

When unselected thymocytes (sorted $CD3^-$ thymocytes) of the two Vβ haplotypes ($V\beta^a$-deleted and $V\beta^b$-non-deleted) were compared with regard to their Vβ gene expression, it became apparent that the genomic deletions in the former haplotype had affected TCR repertoire expression among the various Vβ genes (data not shown). Thus, for compensatory reasons and not unexpectely, most of the residual Vβ genes of a Vβ-deleted mouse exhibited a higher expression in this population than the corresponding genes of Vβ-non-deleted mice. Exceptions to this general rule were, however, noted. For example, the Vβ15 gene was, to the contrary, under-expressed in the Vβ-deleted haplotype compared to the Vβ non-deleted haplotype, and Vβ16 was overexpressed to a greater extent than can be explained by compensatory expression. Differences in Vβ gene expression within a Vβ haplotype were also observed; in, for example, the Vβ-non-deleted haplotype, there was a generally lower expression of the Vβ9 and 17 genes. Moreover, the Vβ17a (Vβ3.2) gene was expressed only in the Vβ-deleted haplotype, confirming previous immunofluorescence studies with an anti-Vβ17a antibody (29). Recent studies (50) have indicated that this gene is present in the genome of both Vβ haplotypes but in the Vβ non-deleted haplotype, because of a single base substitution resulting in a termination codon, the level of mRNA from this gene is low either due to the instability of nonfunctional mRNA or to the lack of positive T cell selection with these rearrangements in the thymus. In addition, allelic polymorphisms of Vβ1, 3, 6 and 10, previously noted at the genomic level (21), were also detected in RNAs of the two Vβ haplotypes. Recent preliminary studies (14), cited above, suggested that the Vβ6 allele of the $V\beta^b$ haplotype is necessary for responses to collagen and development of arthritis in mice of the appropriate $H2^q$ background. Further studies on the relationship of these Vβ (and Vα) allelic variants to responsiveness against foreign and self molecules and to the development of diseases, including autoimmune diseases, is therefore warranted, as is the definition of their primary structure.

C. Tolerance- or Negative Selection-Related TCR Vβ Repertoire Modifications

Because the germline T (and B) cell repertoire is immense and, therefore, capable of recognizing essentially any antigenic determinant, negating mechanisms must be in place by which highly self-reactive lymphocyte clones are eliminated, inactivated or otherwise suppressed to create a tolerant state. With regard to B cells, recent studies (51) with double transgenic mice expressing a neo-self antigen (hen egg lysozyme) and a high affinity anti-lysozyme antibody have suggested that B cell tolerance is primarily mediated by an antigen receptor inactivation process, but contribu-tions of clonal elimination mechanisms have not been ruled out. With regard to T cells, in spite of the extensive literature on suppressor cells and immunologic networks, there has been persistent support for the notion that there is a major censorship function exercised in the thymus itself. This censorship or negative selection prevents autoaggressive (high affinity anti-self) T cells from maturing and migrating, but allows cells with the capacity to recognize a foreign antigen in association with an MHC restriction element to pass this barrier.

Definitive evidence for the clonal deletion of T cells expressing products of certain Vβ genes exhibiting high reactivity to self I-E and/or Mls determinants has recently been obtained by utilizing monoclonal anti-V specific antibodies to demonstrate that T cells expressing self-reacting receptors are absent from the pool of medullary thymocytes and peripheral T cells, but present among cortical, as yet unselected, thymocytes. Thus, I-E-(probably associated with an unknown B cell-specific self-peptide) restricted thymic clonal elimination of mature T cells expressing the Vβ17a (Vβ3.2) gene product was initially documented by Kappler et al. (29) in certain types ($V\beta^a$ haplotype, $I\text{-}E^+$) of mice (C57BR) that encompass this gene in their germline repertoire. Further tolerance-related clonal eliminations of Vβ6- (31) and Vβ8.1- (30) expressing mature T cells were subsequently identified in $I\text{-}E^+$ mice bearing Mls^a determinants.

The Mls antigens (reviewed in 52,53), primarily expressed on B cells, are defined by their ability to stimulate unidirectional strong primary T cell proliferative responses in mixed lymphocyte reactions involving MHC-identical strains. They appear to be encoded by at least two loci, Mls1 and Mls2. The Mls1 locus is on chromosome 1 and has two alleles, the a (active) and the b (null) allele. The chromosomal location of Mls2 locus is unknown, but it determines the Mls^c (active) haplotype. Strains expressing

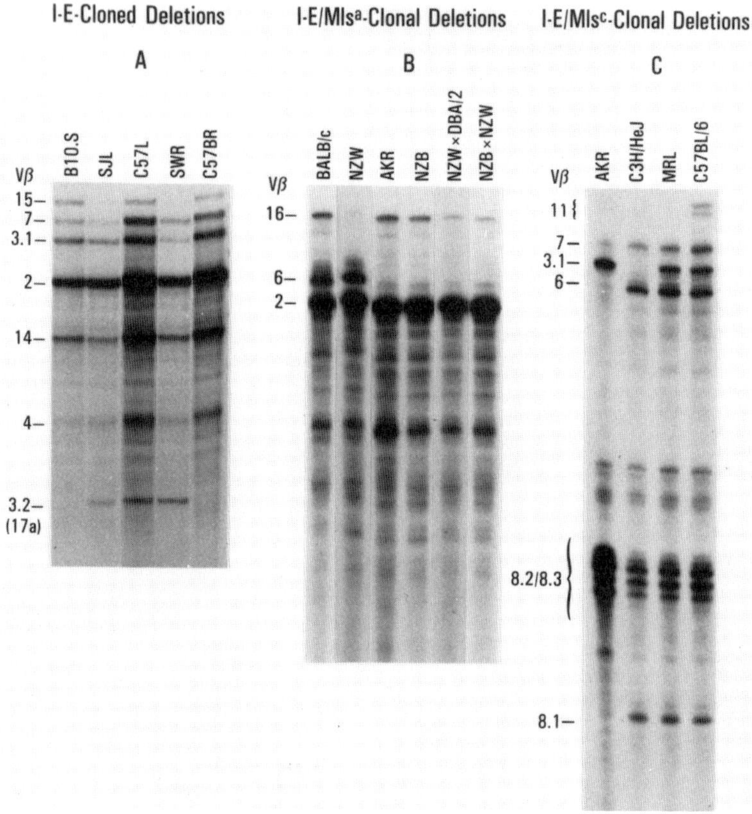

Fig. 7. Confirmation by the RNAse protection assay of the tolerance-related clonal deletions of Vβ17a (Vβ3.2)- (I-E-related, panel A), Vβ6-(I.E/Mls^a-related, panel B), and Vβ8.1- (I-E/Mls^a-related, panel C) expressing splenocytes (see text).

both Mls^a and Mls^c have previously been referred to as Mls^d. In general, Mls^b T cells respond to each of the three other Mls types, but do not stimulate any of these cells. In contrast, Mls^d cells stimulate T cells of each of the other Mls types, but do not respond to any Mls type. Finally, only one combination of mutual stimulation is seen between Mls^a and Mls^c, although in all cases, Mls^c reactivity is weaker. The Mls genes themselves and their products are unknown.

Utilizing the above-described multi-probe RNAse protection assay, we verified the above findings at the RNA level, thus further documenting clonal deletion as a means of tolerance induction. Thus, as depicted in Fig. 7A, Vβ17a-specific mRNA is present in spleens of the I-E⁻ SJL, C57L and SWR strains, but absent in spleen RNAs of the $I-E^+$ C57BR strain. Furthermore (Fig. 7B), no protected Vβ6 bands are seen in spleen mRNAs of strains such as AKR (Mls^a) or NZB and DBA/2 (Mls^d), and this phenomenon is dominantly expressed in crosses of Mls^d mice (NZB or DBA/2) with an Mls^c (NZW) mouse. Moreover, Vβ8.1 mRNA is lacking in spleens of the Mls^a AKR mouse, but is present in spleens of Mls^b (MRL, C57BL/6) or Mls^c (C3H) mice (Fig. 7C).

Following the above confirmation, we then proceeded to utilize our four probe set RNAse protection assay and RNAs of thymocytes and spleen cells of various murine strains hoping to identify abnormalities or additional tolerance-related phenomena that might be relevant to the expression of autoimmune syndromes. The results with probe set A (Vβ15,7,3.1,2, and 14) indicated the absence of Vβ3.1 mRNAs in spleens of NZB, NZW and C3H mice, and Vβ7 in NZB and AKR mice (Fig. 8A). With probe set B (Vβ5.1,16,6), the expression of Vβ5.1 and Vβ16 was found to be very low or absent in spleen RNAs of MRL, NZB and C3H mice as well as in the $(NZBxNZW)F_1$ and $(NZWxDBA/2)F_1$ crosses, but present in spleen RNAs of a number of other strains tested (Fig. 8B). Finally, the results with probe set C+D (Vβ10,11,12; data not shown) indicated that in addition to the genomically imposed complete deletions of Vβ11 and 12 in SJL and SWR

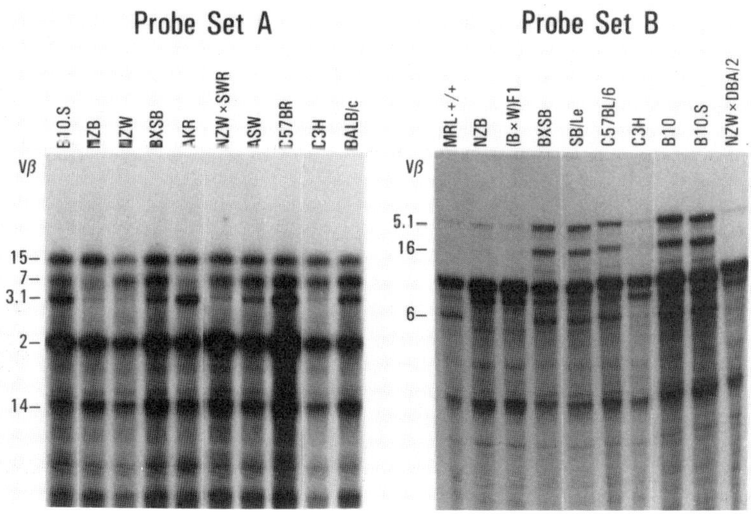

Fig. 8. Clonal deletion of Vβ7 and 3.1 (probe set A) and Vβ5.1, 16 and 6 (panel B) identified by the RNAse protection assay (see text).

mice, partial reduction of Vβ11 and Vβ12 expression was detected in NZW and two of its crosses, as well as in a number of other laboratory strains.

As discussed above, the studies of Kappler et al. (29) demonstrated that the Vβ17a (Vβ3.2) clonal deletion is I-E-mediated, and the studies of McDonald et al. (31) and Kappler et al. (30) demonstrated that the Vβ6 and Vβ8.1 deletions, respectively, are I-E/Mls^{a}-related. The correlations with I-E and Mls of the new deletions (Vβ3.1,7,5.1,11,12, 16) identified in our studies were, therefore, investigated.

TABLE II. Correlation of Vβ3.1 Deletion with Mls^{c} and of Vβ7 Deletion with Mls^{a}

Strain	H-2	I-E	Mls* a	Mls* b	Mls* c	Expression of Vβ3.1	Expression of Vβ7
DBA/2	d	+	+		+	-	-
NZB	d	+	+		+	-	-
BALB/c	d	+			+	-	++
C3H/HeJ	k	+			+	-	++
NZW	z	+			+	-	++
PL/J	u	+			+	-	++
C57BR	k	+		+		+++	++
C57L	b	-		+		+++	++
SJL	s	-			+	++	++
SWR	q	-	+**		+	++	++
AKR	k	+	+			++	-
MRL-+/+	k	+		+		++	++
C57BL/6	b	-		+		++	++
B10.S	s	-		+		++	++
A.SW	s	-			+	+	++

* Mls typings derived from the literature or inferred from Vβ clonal deletions.
**Deduced from an SWR (I-E^{-})xNZW (I-E^{+}) cross that exhibited Vβ6 deletion.

As depicted in Table II, based on published Mls typings and inferred Mls typings derived from this and the above-cited tolerance-related clonal deletion studies, it appears that the Vβ3.1 deletion is most likely mediated by recognition of self I-E in conjunction with Mls^{c}. Thus, all I-E^{+}/Mls^{c} (or Mls^{d}) mice analyzed failed to express Vβ3.1 in their peripheral (spleen) T cells, whereas I-E^{-}/Mls^{c} (or Mls^{d}) strains, such as SJL, SWR and A.SW, did not exhibit

TABLE III. Correlation of Vβ5.1, 11, 12 and 16 Deletion with I-E

Strain	I-E	Vβ5.1/16 Expression	Strain	I-E	Vβ11/12 Expression
SJL	-	+++	C57BL	-	+++
SWR	-	+++	B10.A(4R)	-	+++
C57L	-	+++	BXSB	-	+++
			A.SW	-	+++
C57BL/6	-	++			
B10.A(4R)	-	++	BALB/c	d	++
B10.GD	-	++	NZB	d	++
BXSB	-	++			
A.SW	-	++			
C57BR	k	+	(BxW)F_1	d/z	+
DBA/2	d	+/-	NZW	z	+
NZB	d	+/-	PL/J	u	+
NZW	z	+/-	C3H	k	+
PL/J	u	+/-	MRL-+/+	k	+
C3H	k	+/-	B10.A(2R)	k	+
MRL-+/+	k	+/-			

this clonal deletion. On the other hand, Vβ7 deletion appears to be I-E/Mls^a-related (like Vβ6 and 8.1). Moreover, deletions of Vβ5.1, 11, 12 and 16 appear to be unrelated to Mls, but required I-E (Table III). For example, the I-E$^+$ MRL-+/+ mice do not show Mls-related deletions and, therefore, are presumed to be Mls^b. Nonetheless, they do delete the Vβ5.1, 11, 12 and 16. These observations indicate that clonal modifications imposed by self-I-E recognition extend beyond the originally described Vβ17a deletion in the C57BR mouse, and are, therefore, of broader significance.

The deletions of Vβ6- and Vβ8.1-expressing peripheral T cells have been considered to occur at the double-positive stage of thymic differentiation. This conclusion is based on the fact that cells bearing TCRs that confer autoreactivity to class II MHC ligands (such as Vβ17a for self-I-E and Vβ6 or Vβ8.1 for self-I-E/Mls^a) are deleted not only from the class II MHC-specific CD4$^+$8$^-$ subset, but also from the class I MHC-specific CD8$^+$4$^-$ subset (31,36,37). However, with regard to Vβ11 and 12 deletions, we found that they were more pronounced in the CD4$^+$8$^-$ than in the CD4$^-$8$^+$ thymocyte subset (data not shown), suggesting that negative selection of these Vβs might continue after the conversion of the double-positive cells to the single-positive type, presumably commensurate to increased affinity of TCR-MHC interactions associated with acquisition of higher TCR density.

D. Origin of *lpr* and *gld* Cells

The *lpr* and *gld* autosomal recessive mutations are prime examples of single-gene defects associated with a massive expansion of a unique, phenotypically similar, lymphocyte subset that appears to be responsible for the heightened polyclonal and autoimmune responses observed in mice of varying genetic backgrounds homozygous for these mutations (reviewed in 54,55). The appearance of this expanded population has been shown to be thymus dependent (1,2). Initial immunofluorescent and cytotoxicity studies demonstrated that >90% of the cells in the enlarged lymph nodes of *lpr* or *gld* homozygous mice are positive for Thy-1 antigen and express low levels of the Ly-1 (CD5) antigen. Additional studies demonstrated that the expanded *lpr* and *gld* Thy-1$^+$, dull CD5$^+$ lymph node cells were negative for both T cell subset markers CD4 and CD8, but expressed other cell surface antigens including Ly-5 (B220), Ly-6C, Ly-22, Ly-24 (Pgp-1), PC1 and an abundance of the so-called *l* K$^+$ channels. Some of the proliferating lymph node cells (30-40%) also express one of the heat-stable antigens (HSA) detected by the monoclonal antibody J11d, but they are IL2-R$^-$. These double-negative (CD4$^-$8$^-$) cells also show rearrangement and significant expression of full-length TCR α- and β-chain transcripts and bear surface TCR α:β and CD3, but at reduced density from that of normal T cells. Finally, Southern blotting (56-58) and analysis of cDNA clones (59) have indicated the polyclonal nature of the *lpr* and *gld* cells, with a predominant expression (65% of cDNA clones) of Vβ8.2 and 8.3 gene products (59). A striking feature that has emerged from these combined findings is that the *lpr/gld* cells express both mature (TCR α:β) and immature (CD4$^-$8$^-$, CD5^{low}) T cell markers. Because of this, the relationship of these cells to the known normal T cell subsets has been difficult to establish.

The recognition of the thymic differentiation pathways and of the I-E/Mls-related clonal deletions outlined above have provided valuable new tools to further address the issue of *lpr* and *gld* cell origin. The concept we tested was whether these abnormally expanded double-negative TCR $\alpha:\beta$-bearing cells had been subjected to the I-E/Mls-imposed T cell repertoire negative selection, as outlined above. RNA was extracted from sorted populations of $CD4^-8^-$ T cells taken from the enlarged lymph nodes of the AKR-, MRL-, C3H- and C57BL/6-*lpr/lpr* mice and C3H-*gld/gld* mice and characterized for Vβ mRNA expression by protection analysis. The results of this analysis (Fig. 9) revealed essentially the identical set of tolerance-related clonal deletions as found in mature peripheral (spleen) T cells of the non-*lpr/gld* congenic strains (deletions of Vβ6, 7, 8.1 and 11 in $I\text{-}E^+/Mls^a$ AKR mice; Vβ3.1 and 11 in $I\text{-}E^+/Mls^c$ C3H mice, and Vβ11 in $I\text{-}E^+/Mls^b$ MRL mice). Low expression of Vβ5, 12 and 16 were also seen in all $I\text{-}E^+$ *lpr/gld* and normal congenics (not shown).

These findings, taken together with evidence indicating the requirement for CD4 participation in I-E- (36) and I-E/Mls^a- (37) induced clonal deletions as well as for CD8 participation in class I-restricted clonal deletions (60), point strongly to the existence of a previously unrecognized pathway of late thymic differentiation.

Simply stated, it appears that thymocytes destined for the lineage giving rise to *lpr/gld* (and probably to a subset of the heterogeneous normal double-negative TCR $\alpha:\beta^+$ cells) have at least passed through the double-positive stage in which tolerance-related clonal deletions occur and, subsequently, are somehow induced to downregulate their accessory molecules and thereby effectively becoming "secondary" double-negative, but TCR $\alpha:\beta^+$, cells. The derivation of these cells through this loss of the CD4/CD8 pathway is further supported by a recent report (8, cited above) in which *in vivo* treatment of MRL-*lpr/lpr* mice with anti-CD4 antibody inhibited accumulation of the abnormal $CD4^-8^-$, TCR $\alpha:\beta^+$ cells

We can envisage two possible mechanisms by which downregulation of accessory molecules can occur in these cells, as depicted diagrammatically in Fig. 2; 1) if programmed downregulation of CD4/CD8 is the rule for non-positively selected $CD4^+8^+$ cells (followed by cell death), then double-negative TCR $\alpha:\beta^+$ cells could represent a short-lived intermediate cell type in this process; and 2) a second possibility, which we currently favor and which is supported by some highly suggestive, although indirect, evidence, is the involvement of a novel back-up form of tolerance induction, perhaps directed at some thymocytes expressing moderately autoreactive TCRs. Such moderately autoaggressive cells might be present at the double-positive stage and

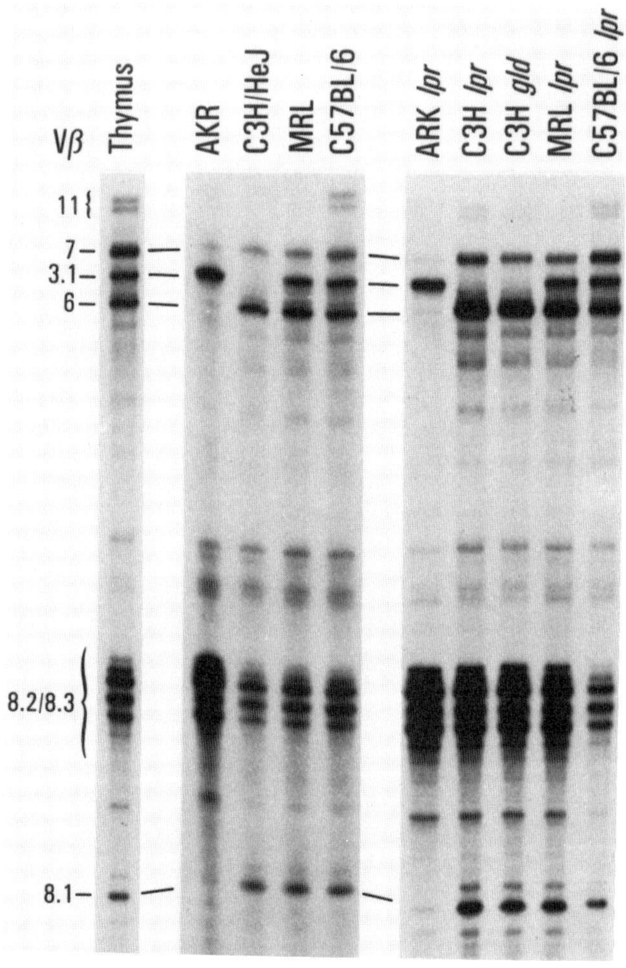

Fig. 9. Demonstration of tolerance-related clonal deletions in splenocytes (left panel) and double-negative (CD4⁻8⁻) abnormally expanded lymph node cells of lpr and gld congenic mice (right panel). RNA from total thymocytes of BALB/c mice is included for comparison.

converted to double-negative cells via the so-called "primary" negative selection process, wherein the highly autoaggressive clones are deleted. Alternatively, such cells might be generated during a postulated "secondary" negative-selection process exerted on single-positive cells that changed via maturation and higher receptor level expression from low to moderate/high affinity autoreactive cells; the highly reactive cells will be eliminated, while some of the moderately reactive cells may escape deletion, but still downregulate their CD4/8 molecules. The recently reported findings of Kisielow et al. (60) using transgenic mice expressing a self-reactive TCR specific for the male HY antigen suggest that CD4/8 loss may indeed be such a tolerance-related event. In this investigation, the peripheral transgene-expressing T cell population in male (i.e., autoreactive) mice, but not in female (non-autoreactive) mice, was found to be composed almost entirely of cells that had lost the CD8 accessory molecule required for efficient HY antigen recognition; most of these cells (58%) were of the double-negative phenotype, with the remainder being $CD4^{+}8^{low}$ (35%) or $CD4^{+}8^{-}$ (7%). We interpret such cells to represent probable escapees from clonal elimination that were "tolerized" by accessory molecule downregulation before being allowed to exit to the periphery.

Based on the above schemes, it indeed seems plausible that the *lpr* and *gld* cells represent a magnified and otherwise modified version of a subset of the heterogeneous minor normal double-negative TCR $\alpha:\beta^{+}$ thymocyte population. In the normal setting, self-reactive double-negative cells that escape deletion will slowly accumulate in the thymus to constitute the late-appearing double-negative TCR $\alpha:\beta^{+}$ subset. Some of these cells might migrate to the periphery, but the majority would be expected to eventually die intrathymically due to their lack of accessory molecules and resultant inability to efficiently fulfill their function. In contrast, *lpr* and *gld* mice, due to undefined modifications introduced by these mutations, produce a high number of such cells in the thymus, a large proportion of which leak into the periphery, populate lymph nodes and spleen and continue to proliferate.

In advancing this concept, it might therefore be suggested that double-negative TCR $\alpha:\beta^{+}$ cells (normal or *lpr/gld*) express essentially autoreactive TCRs. If such cells are exported in large numbers into the periphery, as in *lpr* and *gld* homozygous mice, autoimmune manifestations can clearly ensue. For example, such double-negative cells might retain sufficient autoreactivity in spite of their lack of CD4/CD8 and induce or accelerate autoimmunity by secretion of appropriate B cell differentiation/promoting lymphokines (61). Alternatively, a portion of these cells may reacquire accessory molecules and become fully functional and autoreactive. Indeed, reacquisition of accessory molecules by *lpr* and normal double-negative T cells cultured *in vitro* has been demonstrated (62-65).

The above-postulated autoreactive potential for double-negative TCR $\alpha:\beta^+$ cells is further supported by several other studies. Thus, double-negative splenic T cells isolated from normal (BALB/c, DBA/2) mice upon ConA activation reacquired CD4 and, in contrast to other ConA-stimulated T cell subsets, induced syngeneic B cells to proliferate and differentiate into Ig-secreting cells at high levels (65), a situation not unlike that seen spontaneously with the constitutively activated *lpr* cells (61). Such activated peripheral double-negative TCR $\alpha:\beta^+$ normal lymphocytes also proliferated upon incubation with syngeneic dentritic cells and were inhibited by anti-class II antibodies, further documenting their autoreactive potential (64,65). Induction of autoimmune disease by transfers of double-negative, $Thy1^+$-$Ly1^{low}$ spleen cells from normal BALB/c mice (66), or thymic cells from cyclosporin-treated mice (67) severely depleted of $CD4^+8^-$ and $CD8^+4^-$ cells into syngeneic nude mice has also been documented. Furthermore, in $(NZBxW)F_1$ lupus mice (68), and in humans with lupus (S.K. Datta, personal communication), helper *in vitro* activity for anti-DNA production was found not only in $CD4^+8^-$ but also, surprisingly, at an equal, if not higher, degree in $CD4^-8^-$ spleen and peripheral T cells, respectively. Interestingly, studies in mice suggest that the frequency of double-negative TCR $\alpha:\beta^+$ cells in thymuses and spleens differ in various genetic backgrounds (22,65) and thus may be genetically controlled. Such genetically imposed expansions of these *bona fide* autoreactive double-negative TCR $\alpha:\beta^+$ cells may contribute in an important way to the induction of murine, and even human, systemic autoimmune diseases.

V. CONCLUSIONS

To summarize, the above studies addressing the TCR germline and expressed repertoire of autoimmune and other laboratory mice indicate the following:

1) There is no unique autoimmunity-associated α or β TCR gene haplotype, and the germline TCR repertoire in autoimmune mice is similar to that of normal mice.

2) The inherent program of Vβ gene expression in unselected thymocytes is related to Vβ genomic organization, and imparts a significant skewing effect on the Vβ repertoire that, in general, persists in the mature T cell population.

3) All readily detectable tolerance-related Vβ clonal elimination phenomena can apparently be attributed to either I-E or Mls reactivity, including deletion of Vβ3.2 (17a) in $V\beta^a$ haplotype-$I\text{-}E^+$ mice, deletion of Vβ6, 7 and 8.1 in $I\text{-}E^+/Mls^a$ mice, deletion of Vβ3.1 expressing cells in $I\text{-}E^+/Mls^c$ mice, and deletions of Vβ5.1, 11, 12 and 16 in $I\text{-}E^+$ strains.

4) Most of the above clonal deletions occur at the double-positive stage ($CD4^+8^+$) of thymic differentiation, but some might continue after conversion to the single-positive ($CD4^+8^-$ or $CD8^+4^-$) phenotype.

5) The abnormally proliferating TCR $\alpha:\beta^+$, $CD4^-8^-$ *lpr* and *gld* lymph node cells, based on tolerance-related deletion studies, are postulated to derive from autoreactive thymocytes that have escaped deletion, but lost their CD4 and CD8 accessory molecules. These cells are similar to a subset of the heterogeneous double-negative TCR $\alpha:\beta$ minor normal T cell population. Exportation and expansion of these cells in the periphery may be important in the development of systemic autoimmunity.

6) Lupus-prone mice show no generalized defect in the expression of tolerance-related clonal elimination. However, unique patterns of Vβ gene expression may be identifiable, which in themselves or in combination with other genes (i.e., MHC) might allow the development of autoimmunity.

ACKNOWLEDGEMENTS

The authors would like to thank Robert S. Balderas, Robert J. McEvilly and Michael Bobardt for expert technical assistance, and M. Kat Occhipinti for editing and manuscript production.

References

1.) Theofilopoulos, A.N., Balderas, R.S., Shawler, D.L., Lee, S., and Dixon, F.J. (1981). J. Exp. Med. 153:1405.

2.) Steinberg, A.D., Roths, J.B., Murphy, E.D., Steinberg, R.T. and Raveche, E.S. (1980). J. Immunol. 125:871.

3.) Mihara, M., Ohsugi, Y., Saito, K., Miyai, T., Tagashi, M., Ono, S., Murakami, S., Dobashi, K., Hirayama, F., and Hamaoka, T. (1988) J. Immunol. 141:85.

4.) Zamvil, S., Nelson, P., Trotter, J., Mitchell, D., Knobler, R., Fritz, R., and Steinman, L. (1985) Nature 317:355.
5.) Maron, R., Zerubavel, R., Friedman, A., and Cohen, I.R. (1983) J. Immunol. 131:2316.
6.) Holmdahl, R., Klareskog, L., Rubin, K., Larsson, E., and Wigzell, H. (1985) Scand. J. Immunol. 22:295.
7.) Wofsy, D., and Seaman, W.E. (1985) J. Exp. Med. 161:378.
8.) Santoro, T.J., Portanova, J.P., and Kotzin, B.L. (1988) J. Exp. Med. 167:1713.
9.) Koiki, T., Itoh, Y., Ishii, T., Ito, I., Takabayahsi, K., Maruyama, N., Tomioka, H., and Yoshida, S. (1987) Diabetes 36:539.
10.) Shizuru, J.A., Taylor-Edwards, C., Banks, B.A., Gregory, A.K., and Fathman, C.G. (1988) Science 240:659.
11.) Ranges, G.E., Sriram, S., and Cooper, S.M. (1985) J. Exp. Med. 162:1105.
12.) Waldor, M.S., Sriram, S., Hardy, R., Herzengerg, L.A., Lanier, L., Lim, M., and Steinman, L. (1985) Science 227:415.
13.) Christadoss, P., and Dauphinee, M.J. (1986) J. Immunol. 136:2437.
14.) Haggi, R.M., Banerjee, S., Behlke, M.A., Dungeon, G., Loh, D.Y., Stuart, J., Luthra, H.S., and David, C.S. (1988) FASEB J. 2:661 (Abstract).
15.) Zamvil, S.S., Mitchell, D.J., Lee, N.E., Moore, A.C., Waldor, M.K., Sakai, K., Rothbard, J.B., McDevitt, H.O., Steinman, L., and Acha-Orbea, H. (1988) J. Exp. Med. 167:1586.
16.) Urban, J.L., Kumar, V., Kono, D.H., Gomez, C., Horvath, S.J., Clayton, J., Ando, D.G., Sercarz, E.E., and Hood, L. (1988) Cell 54:577.
17.) Acha-Orbea, H., Mitchell, D.J., Timmermann, L., Wraith, D.C., Tausch, G.S., Waldor, M.K., Zamvil, S.S., McDevitt, H.O., and Steinman, L. (1988) Cell 54:263.
18.) Allison, J.P., and Lanier, L.L. (1987) Ann. Rev. Immunol. 5:503.
19.) Davis, M.M., and Bjorkman, P.J. (1988) Nature 334:395.
20.) Kronenberg, M., Siu, G., Hood, L.E., and Shastri, N. (1986) Ann. Rev. Immunol. 4:529.
21.) Behlke, M.A., Chori, H.S., Huppi, K., and Loh, D.Y. (1986) Proc. Natl. Acad. Sci. USA 83:767.
22.) Fowlkes, J., and Pardoll, D.M. (1988) Adv. Immunol. (In Press).
23.) Janeway, C.A. (1988) Nature 335:208.
24.) Marrack, P., and Kappler, J. (1988) Immunol. Today 9:308.

25.) Sprent, J., and Webb, S.R. (1987) Adv. Immunol. 41:39.
26.) Teh, H.S., Kisielow, P., Scott, B., Kishi, H., Uematsu, Y., Bluthmann, H., and von Boehmer, H. (1988) Nature 335:229.
27.) Kisielow, P., Teh, H.S., Bluthmann, H., and von Boehmer, H. (1988) Nature 335:730.
28.) Sha, W.C., Nelson, C.A., Newberry, R.D., Kranz, D.M., Russell, J.H., and Loh, D.Y. (1988) Nature 335:271.
29.) Kappler, J.W., Roehm, N., and Marrack, P. (1987) Cell 49:273.
30.) Kappler, J.W., Staerz, U., White, J., and Marrack, P.C. (1988) Nature 332:35.
31.) MacDonald, H.R., Schneider, R., Lees, R.K., Howe, R.C., Acha-Orbea, H., Festenstein, H., Zinkernagel, R.M., and Hengartner, H. (1988) Nature 332:40.
32.) Pullen, A.M., Marrack, P., and Kappler, J.W. (1988). Nature 335:796.
33.) Abe, R., Vacchio, M.S., Fox, B., and Hodes, R.J. (1988) Nature 335:827.
34.) Lo, D., and Sprent, J. (1986) Nature 318:672.
35.) Sprent, J., Lo, D., Er-Kai, G, and Ron, Y. (1988) Immunol. Rev. 101:173.
36.) Fowlkes, B.J., Schwartz, R.H., and Pardoll, D.M. (1988). Nature 334:620.
37.) MacDonald, H.R., Hengartner, H., and Pedrazzini, T. (1988). Nature 335:174.
38.) Fowlkes, B.J., Kruisbeek, A.M., Ton-That, H., Weston, M.A., Coligan, J.E., Schwartz, R.H., and Pardoll, D.M. (1987) Nature 329:251.
39.) Scollay, R., Wilson, A., D'Amico, A., Kelly, K., Egerton, M., Pearce, M., Li, W., and Shortman, K. (1988) Immunol. Rev. 104:81.
40.) Crispe, I.N., Moore, M.W., Husmann, L.A., Smith, L., Bevan, M.J., and Shimonkevitz, R.P. (1987) Nature 329:336.
41.) Ceredig, R., Lynch, F., and Newman, P. (1987) Proc. Natl. Acad. Sci. USA 84:8578.
42.) Noonan, D.J., Kofler, R., Singer, P.A., Cardenas, G., Dixon, F.J., and Theofilopoulos, A.N. (1986) J. Exp. Med. 163:644.
43.) Kotzin, B.L., Barr, V.L., and Palmer, E. (1985) Science 229:167.
44.) Yanagi, Y., Hirose, S., Magasawa, R., Shirai, T., Mak, T.W., and Tada, T. (1986) Eur. J. Immunol. 16:1179.
45.) Singer, P.A., McEvilly, R.J., Bobardt, M., McConahey, P.J., Dixon, F.J., and Theofilopoulos, A.N. (1988) FASEB J 2:A1670 (Abstract).

46.) Kotzin, B.L., and Palmer, E. (1987) J. Exp. Med. 165:1237.
47.) Lai, E., Barth, R.K., and Hood, L. (1987) Proc. Natl. Acad. Sci. USA 84:3846.
48.) Singer, P.A., McEvilly, R.J., Balderas, R.S., Dixon, F.J., and Theofilopoulos, A.N. (1988) Proc. Natl. Acad. Sci. USA 85:7729.
49.) Melton, D.A., Krieg, P.A., Rebagliati, M.R., Maniatis, T., Zinn, K., and Green, M.R. (1984) Nuc. Acids. Res. 12:7035.
50.) Wade, T., Bill, J., Marrack, P.C., Palmer, E., and Kappler, J.W. (1988) J. Immunol. 141:2165.
51.) Goodnow, C.C., Crosbie, J., Adelstein, S., Lavoie, T.B., Smith-Gill, S.J., Brink, R.A., Pritchard-Briscoe, H., Wotherspoon, J.S., Loblay, R.H., Raphael, K., Treyt, R.J., and Basten, A. (1988) Nature 334:676.
52.) Abe, R., and Hodes, R.J. (1988) Immunol. Today 9:230.
53.) Janeway, C.A., Fischer-Lindahl, K., and Hammerling, U. (1988) Immunol. Today 9:125.
54.) Theofilopoulos, A.N., and Dixon, F.J. (1985) Adv. Immunol. 37:269.
55.) Singer, P.A., and Theofilopoulos, A.N. (To be submitted)
56.) Nemazee, D.A., Studer, S., Steinmetz, M., Dembic, Z., and Kiefer, M. (1985). Eur. J. Immunol. 15:760.
57.) Davidson, W.F., Dumont, F.J., Bedigian, H.G., Fowlkes, B.J., and Morse, H.C. III. (1986) J. Immunol. 136:4075.
58.) Miescher, G.C., Budd, R.C., Lees, R.K., and MacDonald, H.R. (1987) J. Immunol. 138:1959.
59.) Singer, P.A., McEvilly, R.J., Noonan, D.J., Dixon, F.J., and Theofilopoulos, A.N. (1986) Proc. Natl. Acad. Sci. USA 83:7018.
60.) Kisielow, P., Bluthmann, H., Staerz, U.D., Steinmetz, M., and von Boehmer, H. (1988). Nature 333:742.
61.) Prud'homme, G.J., Park, C.L., Fieser, T.M., Kofler, R., Dixon, F.J., and Theofilopoulos, A.N. (1983) J. Exp. Med. 157:730.
62.) Budd, R.C., MacDonald, H.R., Lowenthal, J.W., Davignon, J.-L., Izui, S., and Cerottini, J.-C. (1985) J. Immunol. 135:3704.
63.) Gause, W.C., Mountz, J.D., and Steinberg, A.D. (1988) J. Immunol. 140:1.
64.) Reimann, J., Bellan, A., and Conradt, P. (1988). Eur. J. Immunol. 18:989.
65.) deTalance, A., Regnier, D., Spinella, S., Morisset, J., and Seman, M. (1986). J. Immunol. 137:1101.
66.) Sakaguchi, S., Fukuma, K., Kuribayashi, K., and Masuda, T. (1985). J. Exp. Med. 161:72.

67.) Sakaguchi, S., and Sakaguchi, N. (1988) J. Exp. Med. 167:1479.
68.) Datta, S.K., Patel, H., and Berry D. (1987) J. Exp. Med. 165:1252.

STRUCTURE OF THE HUMAN INTERLEUKIN 2 RECEPTOR AND THE BIOCHEMICAL BASIS FOR ITS REGULATION

Dean W. Ballard
Marion R. Fung
Ernst Böhnlein
Warner C. Greene

Howard Hughes Medical Institute
Departments of Medicine and Microbiology/Immunology
Duke University Medical Center
Durham, North Carolina 27710

I. INTRODUCTION

The proliferation of human T lymphocytes is controlled by the coordinate activation of two genes, one encoding the lymphokine interleukin 2 (IL-2) and the other encoding its membrane receptor (IL-2R) (2-4). IL-2R expression is induced by a variety of stimuli including antigens, antibodies specific for the T-cell antigen receptor complex, the HTLV-1 derived transactivator (tax) protein, cytokines, and nonspecific mitogens such as phytohemagglutinin (PHA) and phorbol 12-myristate 13-acetate (PMA). The binding of IL-2 to its functional high affinity membrane receptor allows for the rapid clonal expansion of cells originally reacting with antigen or mitogen (1-4). The subsequent decline in production of both IL-2 and high affinity IL-2R appears to contribute to the physiological termination of the T cell immune response.

II. STRUCTURE OF THE HUMAN IL-2 RECEPTOR

A. The IL-2 Receptor Exists in Multiple Affinity Forms

Three different types of human IL-2R have now been identified which display differing affinities (high, intermediate and low) for ligand. The high affinity IL-2R appears to correspond to a membrane receptor complex composed of at least two different IL-2 binding subunits, including the well-characterized 55 kD Tac antigen (p55, IL-2Rα) (5-7) and the recently recognized 70-75 kD subunit (p70, IL-2Rβ) (8-12). High affinity receptors interact with IL-2 with an apparent K_d of 2-50 pM and represent the primary receptor form responsible for mediating the growth promoting response to physiological concentrations of IL-2 (13,14). The intermediate affinity IL-2R corresponds to expression of the IL-2Rβ subunit alone (9-12). This receptor binds ligand with an apparent K_d of 0.5 to 1.0 nM and in the presence of high concentrations of ligand appears capable of transducing intracellular signals including the induction of IL-2Rα gene expression (15). Low affinity IL-2R binds IL-2 with an apparent K_d of 10-20 nM and represent IL-2Rα protein expressed in the absence of the IL-2Rβ subunit (16).

Recent studies indicate that the IL-2Rα and IL-2Rβ proteins interact with different epitopes on the IL-2 molecule thus providing a logical explanation for high affinity binding by the α/β heterodimeric complex (11,17). Specifically, the N-terminus of IL-2 appears essential for IL-2Rβ interactions, as anti-IL-2 peptide antibodies specific for residues 8-27 block IL-2 binding to IL-2Rβ but not to IL-2Rα. In addition, site directed mutagenesis of residue 20 in the IL-2 molecule (aspartic→lysine) completely abrogates IL-2Rβ binding activity but does not alter IL-2Rα binding. Antibody blocking studies suggest that residues between amino acids 33-53 in IL-2 are involved in IL-2Rα binding, however, these antibodies also modestly affect ligand binding to IL-2Rβ (11).

B. Contrasting Kinetics of IL-2 Binding to the IL-2Rα and IL-2Rβ Subunits

Recent studies have revealed that the kinetics of ligand association and dissociation from the IL-2Rα and IL-2Rβ subunits are strikingly different (18,19). Specifically, IL-2 rapidly binds to the IL-2Rα chain with a $t_{1/2}$ of approximately 5 sec. However, after binding, the ligand also rapidly dissociates with a $t_{1/2}$ of 5-10 seconds, thus explaining its overall low affinity. In sharp contrast, IL-2 associates with the IL-2Rβ subunit much more slowly with a $t_{1/2}$ of 40-50 minutes at 4° C. This slow rate of ligand binding suggests that this process may not be solely limited by the diffusion of IL-2 but rather may involve conformational changes in receptor structure. However, once IL-2 has bound to the IL-2Rβ protein, it dissociates very slowly with a measured $t_{1/2}$ of 4-5 hours. These findings explain the resultant intermediate affinity of the IL-2Rβ binding sites. Interestingly, the high affinity IL-2R complex exhibits a composite of these association and dissociation kinetics. The rate for IL-2 binding to the high affinity receptor occurs with a $t_{1/2}$ of approximately 30 seconds, resembling the rapid rate of ligand association characteristic of the IL-2Rα chain. In contrast, the rate of IL-2 dissociation from the high affinity receptor is very slow, occurring with a $t_{1/2}$ of approximately 4 hours. This value is virtually identical to the slow dissociation kinetics characteristic of the IL-2Rβ chain. These findings suggest that the IL-2Rα chain primarily controls association while the IL-2Rβ subunit regulates ligand dissociation. These results also underscore the important contributions of each individual subunit to the assembly of a receptor complex uniquely able to rapidly bind and retain its ligand.

C. Evidence for a Stable α-β Heterodimeric Complex

Previous studies have revealed that the IL-2Rβ protein by itself is capable of mediating rapid endocytosis of ligand (20) with kinetics essentially identical to that found for the high affinity receptor (21,22). In contrast, the IL-2Rα protein lacks the ability to internalize IL-2. As the intracytoplasmic domains of proteins largely regulate such endocytotic processes, these findings suggest that the cytoplasmic segment of the IL-2Rβ subunit may be larger than the 13 residues present in the IL-2Rα chain. The differences in IL-2 binding kinetics to the IL-2Rα and IL-2Rβ subunits noted above, coupled with our inability to clearly detect a stable ternary receptor complex composed of the α and β subunits and IL-2, raised the possibility that the IL-2Rα subunit served only to bind and transfer IL-2 to the IL-2Rβ chain rather than participating in the formation of a stable heterodimeric receptor complex. However, in recent studies, we have demonstrated that the IL-2Rα subunit does stably associate with the IL-2Rβ subunit (23). In the presence of IL-2, the ternary complex composed of IL-2/IL-2Rα/IL-2Rβ is internalized as a single unit. In the human system, it remains unknown whether IL-2 is needed to initiate assembly of the complex or, alternatively, to trigger the internalization of a preassembled α/β receptor complex.

D. Signal Transduction Through the IL-2Rβ Subunit

Constitutive surface expression of the IL-2Rβ protein in the absence of the IL-2Rα subunit has been detected in resting T cells and natural killer cells (12,15,24-26). Furthermore, the IL-2Rβ receptor subunit alone appears able to transduce intracellular signals that lead to the activation of resting T cells and increased cytolytic activity within the natural killer cell populations (15,25,26). Interestingly, with both cell types, IL-2 binding to the IL-2Rβ triggers the expression of a variety of early activation genes including c-myc and c-myb (15) as well as induction of the IL-2Rα gene expression which ultimately permits the assembly of high affinity IL-2R (15).

Recent studies performed with Dr. Gordon Mills (Toronto) and Richard Robb (Glenolden), have revealed that IL-2 binding promotes tyrosine specific phosphorylation of the IL-2R complex, likely involving the IL-2Rβ subunit. It remains unclear whether this event reflects autophosphorylation or, alternatively, involves the participation of a receptor-associated tyrosine kinase. These findings have potentially important implications for the mechanism of signal transduction occurring via the high affinity IL-2R complex. Ultimately, the isolation of IL-2Rβ specific monoclonal antibodies and the cloning of IL-2Rβ cDNAs will be required to unravel the structure and mechanism of action of the high affinity human IL-2R.

III. REGULATION OF IL-2Rα GENE EXPRESSION

A. Identification of Cis-Acting Regions Involved in IL-2Rα Promoter Activation

Recently, our investigations have focused on the biochemical basis for activation of the IL-2Rα gene as the rapid induction of this receptor subunit during T cell activation plays a critical role in the assembly of high affinity IL-2R. The 5′ flanking region of the IL-2Rα gene has been cloned, sequenced and studied both for the presence of cis-acting sequences involved in mitogen activation and the binding of transacting nuclear proteins required for induction of gene expression. To define sequences involved in mitogen activation, a nested series of 5′ deletion mutants of the IL-2Rα promoter were prepared with Bal 31 exonuclease and linked to the chloramphenicol acetyl transferase (CAT) reporter gene (27). These IL-2Rα-CAT expression plasmids were then transfected into various cell populations and the cultures activated with different stimulatory agents. In Jurkat leukemic T cells, we observed that deletion of IL-2Rα promoter nucleotides 3′ of base -281 was associated with a pronounced decline in activation mediated by PHA, PMA or tumor necrosis factor-α (TNF-α) (27,28, Lowenthal et al., manuscript submitted). In contrast, despite deletion to nucleotide -266, the IL-2Rα promoter remained highly inducible by the transactivator (tax) protein from the type 1 human T cell leukemia virus (HTLV-1) (27,29,30). Thus, the requisite cis-sequences appear to differ depending upon the nature of the inducing signal. Recently, we have confirmed these differing patterns of activation in primary human T cells (Lowenthal et al., manuscript submitted).

B. Analysis of DNA-Protein Interactions Involved in IL-2Rα Promoter Activation

To study the potential interaction of inducible transacting factors with cis-sequences in the IL-2Rα promoter, oligonucleotide duplexes spanning the functionally important region between nucleotides -291 and -245 were prepared. After radiolabeling with ^{32}P, these probes were used for gel retardation assays with nuclear extracts isolated from unstimulated and PMA, tax, (27,28,31) or TNFα (Lowenthal et al., manuscript submitted) induced Jurkat and peripheral blood T cells. Nuclear proteins extracted from uninduced cells failed to support the formation of electrophoretically retarded DNA-protein complexes. In sharp contrast, extracts from PMA, tax or TNFα induced cells yielded two discrete DNA-protein complexes. The formation of these complexes reflected sequence specific DNA protein interactions, as the addition of unlabeled homologous probe, but not unrelated probes, blocked their formation.

To further define the site of protein binding to the IL-2Rα promoter, serial 3-base mutations were introduced and the probes analyzed for direct binding and competitive activity in the gel retardation assays (31). These studies localized the binding site for one or more factors to a region bounded by bases -267 and -256. These results were independently confirmed in 1, 10-phenanthroline copper footprinting and methylation interference assays which mapped protein contact sites to residues -266 to -256 (28, and unpublished data). Studies were next performed to investigate whether this 12 base pair IL-2Rα promoter binding site was required for IL-2Rα promoter induction in T cells. Site-directed mutagenesis was employed to selectively remove this 12 base pair binding site within the context of a fully active -317 promoter construct. When transfected into primary human T cells or Jurkat T cells, this internal deletion mutant was not induced by PMA, tax, or TNFα. These findings thus support a critical role for this promoter binding site in mitogen induction of the IL-2Rα gene.

To examine whether this IL-2Rα promoter element was alone sufficient to impart mitogen inducibility, 18 bp oligonucleotides spanning this site were inserted upstream of the Herpes simplex thymidine kinase (TK) promoter linked to the CAT gene (27,28,31). Transfection of these recombinant TK-CAT plasmids revealed that the presence of the IL-2Rα promoter element was sufficient to impart PMA, TNFα and tax inducibility to this normally unresponsive heterologous promoter unit. Furthermore, the IL-2Rα element was found to function in either orientation and multiplicative effects were obtained when the binding site was reiterated. Thus, this IL-2Rα promoter element appears to exhibit enhancer-like properties and is both necessary and sufficient to support mitogen inducibility. These findings, however, do not exclude a role for other control regions in the overall activation of the receptor gene induced by T cell mitogens.

C. The IL-2Rα Promoter Binding Site Shares Homology with the HIV-1 Enhancer

Comparison of the sequence of this 12 bp IL-2Rα promoter element with other known DNA binding sites revealed a striking similarity to the κB enhancers present in a variety of viral and cellular genes, including the long terminal repeat of the type-1 human immunodeficiency virus (HIV-1) and κ light chain immunoglobulin gene intron (31). These two enhancer binding sites have been reported to interact with a factor termed NF-κB (32). The homology of the IL-2Rα promoter binding site with the HIV-1 enhancer was particularly intriguing as we and others had previously demonstrated that the HIV-1 LTR is responsive to a variety of T cell activation signals (PHA, PMA, <u>tax</u>) (32-35). Furthermore, deletion analysis of the HIV-1 LTR had supported a central role for the viral enhancer in these inductive responses. The sequence homology between the HIV-1 enhancer and IL-2Rα promoter element proved functionally significant as unlabeled HIV-1 enhancer oligonucleotides completely blocked the interaction of proteins with the IL-2Rα promoter binding site (31). Similarly, unlabeled IL-2Rα promoter oligonucleotides containing this binding site blocked the formation of at least two inducible DNA complexes with the HIV-1 enhancer.

D. Characterization of Proteins That Specifically Bind to the IL-2Rα κB element

Direct evidence for the binding of at least one common inducible nuclear protein by both the IL-2Rα and HIV-1 enhancer was obtained using DNA affinity precipitation assays (31). Briefly, nuclear proteins from PMA induced or uninduced Jurkat T cells were radiolabeled with ^{35}S-methionine and then incubated either with biotinylated wild type or mutant oligonucleotide probes from the IL-2Rα promoter and HIV-1 enhancer. The resultant DNA-protein complexes were recovered by incubation with avidin-agarose, the proteins were then eluted and analyzed on high resolution 2-dimensional polyacrylamide gels. Both the HIV-1 enhancer and the IL-2Rα promoter wild type oligonucleotides were found to specifically bind the same 86 kD inducible protein termed HIVEN86A (37). In contrast, HIV-1 enhancer or IL-2Rα promoter oligonucleotides mutated within the κB site failed to interact with this inducible nuclear protein. Similarly, the HIVEN86A protein was detectable in Jurkat-<u>tax</u>, but not Jurkat anti-<u>tax</u> cells (28). These findings thus confirmed that both the HIV-1 enhancer and IL-2Rα promoter shared the capacity to bind at least one common nuclear protein inducible by PMA or <u>tax</u>. These results, however, did not exclude the binding of yet other proteins perhaps poorly labeled in the protocol used for DNA affinity precipitation. To evaluate independently the potential binding of other proteins to the κB element, photoreactive DNA probes were prepared for use in ultraviolet light-induced DNA-protein crosslinking studies. These experiments revealed the binding of at least two major proteins to the IL-2Rα promoter binding site. These proteins included an 80-90 kD and a 50-55 kD species, (Ballard et al., manuscript submitted, Lowenthal et al., manuscript submitted). It is possible that these T cell proteins correspond to the 86 kD HIVEN86A polypeptide (37) and the 51 kD NF-κB protein recently purified by Kawakami and coworkers from human Burkitt B cells (38). Recent studies indicate that the induction of both of these polypeptides is controlled at a post-translational level as their induced expression occurs in the presence of cycloheximide or anisomycin at concentrations sufficient to block >97% of *de novo* cellular protein synthesis (Bohnlein et al., manuscript submitted).

The relationship of the 80-90 kD and 50-55 kD protein species remains undefined. Interestingly, we have found that treatment of both the 80-90 kD and 50-55 kD crosslinked species with staphylococcus V8 protease yields a series of 15-20 kD DNA binding domains. It is possible that these polypeptides are the products of distinct genes. Alternatively, these proteins may be derived from the same gene but reflect different polypeptides produced by differences in post-transcriptional or post-translational processing.

E. Different Sequence Requirements for IL-2Rα Promoter Activation by Phorbol Esters, TNFα and the *tax* Protein of HTLV-1

When compared, the IL-2Rα promoter sequence requirements for PMA and TNFα activation of the IL-2Rα promoter proved consistently different from *tax* (27-29, Lowenthal et al., manuscript submitted). Specifically, residues 5′ of the κB element located between nucleotides -281 and -267 were needed for optimal PMA and TNFα induction but were fully dispensable when *tax* was used as the activating agent. Site-directed mutagenesis of the 5′ flanking region confirmed these functional differences. Thus, a second regulatory element important for PMA and TNFα activation appears to be located immediately 5′ of the κB element. Despite extensive study, no protein interactions at this site could be detected by gel retention, footprinting or methylation interference. However, using a solution exonuclease III protection assay, we have recently detected the binding of a protein that produces an exonuclease stop approximately 10 bp 5′ of the κB site (Ballard et al., manuscript submitted). This termination site reflected the specific binding of protein within this flanking region as wild type probes but not the 5′ mutant probes competed for detection of this upstream interaction. Interestingly, this protein is constitutively produced in resting T cells. DNA affinity precipitation assays have permitted preliminary identification of two candidate proteins for this activity, including a 56 kD and a 90 kD species. Thus, PMA and TNFα induction of the IL-2Rα promoter appear to require the upstream binding of this constitutive factor(s) in addition to the inducible κB binding proteins, while tax activation circumvents the requirement for this constitutive factor.

IV. SUMMARY

The growth of human T cells depends upon the expression of high-affinity IL-2 receptors which are composed of at least two different subunits. The IL-2Rβ (p70-75) protein binds IL-2 with intermediate affinity, plays an important role in signal transduction, and is constitutively expressed on the surface of resting T and NK cells. The IL-2Rα subunit binds IL-2 with low affinity, stably interacts with the IL-2Rβ subunit to form high-affinity IL-2R and is readily induced by a variety of T cell activation signals including antigen, phorbol esters, mitogenic lectins, TNFα and the tax protein of HTLV-1. The induction of IL-2Rα gene expression by each of the agonists involves the post-translational activation of at least two DNA binding proteins (80-90 kD, 50-55 kD) that interact with a κB -like sequence located in the IL-2Rα promoter. This binding site exhibits enhancer-like properties and is required for IL-2Rα promoter activation in both Jurkat T cells and primary T cells. Furthermore, this κB element alone is sufficient to impart inducible properties to a normally unresponsive heterologous promoter. Of note, this IL-2Rα promoter element markedly resembles the HIV-1 enhancer which is simlarly inducible by PMA, tax, and TNF-α. These findings have potentially important implications for HTLV-1/HIV-1 interactions in dually infected patients and for the role that T cell activation may play in the induction of HIV-1 replication in T cells latently infected with this pathogenic human retrovirus.

REFERENCES

1. Smith, K.A. (1984). Interleukin 2. Ann. Rev. Immunol. 2:319.
2. Taniguchi, T., Matsui, H. Fujita, T., Hatakeyama, M., Kashima, N., Fuse, A., Hamuro, J., Nishi-Takaoka, C. and Yamada, G. (1986). Prog. Hematol. 14:283.
3. Greene, W.C., Leonard, W.J. and Depper, J.M. (1986). Prog. Hematol. 14:283.

4. Weiss, A. and Imboden, J.B. (1987). Adv. Immunol. 41:1.
5. Leonard, W.J., Depper, J.M., Robb, R.J., Waldmann, T.A. and Greene, W.C. 1982). Nature 300:267.
6. Leonard, W.J., Depper, J.M., Crabtree, G.R., Rudikoff, S., Pumphrey, J., Robb, R., Krönke, M., Svetlik, P.B., Peffer, N.J., Waldmann, T.A. and Greene, W.C. (1984). Nature 311:626.
7. Robb, R.J. and Greene, W.C. (1983). J. Exp. Med. 158:1332.
8. Sharon, M., Klausner, R.D., Cullen, B.R., Chizzonite, R. and Leonard, W.J. (1986). Science 234:859.
9. Tsudo, M., Kozak, R.W., Goldman, C.K. and Waldmann, T.A. (1986). Proc. Natl. Acad. Sci. 83:9694.
10. Teshigawara, K., Wang, H.M., Kato, K. and Smith, K.A. (1987). J. Exp. Med. 165:223.
11. Robb, R.J., Rusk, C.M., Yodoi, J. and Greene, W.C. (1987). Proc. Natl. Acad. Sci. 84:2002.
12. Dukovich, M., Wano, Y., Thuy, L., Katz, P., Cullen, B.R., Kehrl, J.H. and Greene, W.C. (1987). Nature 327:518.
13. Robb, R.J., Munck, A., and Smith, K.A. (1981). J. Exp. Med. 154:1455.
14. Robb, R.J., Greene, W.C. and Rusk, C.M. (1984). J. Exp. Med. 160:1126.
15. Le thi Bich-Thuy, Dukovich, M., Peffer, N.J., Fauci, A.S., Kehrl, J.H. and Greene, W.C. (1987). J. Immunol. 139:(5):1550.
16. Greene, W.C., Robb, R.J., Svetlik, P.B., Rusk, C.M., Depper, J.M. and Leonard, W.J. (1985). J. Exp. Med. 162:363.
17. Collins, L., Tsien, W-H., Seals, C., Hakimi, J., Weber, D., Bailon, P., Hosking, J., Greene, W.C., Toome, V. and Ju, G. (1988). Proc. Natl. Acad. Sci. USA 85:7709.
18. Lowenthal, J.W. and Greene, W.C. (1987). J. Exp. Med. 166:1156.
19. Wang, H-M. and Smith, K.A. (1987). J. Exp. Med. 166:1055.
20. Robb, R.J. and Greene, W.C. (1987). J. Exp. Med. 165:1202.
21. Fujii, M., Sugamura, K., Sano, K., Nakai, M., Sugita, K. and Hinuma Y. (1986). J. Exp. Med. 163:550.
22. Weissman, A.L., Harford, J.B., Svetlik, P.B., Leonard, W.J., Depper, J.M., Waldmann, T.A., Greene, W.C. and Klausner, R.D. (1986). Proc. Natl. Acad. Sci. USA 83:1463.
23. Fung, M.R., Ju, G. and Greene, W.C. (1988). J. Exp. Med. 168:1923.
24. Tsudo, M., Goldman, C.K., Bonbiovanni, K.F., Chan, W.C., Winton, M. Yagita, Grimm, E.A. and Waldmann, T.A.

(1987). Proc. Natl. Acad. Sci. USA 84:5394.
25. Siegel, J.P., Sharon, M., Smith, P.L. and Leonard, W.J. (1987). Science 238:75.
26. Kehrl, J.H., Dukovich, M., Whalen, G., Katz, P., Fauci, A.S. and Greene, W.C. (1988). J. Clinical Invest. 81:200.
27. Lowenthal, J.W., Böhnlein, E. and Greene, W.C. (1988). Proc. Natl. Acad. Sci. USA 85:4468.
28. Ballard, D.W., Böhnlein, E., Lowenthal, J.W., Wano, Y., Franza, R.B. and Greene, W.C. (1988). Science 241:1652.
29. Cross, S.L, Feinberg, M.B., Wolf, J.B., Holbrook, N.J., Wong-Staal, F. and Leonard, W.J. (1987). Cell 49:47.
30. Maruyama, M., Shibuya, H., Harada, H., Hatakeyama, M., Seiki, M., Fujita, T., Inoue, J., Yoshida, M. and Taniguchi, T. (1987). Cell 48:343.
31. Böhnlein, E., Lowenthal, J.W., Siekevitz, M., Franza, B.R. and Greene, W.C. (1988). Cell 53:827.
32. Nabel, G. and Baltimore, D. (1987). Nature 326:711.
33. Siekevitz, M., Josephs, S.F., Dukovich, M., Peffer, N., Wong-Staal, F. and Greene, W.C. (1987b). Science 238:1575.
34. Siekevitz, M., Feinberg, M.B., Holbrook, N., Yodoi, J., Wong-Staal, F. and Greene, W.C. (1987a). Proc. Natl. Acad. Sci. 84:5389.
35. Kaufman, J.D., Valandra, G., Rodriguez, G., Bushar, G., Giri, C. and Norcross, M.D. (1987). Molec. Cell. Biol. 7:3759.
36. Tong-Starksen, S.E., Luciw, P.A. and Peterlin, B.M. (1987). Proc. Natl. Acad. Sci. 84:6845.
37. Franza, R.B., Josephs, S.F., Gilman, M.Z., Ryan, W. and Clarkson, B. (1987). Nature 330:391.
38. Kawakami, K., Scheiderest, C. and Roeder, R.G. (1988). Proc. Natl. Acad. Sci. USA 85:4700.

VIRUSES AS A TRIGGERING FACTOR OF AUTOIMMUNE TYPE I DIABETES

Ji-Won Yoon
Sung-Hee Ihm

Division of Virology
Department of Microbiology and Infectious Diseases
and
Laboratory of Viral and Immunopathogenesis of Diabetes
Julia McFarlane Diabetes Research Centre
The University of Calgary
Calgary, Alberta
Canada T2N 4N1

Robert G. McArthur

Department of Pediatrics

INTRODUCTION

Type I diabetes is characterized by pancreatic beta cell destruction which leads to hypoinsulinemia, hyperglycemia, polyuria, polydipsia, and polyphagia. It is believed that a variety of etiological factors such as genetic factors and environmental factors lead to this common pathologic picture. In fact, the familial occurrence of diabetes, or at least the tendency to develop the disease, has been observed and described for such a long time that it is considered to be a fact. However, the true nature of the genetic mechanisms governing the transmission of the diabetic trait is not well understood. Concordance for IDDM between identical twins approaches 50%, suggesting that besides genetic factors, non-genetic factors such as triggering factors can also influence the clinical expression of genetic susceptibility. As triggering factors affecting the induction of diabetes, diabetogenic viruses, chemicals, diet, and toxins are likely candidates as either primary injurious agents for pancreatic beta cells or inducing agents for autoimmunity in man and animals (1,2). Several mechanisms by which viruses can trigger autoimmunity have been suggested (3,4). These include: (a) The virus tenders the infected cell or some component of it foreign to the host (5). This may occur if the virus incorporates host antigens into its envelope or modifies the host antigens by virus infection. Certain viruses may induce aberrant expression of Ia antigens on the host cells (6,7). (b) The virus triggers autoimmunity by acting on the immunoregulatory system. Certain viruses may destroy subpopulations of lymphocytes (e.g. helper or suppressor T cells) or stimulate them, resulting in unbalance of immune system. (c) The virus can trigger an autoimmune response through molecular mimicry. Antibodies made against certain viral antigens may cross react with normal host cell antigens.

Recently, it has been shown that rubella virus and reovirus seem to be associated with autoimmunity in the pathogenesis of diabetes in neonatal golden Syrian hamsters (8) and suckling SJL/J mice (9,10), respectively. Recently, we have found that beta cell specific expression of endogenous retrovirus is closely associated with the development of insulitis and diabetes in NOD mice (11). In man, congenital rubella syndrome provides some evidence that viral infection can be associated with the subsequent development of autoimmune type I diabetes (12,13). In addition to the congenital rubella syndrome, persistent cytomegalovirus infection appears to be associated with autoimmune type I diabetes (14). In this brief review, we would like to summarize some of the experimental results carried out in our laboratory and the current state of knowledge on the association of virus infection with autoimmune type I diabetes in man and animals.

I. ANIMAL MODELS

Since the first report on virus-induced diabetes in mice (15), there have been extensive studies using animal models to elucidate the role of viruses in the pathogenesis of type I diabetes. A group of viruses including encephalomyocarditis (EMC) virus, mengovirus 2T, and Coxsackie B viruses can cause diabetes in susceptible mice through acute cytolytic infection of the beta cells. In contrast, rubella virus, retrovirus and reovirus seem to be associated with autoimmune type I diabetes.

1. Rubella Virus

The congenital rubella syndrome (CRS) provides one of the best documentations in man that a viral infection is associated with the subsequent development of autoimmune IDDM. Thus, an animal model of rubella virus-induced diabetes could be an important tool in studies of diabetes following CRS in man. Recently, we have developed an animal model for rubella virus-induced diabetes in neonatal golden Syrian hamsters, which closely parallels the diabetes observed with CRS in man (8). Seven to 10 day old male LVG strain golden Syrian hamsters were inoculated with rubella virus passaged in beta cells; all hamsters developed hyperglycemia and hypoinsulinemia. Histopathologic examination revealed marked mononuclear cell infiltration in 34.5% of islets from infected hamsters 21 days following rubella virus inoculation. Rubella virus-specific antigen could be detected by indirect immunofluorescence in beta cells isolated 14-21 days after infection in 8 out of 10 hamsters tested. In addition, very weak cytoplasmic islet cell antibodies were present in 8 out of 20 infected animals. We also have preliminary data indicating that administration of the passaged variant of rubella virus to fetal hamsters, during the first trimester of gestation, causes development of congenital anomalies similar to those of congenital rubella syndrome in humans (absent hind limbs) as well as diabetes.

However, the mechanism of rubella virus-induced diabetes is not known. In contrast to EMC virus, rubella virus is not highly lytic. Our preliminary data -- insulitis in 34.5% of hamster islets and measurable circulating islet cell antibodies -- is somewhat compatible with an autoimmune process. Rubella virus belongs to the togavirus family. This enveloped virus is surrounded by a lipoprotein coat derived when the maturing virus buds through the host cell membrane (16). Thus, rubella virus might insert, expose or alter antigens in the plasma membrane of the host cell during intracellular infection (17). Alternatively, the virus might induce an autoimmune syndrome by disturbances in T-cell subpopulations (helper or suppressor T-cells) that regulate the immune response of the host (18,19). However, the precise mechanism(s) of the rubella virus-induced diabetes-like syndrome in hamsters remains to be determined.

2. Retrovirus

The mouse carries genomic information for producing type A, B, and C retroviruses distinguishable on morphologic, serologic, and biochemical criteria. The expression of these retroviral genes in pancreatic beta cells of mice may be of pathogenic significance in the development of both chemically and genetically induced diabetes. Appel et al. noted that multiple injections of streptozotocin in CD-1 mice resulted in the induction of endogenous type C retrovirus and intracisternal type A virus in pancreatic beta cells followed by diabetes in these animals (20). Intracellular type C particles have also been reported sequestered within the RER in beta cells of the non-obese diabetic (NOD) mouse (21). Leiter et al. suggested that production of intracisternal type A virus conferred susceptibility to the diabetogenic effect of the db gene in db/db mice of the CBA/LtJ and C57BL/KsJ strains (22). The appearance of increased numbers of morphologically identifiable intracisternal type A particles (IAPs) in beta cells was accompanied by increased intracellular concentrations of p73, a core protein antigen of IAP, and it was postulated that p73 may act as a "neoantigen" to reject the beta cells expressing p73. It was also shown that there is molecular mimicry between insulin and retroviral antigen p73 and that cross-reactive autoantibodies against these molecules develop in the sera of NOD and C57BL/KsJ db/db mice (23). Recently, we have observed that the beta cell specific expression of endogenous retrovirus is associated with the development of insulitis and diabetes in NOD mice (11).

The studies from our laboratory and others revealed that the administration of cyclophosphamide to NOD mice produces a rapid progression to overt diabetes with severe insulitis within 2 to 3 weeks (24,25). Cyclophosphamide significantly increases the incidence of diabetes in NOD mice by either inhibiting suppressor T cells or activating cytotoxic T cells (26). However, the depletion of macrophages by silica treatment resulted in the prevention of insulitis and diabetes in cyclophosphamide-treated NOD mice (24). These findings suggested that macrophages play a major role in the initiation of organ-specific autoimmunities in NOD mice and the presentation of autoantigen(s) on the specific target cells, such as beta cells, by the macrophages would be the initial step in the development of insulitis. Our recent investigation was initiated to determine if there are any specific changes in the beta cells which may lead to the attraction of macrophages for the initiation of beta cell specific autoimmune disease in the cyclophosphamide-treated NOD male mice. When thin sections of islets from NOD male mice, which received silica for the preservation of islets and subsequently cyclophosphamide, were examined under the electron microscope, clusters of endogenous retrovirus particles (A type) were frequently found in the beta cells. In contrast, retrovirus particles were rarely found in the beta cells from NOD male mice which received silica only. Other endocrine cells and exocrine acinar cells did not contain such virus particles. These virus particles were not found in spleen, liver, or kidneys either in cyclophosphamide-treated or untreated NOD male mice. There was a clear correlation between the presence of retrovirus particles in the beta cells and insulitis lesions in the cyclophosphamide treated mice. On the basis of these observations, it is concluded that the beta cell specific expression of endogenous retrovirus is associated with the development of insulitis and diabetes in NOD mice.

The role of beta cell specific expressed retrovirus in the pathogenesis of autoimmune type I diabetes in NOD mice has not been defined. These endogenous retroviruses might induce either an aberrant expression of Class II major histocompatibility complex (MHC) antigen on the beta cells or beta cell specific autoantigen(s). Our preliminary data revealed that beta cells from these NOD mice were not stained by anti-Ia-antibody (Amano, K and Yoon, JW, unpublished data). This result suggests that the retrovirus may not induce Class II antigen in this condition. Work in several laboratories has indicated that retrovirus (e.g. MuLV) gp 70 may be present on the surface of cells without production of detectable infectious virus (27-29). By immunofluorescent techniques, Lerner and his co-workers found a protein similar or identical to the retrovirus (MuLV) gp 70 major envelope glycoprotein on the surface of mouse (127/J) thymocytes in lymphoid tissues and in murine epithelial lining cells (30). Since retroviruses (Xenotropic viruses) were regularly recovered from the mouse tissues, it is believed that these immunofluorescent tests could be detecting viral antigen on the cell surface. Whether the viral antigen or virus-induced autoantigen will express on the beta cells from these animals is presently under investigation.

The presentation of antigen on the target cells by antigen-presenting cells is a critical determinant for the distinction between elicitation of the immune response and immunologic tolerance (31). The immune response to a specific antigen on the target tissue involves the activation of a T-helper subset of lymphocytes. The T-helper cell is activated only when it interacts with the antigen presented on the surface of a macrophage or other antigen-presenting cell. In contrast, the direct exposure of lymphocytes to an antigen in the absence of antigen-presenting cells was shown to induce immunologic tolerance to the specific antigen (32). Since the elimination of antigen-presenting cells resulted in the prevention of insulitis in NOD mice, we can hypothesize that the presentation of autoantigens on the target cells by the macrophages would be the initial step in the development of beta cell specific autoimmune disease in NOD mice. However, the amplification of immune responses by T lymphocytes (e.g. L_3T_4 and Lyt_2) would be required for the clinical expression of overt diabetes in the NOD mice.

3. Reovirus

Since reoviruses produce a variety of lesions in newborn mice, we passaged reovirus type 3 in cultured pancreatic beta cells to see whether the virus can be adapted to the beta cells. When the beta cell-passaged virus was infected into suckling SJL/J male mice, some of the infected animals showed an abnormal response in glucose tolerance tests 10 days after infection (33). By immunofluorescence, specific viral antigens were found in some beta cells as well as in acinar cells. By electron microscopy, viral particles were detected in the cytoplasm of some beta cells. Surviving animals remained mildly hyperglycemic for about three weeks, and then returned to normal.

More recently, mice infected with reovirus type 1, which was passaged in pancreatic beta cell cultures, developed transient diabetes and a runting syndrome (9). The runting syndrome consisted of retarded growth, oily hair, alopecia and steatorrhea. Inflammatory cells and viral antigens as well as virus particles were found in the islets of Langerhans (alpha, beta and delta cells) as well as in the anterior pituitary (growth hormone-producing cells). Examination of sera from infected mice revealed autoantibodies that reacted with cytoplasmic antigens in the islets of Langerhans, anterior pituitary, and gastric mucosa of uninfected mice. The administration of either anti-lymphocyte serum, anti-thymocyte serum, or cyclophosphamide reduced or prevented the development of reovirus-induced diabetes (10). In addition, virus-infected, immunosuppressed mice gained weight at almost the same rate as uninfected controls, and mortality was greatly decreased. Thus, Onodera et al. concluded that autoimmunity does play a role in the pathogenesis of reovirus-induced diabetes (9).

Precisely how reovirus infection triggers the development of autoantibodies is still unclear, but viruses have often been suspected as a cause of autoimmune disease. In contrast to reovirus type 1, reovirus type 3 does not induce autoantibodies in mice and does not infect the pituitary. The critical difference between reovirus type 1 and type 3 seems to reside at the level of the sigma-1 polypeptide responsible for virus tropism. Therefore, it is speculated that a single viral molecule appears to control pituitary infection and autoantibody production. In view of the histopathological changes seen in lymphoid organs of reovirus-infected mice, it could be possible that specific subsets of lymphocytes may have receptors for the virus. Thus, both infection of hormone-producing cells and infection of virus with cells of the immune system may be required to initiate the production of autoantibody (9). The precise relationship between infection of reovirus type 1, the induction of autoantibodies and development of diabetic syndrome remains to be determined.

II. HUMAN SYSTEM

Through several case reports on the possible association of diabetes with relatively slow and/or persistent viral infections, rubella virus, cytomegalovirus and mumps virus have been implicated as the triggers of autoimmune IDDM in man.

1. Rubella Virus

The congenital rubella syndrome (CRS) has emerged as an important human model for type I diabetes. In CRS, the diabetes takes 5 to 20 years to develop (34). Although the diabetes is the most common of the delayed manifestations of CRS, autoimmune thyroid disease (35), Addision's disease (35), and growth hormone deficiency (36) have also been reported. Patients with CRS and diabetes have a significantly increased frequency of HLA DR3 and a significantly decreased frequency of HLA DR2 (37).

Epidemiologic studies have shown that the prevalence of IDDM among CRS patients is significantly high in both the United States and Australia (about 20%) (34,37), whereas other studies in the U.K. have failed to confirm this association (38). However, rubella virus has been isolated from the pancreas in a few cases of congenital infection (39,40) and insulitis with severe beta cell depletion was also reported in the case of an infant with CRS dying of acute onset diabetes (34).

There have been clues that the endocrine abnormalities in CRS might have an autoimmune basis; an increased prevalence of islet cell surface antibody (21% of CRS patients, 50-80% of patients with abnormal carbohydrate metabolism) (12,13), an increased prevalence of antithyroid microsomal and/or antithyroglobulin antibody (26% of CRS Patients) (12,13), an increased prevalence of antiinsulin autoantibody (13% of CRS patients vs. <1% of control) (41). Although the most convincing evidence that a persistent viral infection may cause IDDM and produce autoantibody comes from studies of patients with the CRS, it is not known how rubella virus triggers autoimmunity and IDDM. Animal models of rubella should be useful in elucidating underlying pathogenesis.

2. Cytomegalovirus

A case has been reported that a child with congenital cytomegalovirus infection developed diabetes at the age of thirteen months (42). In another report, characteristic inclusion bodies (20/45 cases) were found in the beta cells of infants and children who died of disseminated CMV infection (43). Insulitis and CMV-like particles have been observed in the pancreas of a particular rodent (Octodon degu), which manifests spontaneous diabetes (44). Recently, we have examined the lymphocytes from newly diagnosed type I diabetic patients for the presence of human CMV genome by molecular hybridizations with human CMV specific genome. The CMV specific viral genome was found in 22% of diabetic patients, but in 2.6% of control subjects. 62% and 69% of CMV genome-positive patients had islet cell antibody (ICA) and cytotoxic beta cell surface antibody (CBSA) in their serum, respectively, suggesting that persistent CMV infections may be relevant to pathogenesis in some cases of type I diabetes (14).

Human CMV infection is ubiquitous and largely subclinical (45). In many persistent viral infections, the initial viral infection takes place before birth or in very early life, although the disease may not appear until later. The infection can be passed through the sperm or ovum if viruses integrate their genomes into the host DNA. Viral infections can also be transmitted transplacentally, perinatally, or postnatally through close contact or breast milk. The immaturity of the immune systems of infants also favours the establishment of persistent viral infections (46).

Nucleic acid hybridization is especially useful in studies of persistent viral infections, since it can detect even inactive or incomplete viral genomes in a cell (47,48). Since persistent viral infections are often local, in-situ hybridization can be used to localize the individual cells that contain the viral genome. Our findings, with both dot and in-situ hybridization techniques, that about 15% of newly diagnosed type I diabetic patients had human CMV specific viral genome in their lymphocytes and islet cell autoantibodies in their sera suggest that autoimmune type I diabetes is sometimes associated with persistent CMV infections (14).

What might be the link between persistent CMV infection and autoimmune type I diabetes? Autoimmune disease could result from an immune response to viral antigens in the host cells or to host-cell-specific antigens that are exposed as a result of infection. If the CMV infection persists in the beta cells and either expresses viral antigens or induces an aberrant expression of class II major histocompatibility complex (MHC) antigen on the cells in certain circumstances, such as particular genetic background and environmental effects (eg., drug, diet, toxins, infections), persistent CMV infection might trigger beta-cell-specific autoimmune disease such as type I diabetes under the given situation. CMV is also known to disturb immunoregulation (49), resulting in loss of self-tolerance (50). However, whether this mechanism is involved in CMV-associated type I diabetes in man remains to be determined.

3. Mumps Virus

Mumps virus has been the virus most frequently reported to be clinically associated with diabetes mellitus since the first report in the last century (51). Gamble has demonstrated that mumps infection apparently precedes the development of diabetes in some newly diagnosed diabetic children (52). Helmke *et al.* have reported that some children may develop islet cell antibody during the phase of parotitis (53). Mumps virus also has been shown to infect cultured human beta cells (54). Although these data suggest that mumps virus can be associated with type I diabetes, recent epidemiologic studies do not support this hypothesis (55).

CONCLUSION

In this review, we discussed several candidate viruses which might trigger autoimmune type I diabetes in animals and man. Under certain circumstances, those viral infections could induce a persistent autoaggression leading to manifestation of diabetes mellitus several years later.

A new model of rubella virus-induced diabetes in hamsters has been shown to share the autoimmune features described in the diabetes in association with human CRS. The CRS has emerged as an important human model for autoimmune-mediated type I diabetes since the clear cut relationship between the clinical diagnosis of CRS and the subsequent development of diabetes mellitus with autoantibody production was noted. Recent our observation of association between increased endogenous retrovirus gene expression and increased severity of insulitis in NOD mice suggests that some endogenous virus might be a trigger of autoimmunity. In humans, there was a case report that a child with congenital cytomegalovirus infection developed diabetes mellitus at the age of thirteen months. Recently we have found that 15% of newly diagnosed type I diabetic patients had human CMV specific viral genome in their lymphocytes and islet cell autoantibodies in their sera suggesting that autoimmune type I diabetes is sometimes associated with persistent CMV infections.

Even though the mechanisms by which viruses can induce autoimmunity are unknown at present, data from animal models and diabetic patients suggest that certain viral infections are causatively linked to the development of autoimmune type I diabetes.

REFERENCES

1. Yoon, J.W., Kim, C.J., Pak, J.Y., McArthur R.G. (1987) Cli. Invest. Med. 10, 457-469.
2. Notkins, A.L., Yoon, J.W., Onodera, T., Toniolo, A. and Jenson, A.B. (1981) Virol. XI, 141-162.
3. Theofilopoulos, A.N., Dixon, F.J. (1982) Am. J. Pathol. 108, 321-341.
4. Notkins, A.L., Onodera, T., Prabhakar, B. (1984) In "Concepts in viral Pathogenesis" (A.L. Notkins, M.B.A. Oldstone, eds.) pp. 210-215. Springer-Verlag Press, New York.
5. Eaten, M.D. (1980) Infect. Immun. 27, 855-861.
6. Massa, P.T., Dorroes R., Ter Meulen V. (1986) Nature 320, 543-546.
7. Bosi, E., Todd, I., Pujol-Borrell, R., Bottazzo, G.F. (1987) Diabetes/Metab. Rev. 3, 893-924.
8. Rayfield, E.J., Kelly, K.J., Yoon, J.W. (1986) Diabetes 35, 1278-1281.
9. Onodera, T., Toniolo, A., Ray, U.R., Jenson, A.B., Knazek, R.A., Notkins, A.L. (1981) J. Exp. Med. 153, 1457-1465.
10. Onodera, T., Ray, U.R., Melez, K.A., Suzuki, H., Toniolo, A., Notkins, A.L. (1982) Nature 297, 66-69.
11. Suenaga, K., Yoon, J.W. (1988) Diabetes 37, 1722-1726.
12. Ginsberg-Fellner, F., Witt, M.E., Yagihashi, S. (1984) Diabetologia 27, 87-89.
13. Ginsberg-Fellner, F., Witt, M.E., Fedun, B. (1985) Rev. Infect. Dis. 7(Suppl. 1) S170-S175.

14. Pak, C.Y., Eun, H.M., McArthur, R.G., Yoon, J.W. (1988) Lancet 2, 1-14.
15. Craighead, J.E., McLane, M.F. (1968) Science 162, 913-914.
16. Schlesinger, M.J., Kaarianen, L. (1980) In "Togavirus" (R.W. Schlesinger, ed.) pp. 371-389, Academic Press, New York.
17. Allison, A.C. (1977) In "Progress in Immunology" (N.E. Mendel, C. Cheers, C.S. Hoskins, I.F.C. McKenzie and H. Nossal, eds.) p. 512. Elsevier, Amsterdam.
18. Fauci, A.C. (1980) J. Allergy Clin. Immunol. 66, 5-17.
19. Reinherz, E.L., Schlossman, S.F. (1980) N. Engl. J. Med. 303, 370-373.
20. Appel, M.C., Rossini, A.A., Williams, R.M., Like, A.A. (1978) Diabetologia 15, 327-336.
21. Fujita, H., Fujino, H., Nonaka, K., Tarui, S., Tochino, Y. (1984) Biomed. Res. 5, 67-70.
22. Leiter, E.H., Kuff, E.L. (1984) Am. J. Pathol. 114, 46-55.
23. Serreze, D.V., Leiter, E.H., Kuff, E.L., Jardieu, P., Ishizaka, K. (1988) Diabetes 37, 351-358.
24. Lee, K.U., Amano, K., Yoon, J.W. (1988) Diabetes 37, 989-991.
25. Harada, M., Makino, S. (1982) Diabetologia 27, 604-606.
26. Harada, M., Sueishi, T., Misaki, R., Makino, S. (1987) Possible role of Lyt 2+ T cells in cyclophosphamide-enhanced diabetes in NOD mice. Presented in International Research Symposium "The Immunology of Diabetes". Oct. 27-30, Woods Hole, Massachusetts.
27. Ikeda, H., Pincus, T., Yoshiki, T., Strand, M., August, J.T., Boyse, E.A., Mellors, R.C. (1974) J. Virol. 14, 1274-1280.
28. Del Villano, B.C., Nave, B., Croker, B.P. (1975) J. Exp. Med. 141, 172-187.
29. Kennel, S.J., Feldman, J.D. (1976) Cancer Res. 36, 200-208.
30. Lerner, R.A., Wilson, C.B., Del Villano, B.C., McCohahey, P.J., Dixon, F.J. (1976) J. Exp. Med. 143, 151-166.
31. Unanue, E.R., Allen, P.M. (1987) Science 236, 551-557.
32. Toews, G.B., Bergstresser, P.R., Streilein, J.W. (1980) J. Immunol. 124, 445-453.
33. Onodera, T., Jenson, A.B., Yoon, J.W., Notkins, A.L. (1978) Science 301, 529-531.
34. Menser, M.A., Forrest, J.M., Bransby, R.D. (1978) Lancet 1, 57-60.
35. Schopfer, K., Matter, L., Flueler, U., Werder, E. (1982) Lancet 2, 159.
36. Preece, M.A., Kearney, P.J., Marshall, W.C. (1977) Lancet 2, 842-844.
37. Rubinstein, P., Walker, M.E., Fedun, B., Witt, M.E., Cooper, L.Z., Ginsberg-Fellner, F. (1982) Diabetes 31, 1088-1091.
38. Smithsells, R.W., Sheppard, S., Marshall, W.C., Peckham, C. (1978) Lancet 1, 439.
39. DePrins, F., VanAssche, F.A., Desmyter, J. (1978) Lancet 1, 439-440.
40. Patterson, K., Chandra, R.S., Jenson, A.B. (1981) Lancet 1, 1048-1049.
41. Ginsberg-Fellner, F., Fedun, B., Cooper, Z. (1987) In "The Immunology of Diabetes Mellitus" (M.A. Jaworski, G.D. Molnar,

R.V. Rajotte, B. Singh, eds.) pp. 279-286. Elsevier, Amsterdam.
42. Ward, K.P., Galloway, W.H., Auchterlonie, I.A. (1979) Lancet 1, 497.
43. Jenson, A.B., Rosenberg, H.S., Notkins, A.L. (1980) Lancet 2, 354-358.
44. Fox, G.J., Murphy, J.C. (1979) Vet. Pathol. 16, 625-628.
45. Ho, M. (1982) Cytomegalovirus: biology and infection. New York Plenum.
46. Haywood, A.M. (1986) N. Engl. J. Med. 315, 939-948.
47. Bornkamm, G.W., Desgranges, C., Gissmann, L. (1983) Curr. Top. Microbiol. Immunol. 104, 287-298.
48. Kulski, J.K., Norval, M. (1985) Arch. Virol. 83, 3-15.
49. Ho, M. (1984) In "CMV: Pathogenesis and prevention of human infection" (S.A. Plotkin, S. Mitchelson, J.S. Pagano, F. Rapp, eds.) p. 131. Alan R. Liss, Inc., New York.
50. Bartholomaeus, W.N., O'Donoghue, H., Foti, D., Lawson, C.M., Shellam, G.R., Reed, W.D. (1988) Immunology 64, 397-405.
51. Harris, H.F. (1899) Boston Med. Surg. J. 440, 465-469.
52. Gamble, D.R. (1980) Br. Med. J. 2, 99-101.
53. Helmke, K., Otten, A., Willems, W. (1980) Lancet ii, 211-212.
54. Ratzman, K.P., Strese, J., Witt, S., Berling, H., Keilacker, H., Michaelis, D. (1984) Diabetes Care 7, 170-173.

MAPPING SUSCEPTIBILITY TO RHEUMATOID ARTHRITIS INTO A CONFORMATIONALLY EQUIVALENT REGION OF MHC CLASS II MOLECULES ENCODED BY DIFFERENT ALLELES

Robert Winchester

Hospital for Joint Diseases and
Division of Rheumatology,
Department of Medicine,
New York University Medical Center
New York, N.Y.

The dominantly expressed genetic susceptibility for the inappropriate immune response that characterizes rheumatoid arthritis is controlled by several alleles of class II DR β chain genes of the major histocompatibility complex (MHC) including those that encode the serologically distinct DR1 and DR4 specificities. This suggests that the disease may originate from one or more immune recognition events initiated by these MHC molecules. Ethnic differences in susceptibility and parallel differences in the organization of the class II haplotypes that encode similar and divergent serologic specificities permit mapping of susceptibility into a polymorphic region of the DR β gene in a manner analogous to a segregation analysis. The evidence was reviewed for the existence of a single complementary conformation in the third diversity region of the DR β gene that localizes the structural determinants of susceptibility into the mid portion of the α helical rim of the class II molecule. The principal was discussed of the conformational and hence functional equivalence of otherwise distinct alleles that share regions of sequence presumably arising from gene conversion events. The existence in rheumatoid arthritis of a consensus amino acid sequence including the absence of negatively charged residues at positions 71 and 74 suggests the conclusion that a unitary immune recognition event underlies the development of the disease.

INTRODUCTION TO THE CONFORMATIONAL EQUIVALENCE HYPOTHESIS

Since the first application of reagent alloantisera that recognized class II specificities to patients with rheumatoid arthritis it was evident that certain sera identified determinants more closely associated with disease susceptibility that one would have expected based on their nominal serologic specificity for standardized class II alleles [1-4]. The complexity of the class II system and the inherent difficulties of working with polyclonal sera prevented significant progress in those early studies, but based on the insights provided by these reagents, the notion was clearly conceptualized that certain alloantigens or epitopes were better indicators of disease susceptibility than standard typing reagents, and that these epitopes were found to be relatively independent from the classic HLA class II specificities [5].

The demonstration that distinct gene products could share structures that functioned equivalently in antigen presentation, even across the genetic distance between mouse and human, and that the function paralleled the presence of a serologically defined epitope, was an important element in the development of the idea of conformational equivalence [6]. Taken together, these observations formed the rationale for the immunochemical [7-9] and molecular biologic studies of the nature and complexity of the DR4 [10], DR1 [11,12] and DRw10 [12] haplotypes in this laboratory and their relationship to defining the molecular basis of susceptibility to rheumatoid arthritis.

Based on these data, on studies from other laboratories on the association of susceptibility to rheumatoid arthritis in various ethnic groups [13-18], and the reported ethnic differences in frequencies of allelic fine specificities of DR4 [19-23], we postulated that an epitope shared by certain DR molecules associated with susceptibility was formed by a specific sequence of amino acids of the third diversity (hypervariable) region and was itself the molecular basis of susceptibility to rheumatoid arthritis [24]. This concept then was designated the shared epitope hypothesis. It was subsequently extended and modified to emphasize that the element that is shared between serologically distinct allelic products should not be viewed so much as an epitope but as a conformationally equivalent structure presumably involved in and perhaps responsible for a critical immune recognition event [25].

This article will be concerned with certain aspects of this background, especially the use of a sort of segregation analysis exploiting ethnic differences in haplotype organization and gene sequencing techniques to map susceptibility into the sequences of the mid-portion of the DR chain third diversity region. The second part of the review deals with a consideration of the sequences involved in forming the conformation and their disease relevance to susceptibility.

The disease association of rheumatoid arthritis with classic HLA specificities: the problem of multiple susceptibility markers differing among ethnic groups: DR4 was found to be increased in many studies of rheumatoid arthritis, but the increase was not of an equivalent intensity in all reports [1-4,13-15]. In particular, certain ethnic groups differed strikingly in the relative risk and percentage of individuals with rheumatoid arthritis accounted for by the presence of DR4, Table I. Most notably, rheumatoid arthritis was not encountered at an elevated frequency among the Jewish people that were positive for DR4.

That genetic differences in the structure of class II gene products were themselves responsible for the lack of homogeneity in the associations with DR4 became evident with studies delineating the subtypes of DR4 recognized by MLC typing [18,19]. Of the five principal subtypes of DR4 readily recognized by this system, Dw4, Dw14, and Dw15 were found to be most prevalent in ethnic groups that exhibited a strong association of rheumatoid arthritis with DR4, while Dw10 and Dw13 were predominant in those populations that had weak or no associations of rheumatoid arthritis with DR4, Table II [21-23,26-27].

In two ethnic groups, East Indians and Jews, DR1 but not DR4 was identified as the predominant DR allele associated with susceptibility [16-18]. Furthermore, among certain stable Caucasian ethnic groups such as in central Germany, DR1 preponders over DR4 as the primary allele associated with rheumatoid arthritis (B. Ruff, G. Burmester, et al., personal communication). Indeed, among the populations with predominant DR4-associated susceptibility, DR1 could be shown to be associated if the effect of DR4 was corrected. However, the association of rheumatoid arthritis with DR1 was also non-homogeneous as reflected by differences in the intensity of the association of disease susceptibility measured by the relative risk, suggesting the possibility of allelic complexity in DR1, Table III.

An important characteristic of the associations of DR alleles with rheumatoid arthritis is that to date no DR allele has been shown to be associated with dominant resistance to disease

Table I

HLA-DR4 and susceptibility to RA: patterns of association in different ethnic groups

	RA	controls	relative risk
N. American Caucasian	70%	28%	3.5
N. American Blacks	36%	10%	5.0
Japanese	71%	42%	3.3
Mexican	77%	38%	5.0
Israeli Jewish	37%	39%	-1.1

TABLE II

Dw Subtyes of DR4 Frequency Defined by MLC Typing

MLC Type	North American Caucasian	Israeli	Japanese
	(percentage of DR4+ people)		
Dw4	**46***	7	9
Dw10	12	42	-
Dw13	10	21	17
Dw14	**26***	5	5
Dw15	-	2	**41***
Blank	6	11	11
KTZ		5	17
SHA		7	-

* Associated with Rheumatoid Arthritis.

Table III
Risk for RA is associated with both DR4 and DR1 haplotypes

	Caucasian - Great Britain			Jewish Caucasian - Israel		
	RA	controls	RR	RA	controls	RR
DR1	28%	20%	1.5	27%	5.9%	5.4
DR4	74%	38%	4.5	37%	39.0%	-1.1

	Asian Indians (Great Britain)		
	RA	controls	RR
DR1	60%	16%	7.0
DR4	17%	14%	1.2

adapted from: Woodrow et al. Brit. Med. J. (1981) 283:1287.
Schiff et al. Ann. Rheum. Dis. (1982) 41:403.

acquisition. The development of disease was largely accounted for by a dominant susceptibility effect of one allele. The absence of a striking dominant resistance effect as has been observed in insulin-dependent diabetes mellitus with certain DQ β chain alleles [28], suggests that entirely distinct kinds of immune recognition events occur in these two diseases, with susceptibility that is MHC-encoded, see below.

Structure of the class II molecule: The structure of the class II molecules and the genetic organization of the region encoding them will be reviewed as a basis for discussing the mapping of disease susceptibility. One of the major advances in recent years has been the description of the conformation of the MHC class I molecule by Bjorkman et al. using crystallography [29]. The analogous features of the class II molecule permitted the ready visualization of a presumptive class II molecule conformation [30,31]. This is depicted in Figure 1 which illustrates the three diversity (hypervariable) regions of the DRβ chain. Two are located in the β pleated sheet floor of the antigen binding cleft and the third is located in the margin of α helix. In the case of the DR molecule, these three regions contain virtually all of the significant polymorphisms because the α chain is monomorphic. There are rather more possible amino acid substitutions in the first two diversity regions (residues 9-37) than in the third, which presumably reflects constraints of the α helix. Table IV depicts some of the principal variable residues that comprise the diversity regions in the special instance of DR1 and DR4 DRβ chain alleles.

The α helix can be separated into four regions that are characterized by different patterns of amino acid variability. A proximal segment extending from 57 to 61 includes the two contiguous inward or upward positions of variability, 57 and 60. The aspartic acid residue at 57 confers the ability to form a salt bridge to the α chain, a bridge which in the analogous position is considered to be important in disease resistance to DQ allele-encoded susceptibility to insulin dependent diabetes mellitus. As illustrated, the Dw15 DR4 allele lacks this aspartate. The third segment of the α helix includes the third diversity region and is highly homologous to class I, extending from 67 to 79. The inwardly facing residues are at position 67 which exhibits constrained variability in that only amino acids with hydrophobic side chains are found. Residues 70 and 71 comprise the next course of amino acids in the upper and inner wall of the antigen binding cleft. In contrast to the previous variable residues, the residues permissible here include hydrophilic or charged amino acids. At position 70 aspartic acid, glutamine or arginine can occur, and presumably they face

TABLE IV

LOCATIONS OF SIGNIFICANT VARIABILITY AMONG DR1 AND DR4 β CHAINS

										10										20										30										40									
DR2 w2	G	D	T	R	P	R	F	L	Q	Q	D	K	Y	E	C	H	F	F	N	G	T	E	R	V	R	F	L	H	R	D	I	Y	N	Q	E	E	D	L	R	F	D	S	D	V	G	E	Y	R	A
DR1									W		L		F													L		E		C		Y	N				S	V									Y		
DR1 NA16									W		L		F													L		E		C		Y	N				S	V									Y		
DR4 w14									E		V		H													F		D		Y		Y	H				Y	V									Y		
DR4 w4									E		V		H													F		D		Y		Y	H				Y	V									Y		
DR4 w13									E		V		H													F		D		Y		Y	H				Y	V									Y		
DR4 w15									E		V		H													F		D		Y		Y	H				Y	V									Y		
DR4 w10									E		V		H													F		D		Y		Y	H				Y	V									Y		

	50										60										70										80										90					
DR2 w2	V	T	E	L	G	R	P	D	A	E	Y	W	N	S	Q	K	D	F	L	E	D	R	R	A	A	V	D	T	Y	C	R	H	N	Y	G	V	G	E	S	F	I	V	Q	R	R	V
DR1								D										L			Q	R			A											V	G									
DR1 NA16								D										L			Q	R			A											G	V									
DR4 w14								D										L			Q	R			A											V	V									
DR4 w4								D										L			Q	K			A											V	G									
DR4 w13								D										L			Q	R			E											V	G									
DR4 w15								S										L			Q	R			A											V	G									
DR4 w10								D										I			D	E			A											V	V									

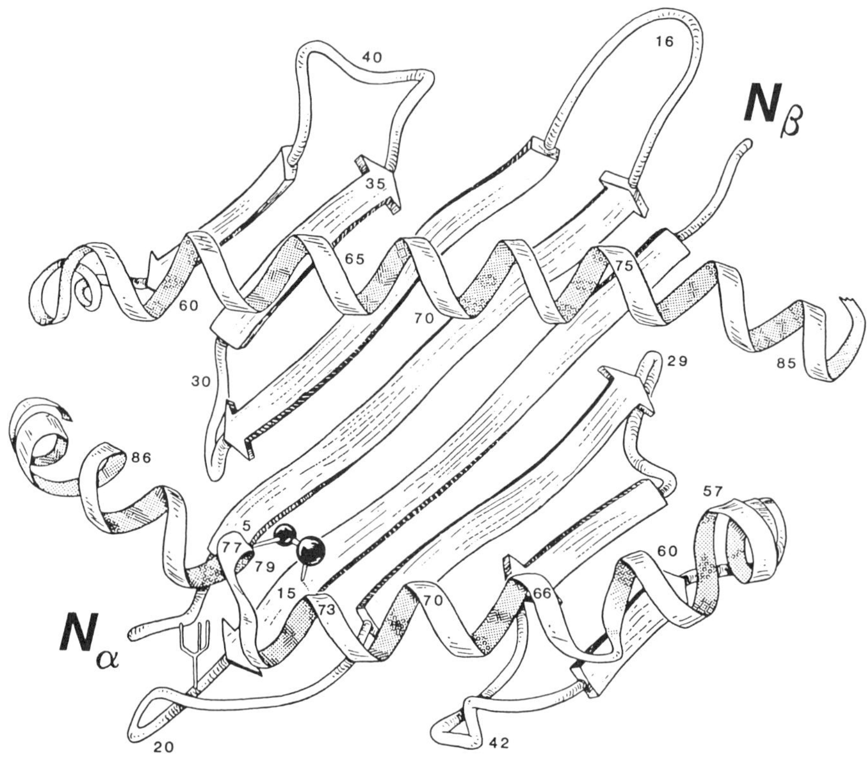

Figure 1. A hypothetical model of the class II antigen-binding domains based on the tertiary structure model of Bjorkman et al. [29] for the class I molecule and the approach to computer projections for secondary structure used by Norcross and Kanehisha. The N terminus of the α chain begins at the lower left and after providing the four left-hand strands of β pleated sheet assumes an α helical structure and forms the upper margin of the antigen binding cleft. The β chain N terminus is at the upper right. This chain provides the β pleated sheet on the right and the lower strand of α helix. A disulfide bond links residues 16 and 79. An oligosaccharide moiety lies just on the other side of the α helix in this region.

TABLE V

Various amino acid substitutions in the first and second diversity regions on the floor of the antigen binding cleft are compatible with susceptibility to rheumatoid arthritis

	1st Diversity Region			2nd Diversity Region				RA
Residue:	9	11	13	28	30	32	37	
Specificity								
DR1 (NS)	W	L	F	E	C	Y	S	+
DR1	W	L	F	E	C	Y	S	+
DR4w14	E	V	H	D	Y	Y	Y	+
DR4w4	E	V	H	D	Y	Y	Y	+
DRw10	E	V	H	D	Y	Y	Y	+?
DR4w13	E	V	F	E	R	H	Y	-
DR4w10	E	V	H	D	Y	Y	Y	-
DR7	E	V	H	D	Y	Y	Y	-
DRw9	W	G	Y	E	L	Y	F	-
DRw53	K	D	F	H	G	Y	N	-
DR2w2	E	A	C	I	Y	Y	Y	-
DR2	Q	D	Y	H	D	Y	D	-
DR3	W	P	R	D	Y	Y	S	-
DR5	E	S	S	D	Y	H	N	-
DRw52	E	Y	S	D	Y	H	Y	-

The boxed residues are not found in either DR1 or DR4 β chain alleles that are associated with susceptibility.

"+" denotes significantly associated with susceptibility to rheumatoid arthritis. "-" denotes the absence of association.

TABLE VI

AMINO ACID SUBSTITUTIONS IN THE THIRD DIVERSITY REGION OF THE DRβ CHAIN α HELIX ASSOCIATED WITH RHEUMATOID ARTHRITIS SUSCEPTIBILITY

	Proximal			Midportion					Distal			
Residue:	57	60	61	67	70	71	74	77	78	82	85	86	
Orientation:	I	U	I	I	UI	I	I	U	I	I	U	I	
Specificity													RA
DR1 (NS)	D	Y	W	L	Q	R	A	T	Y	N	V	G	+
DR1	D	Y	W	L	Q	R	A	T	Y	N	A	V	+
DR4w14	D	Y	W	L	Q	R	A	T	Y	N	V	G	+
DR4w4	D	Y	W	L	Q	K	A	T	Y	N	V	V	+
DRw10	D	Y	W	L	R	R	A	T	Y	N	V	G	+?
DR4w13	D	Y	W	L	Q	R	E	T	Y	N	V	V	-
DR4w10	D	Y	W	I	D	E	A	T	Y	N	V	V	-
DR7	V	S	W	I	D	R	Q	T	V	N	V	G	-
DRw9	V	S	W	F	R	R	E	T	V	N	V	G	-
DRw53	D	Y	W	L	R	R	E	T	Y	N	V	V	?
DR2w2	D	Y	W	F	D	R	A	T	Y	N	V	G	-
DR2	D	Y	W	I	Q	<u>A</u>	A	T	Y	N	A	V	-
DR3	D	Y	W	L	Q	K	<u>R</u>	<u>M</u>	Y	N	V	G	-
DR5	D	Y	W	F	D	R	A	T	Y	N	V	V	-
DRw52	D	Y	W	L	Q	K	<u>Q</u>	<u>M</u>	Y	N	V	G	-

I = Inward facing
U = Upward facing
+ Signifies positively associated
- Means the absence of a significant positive association

Boxed residues signify a negatively charged residue in a third diversity sequence that otherwise is compatible with the consensus sequence. Underlined residues illustrate non-negatively charged residues that are not compatible with the consensus sequence.

upwards towards the T cell, while at position 71 either alanine, arginine, lysine or glutamic acid may be found. The alanine is found in certain DR2 β chains, not illustrated. Residue 72 is an outward-and-downward facing arginine also conserved in class I that forms a salt bridge with an invariant aspartic acid at position 76. Residue 73 is semi-conserved alanine/glycine with alanine occupying the same position, 158, in class I.

The next tier of inward or inward-and-upward facing, highly variable residues is made up of a variable site, position 74, where a leucine, glutamine, arginine, alanine or glutamic acid resides. Only the last two are found in the illustrated sequences. The presence of a glutamic acid at 74 is associated with an arginine at position 71, suggesting the possibility of side chain interactions in certain haplotypes. These alleles, such as DR4 Dw13, are not associated with susceptibility to rheumatoid arthritis. Residue 74 is the most widely variable site in this portion of the α helix with 5 different amino acids observed. At the end of this segment, the upwardly and inwardly facing residues at positions 77 and 78 have limited variability and are hydrophobic residues. The distal segment from residue 80 to 86 has as inwardly or upwardly facing residues, the invariant arginine at position 80, with hydrogen bonding function, and the small hydrophobic residues at positions 85 and 86 which have limited variability including valine or alanine at position 85, and alanine or glycine at 86. These residues may be responsible for adjusting the size and shape of the antigen binding cleft.

Organization of Class II Genes: Figure 2 summarizes the location and number of genes in the class II region.

Use of ethnic differences in the structure of the MHC class II alleles to map the location of susceptibility: While we have used the terms DR4 and DR1 "alleles", more properly, we should have used the term "haplotype" to describe the association data that derive from typing for the serologic specificities. The problem of determining the precise gene likely to encode rheumatoid arthritis susceptibility is complicated by the highly linked series of genes comprising the DR and DQ subregion haplotypes, Fig. 2. The absence of observed recombination in this region of the MHC is a significant obstacle that prevents conventional segregation analysis in families to be used as a tool in mapping susceptibility.

However, the fact that in different ethnic groups susceptibility to rheumatoid arthritis varies in relationship to the particular Dw subtypes of DR4 that are the characteristic of that ethnic group, afforded an opportunity to approach the genetic basis of

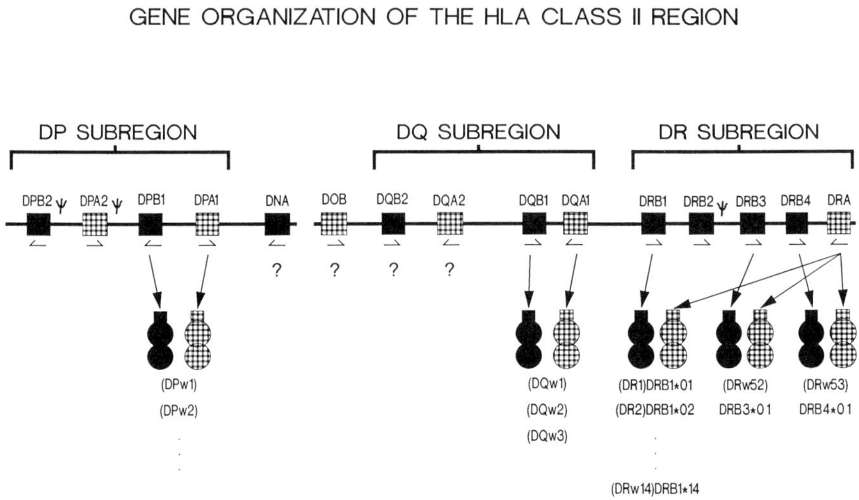

Figure 2. The organization of the class II genes and their products. Both the new and old terminologies are shown. The three subregions each contain an α chain gene and one or more β chain genes. The interaction of the chains encoded in each subregion forms the three principal MHC class II isotypes: DR, DQ and DP molecules. Some allelic series are shown. The B3 gene is intact and expressed in the DRw52 haplotypes, while the B4 gene is intact and expressed in the DRw53 haplotypes.

TABLE VII

Amino acid residues in DR β chain α helix associated with susceptibility to rheumatoid arthritis

Consensus in R.A. DRβ chains		Potential residues excluding susceptibility	
position	**residue**	**residues**	**DRβ chain specificities**
67	leucine	isoleucine	DR4 Dw10, DR7, DR2
		phenylalanine	DRw9, DR2w2, DR5
70	glutamine	<u>aspartic acid</u>	DR4 Dw10, DR7, DR2w2
	arginine ??		DR5
71	arginine	glutamic acid	DR4 Dw10
	lysine	<u>alanine</u>	DR2
74	alanine	<u>glutamic acid</u>	DR4 Dw13, DRw9, DRw53
		<u>glutamine</u>	DR7, DRw52
		<u>arginine</u>	DR3
77	threonine	<u>methionine</u>	DR3 DRw52
78	tyrosine	valine	DR7, DRw9

Underlined residues may be more significant because their presence appears to be critical for excluding susceptibility. Arginine at position 70 is queried because DRw10, which contains this residue, is not reliably shown to be a susceptibility allele.

developing the disease. Accordingly, we set out to analyze DR4 haplotypes at the level of epitopes recognizable by molecular monoclonal antibodies [6-9] and in parallel undertook studies of the gene structure [10-12]. With the anticipation that the structural differences responsible for the different subtypes of DR4 delineated by MLC typing [19] would illuminate the problem of rheumatoid arthritis susceptibility, an extensive effort was made to sequence the relevant DQ and DR subregion genes in the DR4 haplotype [10].

The results of ethnic differences in the haplotypes summarized schematically in Fig. 3 can be used in a sort of segregation analysis to define the locus and its alleles that are most closely associated with susceptibility [25]. As an example, $DQ\beta$ and $DQ\alpha$ chain genes can be excluded because certain identical alleles are shared by DR4 Dw haplotypes, for example Dw4 and Dw10, disparate for association with rheumatoid arthritis. Similarly the $DR\beta_2$ and $DR\alpha$ loci can be eliminated because the lack of polymorphism of DRw53 and $DR\alpha$ alleles does not parallel the presence or absence of disease. The only locus with sufficient allelic heterogeneity to account for the association or lack of association is the $DR\beta_1$ [24,25]. Reciprocally, the identification of this β chain locus greatly diminished the likelihood that gene products other than the known class II MHC products are involved. By way of contrast, this conclusion, taken with the growing knowledge of the complete genomic organization of the DR4 haplotype, renders the oft-invoked hypothesis quite unlikely of a mysterious non-MHC class II-linked polymorphic gene as the responsible agent for susceptibility.

Mapping of susceptibility into the third diversity region of the $DR\beta$ chain gene: By a similar modified segregation analysis using differences in the inferred amino acid sequence of $DR\beta_1$ genes present in the various DR4 subtypes arising through gene conversion events, the intragenic region most likely responsible for susceptibility can be mapped. Tables IV, V and VI illustrate the inferred amino acid sequences of the DR4 β chain variants. The principle of organization of the $DR\beta$ chain alleles is based on two levels of complexity: the first arising through evolutionary relationships [32] primarily evident in the first and second diversity regions responsible for much of the serologic basis by which allelic products are distinguished. The second level results from the exchange of large segments of DNA 3' to codon 57 in the $DR\beta$ chain among different alleles and between loci. For example, essentially the same motif of nucleotides is found in the DRw53 allele of the β_{III} locus, the DRw9 β_I chain and the Drw10 β_I chain genes. The identical amino acids encoded by these nucleotides in the α helical portion of the $DR\beta$ chain specify an epitope recognized by antibody 109d6 that is found on each of the serologically different DR molecules [12]. This emphasizes that large portions of the structure of DRβ chain may be shared by serologically disparate molecules suggesting that function may also be shared [6].

The significant sequence variations in the Dw10 subtype of DR4 that is not associated with rheumatoid arthritis susceptibility was shown to be in the third diversity region. This has two implications, the first of which is that the amino acid sequence of the first and second diversity regions shown in table V for the DR 4 alleles are not in themselves sufficient to confer susceptibility to rheumatoid arthritis. In general the divergence between the sequence of DR1 and DR4 in these diversity regions is marked, and with the exception of positions 28 and 32, there is little homology to suggest that susceptibility is encoded by these regions.

The second implication derives from the changes in the Dw10 DR4 third diversity region that involve the substitution of Ile at position 67 and Asp and Glu respectively at positions 70 and 71. This change from the sequence of the Dw4 prototype third diversity region was a critical finding in suggesting the importance of the third diversity region as a site of special relevance to rheumatoid arthritis. The argument can then be made [24] that the residues in the homologous positions on the Dw subtypes Dw4, Dw14 and Dw15 that are associated with susceptibility are critically involved in determining the immune response underlying rheumatoid arthritis. These residues are: from position 67 <u>Leu</u>-Leu-Glu-<u>Gln</u>-<u>Arg or Lys</u>-Arg-Ala-<u>Ala</u> ending at position 74. A more extensive analysis of the consensus residues and those possibly excluding susceptibility is given in Table VII. The underlined residues are polymorphic and are in either upward or inward facing positions on the α helical portion of the DR molecule. They are either uniquely associated with rheumatoid arthritis susceptibility or required, but not unique, to DR gene products associated with susceptibility. The sequence of the Dw13 allele, not associated with susceptibility, resembles the sequences of Dw4, Dw14 and Dw15 alleles with the important difference that, like the Dw10 allele, there is a highly nonconservative amino acid substitution involving a change from a positively charged amino acid to a negatively charged one. Accordingly, the presence of a negative charge in either position 71 or 74, which occupy contiguous locations in the α helix, appear to prevent the DRβ chain allele from operating as a susceptibility determinant. It is possible that, as discussed above, side chain interactions between residues in position 71 and 74 are critical in forming a configuration of the α-helical rim of the class II molecules that influence disease susceptibility.

Relation of DR1: Inasmuch as DR1 is serologically unrelated to DR4, yet both specificities are associated with rheumatoid arthritis, the structural analysis of the DR1 haplotype affords an important approach to determining whether the interpretation of the molecular basis of susceptibility is a valid notion. The sequence analysis of DR1, including that of a DRβ chain from a rheumatoid arthritis patient, also revealed a surprising identity between the third diversity region of the DR4 subtypes associated with disease susceptibility and DR1 that was unsuspected in view of the serologic differences of molecules that contain either of the two chains [11,12,33], Tables V and VI. This region of shared sequence is identical with that of Dw14 in the third diversity region and strongly supports the conclusions discussed above in the analysis of DR4, as has been presented [11,25].

That the association of susceptibility with DR1 in European Caucasian populations is of a lower intensity as defined by the value of the relative risk (odds ratio) compared to that of DR4 suggests a variety of explanations. One simple hypothesis is that there are different DR1 alleles which share the DR1 serologic specificity, but which differ in their property of conferring disease susceptibility. In support of this possibility, it was therefore of some interest to identify in five patients [11] with rheumatoid arthritis a distinctive variety of the DR1 β_1 chain which indicates the presence of a different allele within the DR1 family, Table IV. It remains to be investigated in a population study whether the unique pattern of sequences at residues 85 and 86 of this DR1 allele confer a higher risk for the development of rheumatoid arthritis than does the common Caucasian DR1 allele [34].

Viewed in this way, susceptibility to rheumatoid arthritis exhibits a dominant mode of inheritance with the conformationally equivalent portions of certain DR4 or DR1 β_1 chain genes defining the molecular basis of the susceptibility, despite the serologic unrelatedness of their products. Examining the sequence of the DRβ chains, this model suggests that DRw10 could also be a susceptibility allele since it contains a similar but not identical sequence in this region. Indeed, DRw10 has been implicated as a possible susceptibility marker in certain situations [12] but a large-scale study has not yet been performed.

Inferences: In attempting to understand the molecular basis of susceptibility to rheumatoid arthritis, one can envision that a specific trimolecular interaction between the T cell receptor of a CD4 helper T cell, a purely hypothetical antigen fragment "X" to which the immune response that underlies rheumatoid arthritis is directed, and the particular MHC class II allele that is capable of presenting antigen "X" to the T cell. According to this speculation, a helper T cell clone or clones that contain receptors capable of recognizing antigen "X" in the context of the particular MHC class II allele would be necessary. The consequence is the production of the specific T cell help for the maturation and expansion of B cells such as those manufacturing rheumatoid factors. Alternatively the role of the class II susceptibility structure could be to act in the formation of the T cell repertoire with the result that T cells are positively selected for which recognize fragments of a particular antigen and can similarly provide help for the differentiation of B cells.

Whether the consensus sequence from residue 67 to 74, Leu-Leu-Glu-Gln/Arg-Arg/Lys-Arg-Ala-Ala in fact encodes a functionally equivalent conformation [35,36] common to all the chains discussed in this review remains the subject for further study. However, taken together, we would emphasize the primacy of DR molecules and the special significance of the third diversity region in determining the molecular basis of disease susceptibility because they are endowed with analogous functional conformations. Accordingly, we would suggest that immune recognition events underlie the initiation of an immune response in rheumatoid arthritis involving either binding of an endogenous antigen fragment, the elusive antigen "X," with subsequent helper T cell receptor binding to the trimolecular complex, or direct interaction of the receptor with the MHC configuration. This determinant selection type of mechanism emphasizes the importance of antigen binding to the development of rheumatoid arthritis. Given the lower degree of specificity but high affinity of peptide binding by MHC class II molecules, antigen "X" could be a set of similar peptides or one peptide distinguished by the presence of negative charges disposed in a manner to interact with the positive charged amino acids in the third diversity region of the DRβ chain. The consensus sequence presumably introduces a set of constraints on the nature of the peptides that could be bound by the susceptibility DR molecule requiring perhaps a critical sequence of negative, hydrophobic and negative charges to fit into the binding site. Of course, the critical event in antigen presentation need not be visualized as simply the presence or absence of a high affinity interaction between peptide and MHC molecule, but could equally well be a difference in orientation in which a peptide is bound.

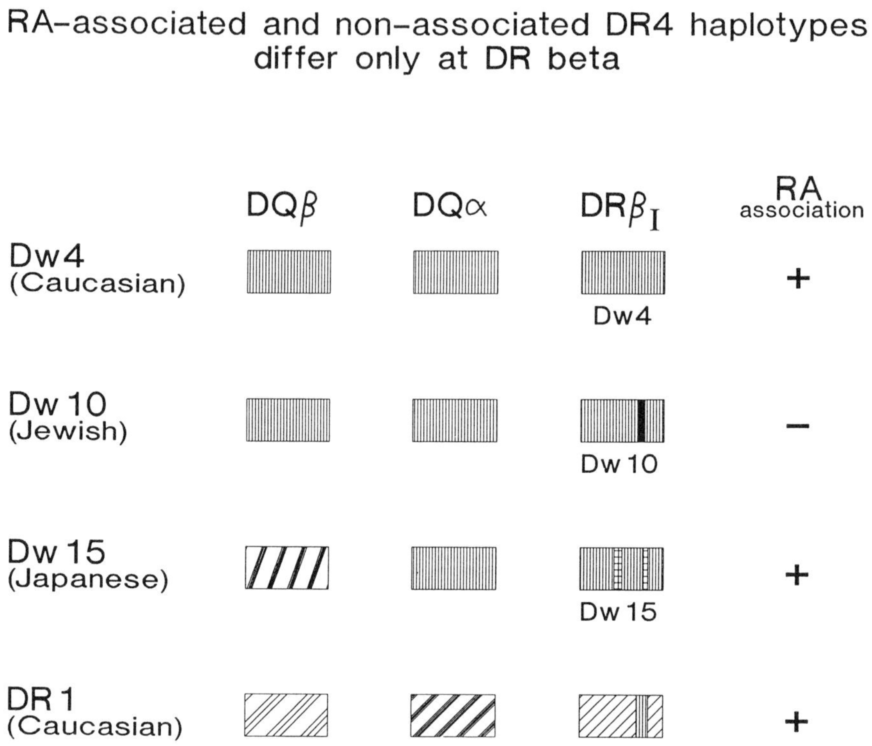

Figure 3. A "segregation" type analysis of susceptibility to rheumatoid arthritis using the presence or absence of an association between disease and structurally distinct haplotypes in different ethnic groups to map sequences likely to be responsible for disease predisposition.

While the absence of a dominant resistance effect such as is seen in insulin-dependent diabetes mellitus suggests a determinant selection model, the possibility of a primary effect on the T cell repertoire cannot be excluded. Here in this alternative view, the conformational equivalency of the third diversity regions would act as a selective conformation in constituting the T cell repertoire.

ACKNOWLEDGMENTS

This work was supported in part by NIH grants AI-19411 and AR-35404.

REFERENCES

1. Winchester, R.J. 1977. B-lymphocyte allo-antigens, cellular expression, and disease significance with special reference to rheumatoid arthritis. Arthritis Rheum. 20:159s.

2. Gibofsky, A., R. Winchester, J. Hansen, M. Patarroyo, B. Dupont, S. Paget, R. Lahita, J. Halper, M. Fotino, E. Yunis, and H.G. Kunkel. 1978. Contrasting patterns of newer histocom patibility determinants in patients with rheumatoid arthritis and systemic lupus erythematosus. Arthritis.Rheum. 21:S134-S138.

3. Stastny, P. 1978. Association of the B-cell alloantigen DRw4 with rheumatoid arthritis. N.Engl.J.Med. 298:869.

4. Gibofsky, A., R.J. Winchester, M. Patarroyo, M. Fotino, and H.G. Kunkel. 1978. Disease associations of the Ia-like human alloantigens. Contrasting patterns in rheumatoid arthritis and systemic lupus erythematosus. J.Exp.Med. 148:1728-1732.

5. Winchester, R., and H.G. Kunkel. 1979. The human Ia system. Adv.Immunol. 28:221-292.

6. Waters, F.J., R.J. Winchester, F. Nagase, and et al.. 1984. Antigen presentation by murine and human cells to a murine T cell hybridoma: Demonstration of a restriction element associated with an MHC class II determinant(s) shared by both species. Proc.Natl.Acad.Sci.USA 81:7559.

7. Toguchi, T., G.R. Burmester, A. Nuñez-Roldan, P. Gregersen, S. Seremetis, S. Lee, I.S. Szer, C.K. Hurley, and R.J. Winchester. 1984. Evidence for the separate molecular expression of four distinct polymorphic Ia epitopes on cells of DR4 homozygous individuals. Hum.Immunol. 10:69-81.

8. Lee, S.H., P.K. Gregersen, H.H. Shen, A. Nuñez-Roldan, J. Silver, and R.J. Winchester. 1984. Strong association of rheumatoid arthritis with the presence of a polymorphic Ia epitope defined by a monoclonal antibody: comparison with the allo-determinant DR4. Rheum.Int. 4:(Suppl):17.

9. Matsuyama, T., R. Winchester, S. Lee, L. Shookster, and A. Nuñez-Roldan. 1988. Identification of the DRw10 DRβ_1 chain allele as encoding a polymorphic class II MHC epitope otherwise restricted to DRβ_2 molecules of the DRw53 type. J.Immunol. 140:537-543.

10. Gregersen, P.K., M. Shen, Q.L. Song, P. Merryman, S. Degar, T. Seki, J. Maccari, D. Goldberg, H. Murphy, J. Schwenzer, C.Y.

Wang, R.J. Winchester, G.T. Nepom, and J. Silver. 1986. Molecular diversity of HLA-DR4 haplotypes. Proc.Natl.Acad.Sci.USA 83:2642-2646.

11. Merryman, P., R. Crapper, S. Lee, P.K. Gregersen, and R.J. Winchester. 1988. MHC class II gene sequences in rheumatoid arthritis: the third diversity regions of both DR $\beta 1$ genes in two DR1,DRw10 individuals specify the same inferred amino acid sequence as the DR $\beta 1$ and DR $\beta 2$ genes of a DR4 (Dw14) haplotype. Arthritis Rheum. 32:251-258.

12. Merryman, P., P.K. Gregersen, S. Lee, J. Silver, A. Nuñez-Roldan, R. Crapper, and R. Winchester. 1988. Nucleotide sequence of a DRw10 β chain cDNA clone; identity of the third D region with that of the DRw53 allele of the β_2 locus and as the probable site encoding a polymorphic MHC class II epitope. J.Immunol. 140:2447-2452.

13. Legrand, L., G.M. Lathrop, B.A. Marcelli, A. Dryll, T. Bardin, N. Debeyre, J.C. Poirier, M. Schmid, A. Ryckewaert, and J. Dausset. 1984. HLA DR genotype risks in seropositive rheumatoid arthritis. Am.J.Hum.Genet. 36:690.

14. Scherak, O., J.S. Smolen, and W.R. Mayr. 1983. HLA DR antigens and disease patterns of rheumatoid arthritis. Rheum.Int. 3:113.

15. Sacha, J.A., and J.R. Kirwan. 1986. Multiple HLA associations and disease susceptibility. Disease Markers 4:13-17.

16. Schiff, B., Y. Mizrachi, S. Orgad, and et al.. 1982. Association of HLA-Aw31 and HLA-DR1 with adult rheumatoid arthritis. Ann.Rheum.Dis. 41:403.

17. Nuñez-Roldan, A., J. Feld, S. Rodriguez de Cordoba, and R.J. Winchester. 1987. Occurrence of specific phytohaemagglutinin-reactive immunoglobulins in the sera of certain individuals. Relevance to the detection of cell surface antigens on phytohaemagglutinin-stimulated cells. Scand.J.Immunol. 25:139-147.

18. Woodrow, J.C., F.E. Nichol, and G. Zaviropoulos. 1981. DR antigens and rheumatoid arthritis: a study of two populations. Br.Med.J. 283:1287.

19. Groner, J.P., A.J. Watson, and F.H. Bach. 1983. Dw/LDrelated molecular polymorphism of DR4 β chains. J.Exp.Med. 157:1687.

20. Reinsmoen, N.L., and F.H. Bach. 1982. Five HLA-D clusters

associated with HLA-DR4. Hum.Immunol. 4:249.

21. Stastny, P. 1976. Mixed lymphocyte cultures in rheumatoid arthritis. J.Clin.Invest. 57:1148.

22. Nepom, G.T., C.E. Seyfried, S.L. Holbeck, K.R. Wilske, and B.S. Nepom. 1986. Identification of HLA-Dw14 genes in DR4+ rheumatoid arthritis. Lancet 2(8514):1002.

23. Zoschke, D., and M. Segall. 1986. Dw subtypes of DR4 in rheumatoid arthritis: evidence for a preferential association with Dw4. Hum.Immunol. 15:118-124.

24. Gregersen, P.K., J. Silver, and R.J. Winchester. 1987. The shared epitope hypothesis -- an approach to understanding the molecular genetics of rheumatoid arthritis susceptibility. Arthritis Rheum. 30:1205-1213.

25. Winchester, R.J., and P.K. Gregersen. 1988. The molecular basis of susceptibility to rheumatoid arthritis: the conformational equivalence hypothesis. Springer Semin.Immunopathol. 10:119-139.

26. Nepom, G.T., P. Byers, C. Seyfried, L.A. Healey, K.R. Wilske, D. Stage, and B.S. Nepom. 1989. HLA genes associated with rheumatoid arthritis. Arthritis Rheum. 32(1):15-21.

27. Ollier, W., D. Carthy, S. Cutbush, R. Okoye, J. Awad, A. Fielder, A. Silman, and H. Festenstein. 1988. HLA-DR4 associated Dw types in rheumatoid arthritis. Tissue Antigens 33:30-37.

28. Todd, J.A., J.J. Bell, and H.O. McDevitt. 1987. HLA DQ β gene contributes to susceptibility to insulin-dependent diabetes mellitus. Nature 329:599-604.

29. Bjorkman, P.J., M.A. Saper, B. Samraoui, W.S. Bennett, J.L. Strominger, and D.C. Wiley. 1988. Structure of the human class I histocompatibility antigen, HLA-A2. Nature 329 8 Oct:506-512.

30. Brown, J.H., T. Jardetzky, M.A. Saper, B. Samroui, P.J. Bjorkman, and D.C. Wiley. 1988. A hypothetical model of the foreign antigen binding site of class II histocompatibility molecules. Nature 332:845-850.

31. Winchester, R.J. 1989. The major histocompatibility complex. In Textbook of Rheumatology, 3rd ed. W.N. Kelley, E.D. Harris, S. Ruddy and C.B. Sledge, eds. W.B.Saunders Co., Philadelphia, P.101.

32. Gregersen, P.K., T. Moriuchi, R.W. Karr, F. Obata, J. Moriuchi, J. Maccari, D. Goldberg, R.J. Winchester, and J. Silver. 1986. Polymorphism of HLA-DR beta chains in DR4, -7, and -9 haplotypes: implications for the mechanisms of allelic variation. Proc.Natl.Acad.Sci.USA 83:9149-9153.

33. Gorski, J., and B. Mach. 1986. Polymorphism of human Ia antigens: gene conversion between two DR B loci results in a new HLA-D/DR specificity. Nature 322:67-70.

34. Bell, J.I., P. Estess, T. St. John, R. Saiki, D. Waitling, H.A. Erlich, and H.O. McDevitt. 1985. DNA sequence and characterization of human class II major histocompatibility complex β chains from the DR1 haplotype. Proc.Natl.Acad.Sci.USA 82:3405-3409.

35. Merryman P, Gregersen P, Matsuyama T, et al. Nucleotide sequence of MHC class II region genes in a patient with DR4 negative rheumatoid arthritis (RA) from a multiplex family; simulation of a DR4 haplotype by trans complementation of the HV III regions. Arthritis Rheum. 1987;30:4 (supplement):S31. (Abstract)

36. Winchester R, Gregersen PK. The molecular basis of susceptibility to rheumatoid arthritis: the conformational equivalence hypothesis. Springer Semin.Immunopathol. 1988;10:119-139.

IN VITRO MODEL SYSTEMS FOR THE STUDY OF THYROID AUTOIMMUNITY:

Regulation of rat MHC class II antigens*

T.F. Davies, W. Hirose, and D.S. Neufeld

Division of Endocrinology,
Department of Medicine,
Mount Sinai School of Medicine,
New York, New York

1. INTRODUCTION

Major histocompatibility (MHC) class I antigens are widely expressed in many types of cells while the MHC class II antigens have a more restricted degree of expression, principally within the immune system. In addition many non-immune cells can express MHC class II antigens when subjected to appropriate stimuli. A useful example is the thyroid gland which normally shows constitutive expression of MHC class I antigens on thyroid epithelial cells but an absence of MHC class II molecules (1). The original observation that MHC class II antigens are, however, expressed by many thyroid epithelial cells in glands from patients with autoimmune thyroid disease (2,3) has led to much

* Supported in part by grants DK28242 & DK35674 from NIDDKD.

Address all correspondence to: Dr. T.F. Davies, Box 1055, Mount Sinai Medical Center, 100th St & 5th Ave, New York, NY 10029.

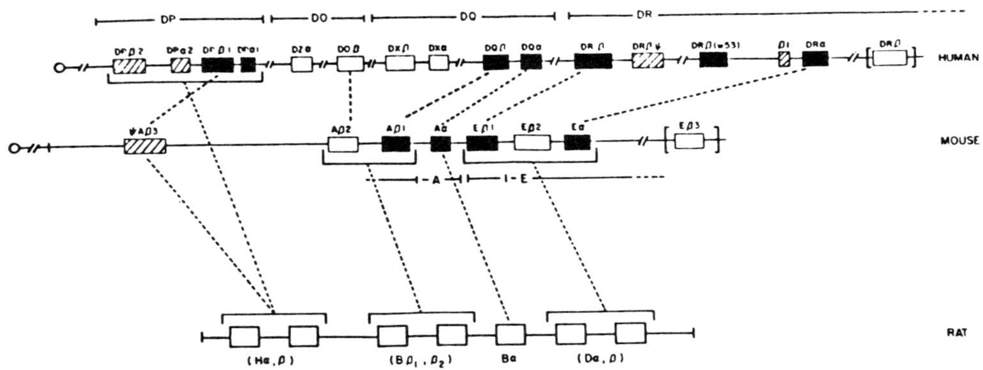

Figure 1. Equivalent class II genes in the human, mouse and rat MHC5.

speculation on the role and importance of such antigens in the initiation and potentiation of the diseases and a search for the important regulatory influences on such gene activation. Our own studies in this area indicate that HLA-DR, DP and DQ antigen expression is secondary to the lymphocytic infiltrate present in human autoimmune thyroid disease (1). More recently we have turned to more predictable in vitro model systems using the available proliferating rat thyroid cells, FRTL-5 and WRT (4,5) which have proven convenient systems for further exploring the cellular and molecular exploration of MHC class II antigen induction and its consequences. This brief paper reviews our studies on the regulation of rat thyroid cell MHC class II genes.

2. THE RAT MHC GENE REGION

The genomic mapping of the rat MHC gene region has only recently been undertaken and shows considerable homology to the murine MHC (6). There are three identified class II genes, RT1.H (which is not expressed), RT1.B and RT1.D all of which map close to the RT1.A (class 1) region (Figure 1). These genes code for antigen molecules consisting of two subunits designated alpha and beta which are part of the immunoglobulin supergene family. The genetic variation within animal populations at the MHC class II region is attributable to the amino acid sequence differences within the polymorphic beta chain of the class II antigens rather than very restricted polymorphisms exhibited by the alpha chains. In humans eight beta chain genes have been identified within the human haploid genome. In contrast, only five beta chain genes have been found in the rat MHC class II region of which only two appear to be commonly expressed.

3. PROLIFERATING RAT THYROID CELL LINES

Human thyroid cells show only limited proliferative potential in vitro (7). Although we have successfully immortalized human thyroid cells using transfection of the adenovirus E1A gene and also the cell fusion technique (8,9), these types of cells have not proven stable in the long term under our care. Hence the availability of proliferating rat thyroid cells lead us to consider their use in pursuing the mechanisms of thyroid cell MHC class II gene regulation. The Fisher rat thyroid line (FRTL-5) is a highly differentiated, immortalized, thyroid epithelial cell which is TSH dependent for growth. We have isolated a clone of the FRTL-5 cells, called 1B-6 (4) which has been subjected to detailed characterization studies (10). The Fisher rat, however, is known to be a poor model for autoimmune thyroiditis, showing no spontaneous thyroid abnormalities and poor responses to thyroid antigen immunization (11). In contrast, the Wistar rat is highly thyroid-antigen responsive and the recent availability of the Wistar rat thyroid cell line (WRT) (5) serves as as interesting contrast for immune studies with the 1B-6 cells. However, the WRT cell is not as dependent on TSH for growth as the FRTL-5 cells and IGF1 is able to maintain adequate proliferative rates.

4. RAT THYROID CELL MHC CLASS II ANTIGENS

A. The Fisher rat thyroid cell line

The Fisher rat 1B-6 clone exhibits many of the characteristics described for human thyroid monolayer cells with regard to MHC class II antigen induction. Rat class II gene transcription and translation showed sensitivity to recombinant rat, but not human, gamma interferon (IF), which was able to induce MHC class II antigen expression in 60-90% of proliferating cells (Figure 2). Furthermore, the effects of rat gamma IF could be mimicked with mitogen-stimulated rat spleen cell supernatants (10). Cells derived from the FRTL line have a unique dependence on TSH for cell growth and replication, while short term human thyroid cells show little (in the absence of serum) or no (in the presence of serum) in vitro growth, with TSH (7). There is growing evidence that proliferating cells from a variety of sources exhibit class II antigen expression during differentiation and may be more susceptible to lymphokine action than non-dividing cells. However, we have observed an anti-proliferative effect of gamma IF on rat thyroid cells at physiological concentrations of TSH (10μU/ml) was also observed but only at high concentrations (12).

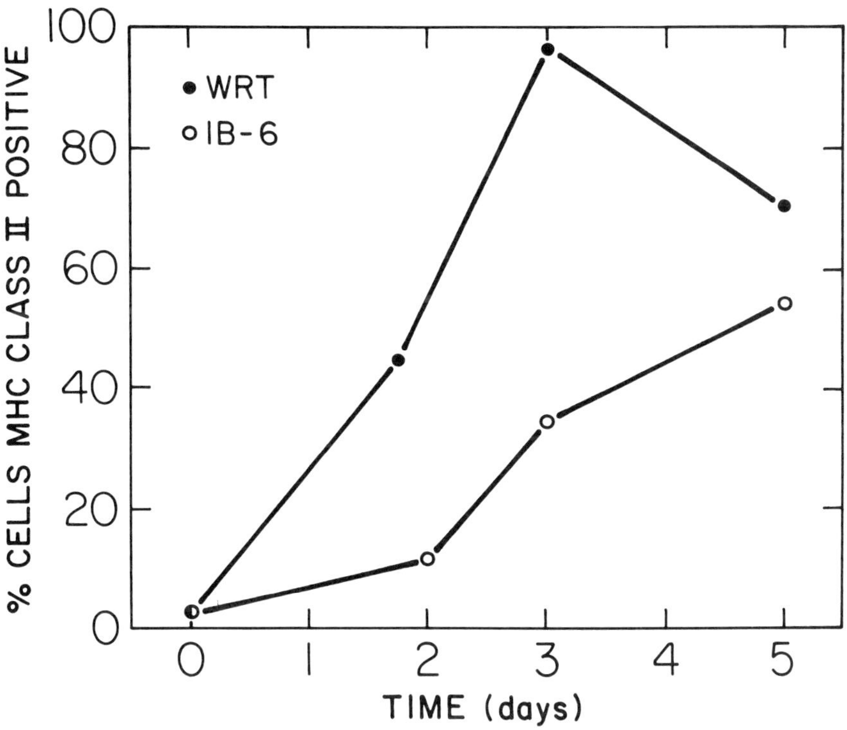

Figure 2. Comparison of WRT and 1B-6 rat thyroid cell responses to 100U/ml rat gamma interferon.

B. The Wistar rat thyroid cell line

The WRT cell has similar TSH receptor responses to TSH as the 1B-6 cell when assessed as cyclic AMP responsiveness. However, these cells have a reduced dependence on TSH for growth and proliferation. We have recently noted that the kinetics and sensitivity of the MHC class II antigen response to rat gamma IF are markedly different from the 1B-6 cells. The WRT cell shows both an earlier and greater MHC class II antigen response to gamma IF such that almost all cells are class II antigen positive 3 days after exposure to 100 U/ml gamma IF (Figure 2).

C. Studies on short-term preparations of rat thyroid monolayer cells

The marked contrast between the MHC class II responsiveness of the 1B-6 and WRT cells lead us to hypothesize that susceptibility to thyroiditis in the rat may be related to enhanced expression of thyroid cell MHC class II antigens. To further explore this possibility we compared a different rat strain, Buffallo, which is also highly responsive to thyroid antigen and has a considerable incidence of spontaneous thyroiditis, with the Fisher rat. In these experiments we utilized freshly prepared thyroid cell monolayers cultured in vitro with increasing concentrations of gamma IF (13). Similar results were obtained, with the Buffallo rat thyroid cell monolayers showing enhanced and earlier MHC class II antigen expression than the Fisher rat (Figure 3).

5. RAT THYROID MHC CLASS II (RT1.D) TRANSCRIPTS

In initial experiments we had utilized a probe to the HLA-DR non-polymorphic alpha chain region which cross-hybridized to the rat class II transcripts. Using this probe, we were unable to detect basal transcription of the class II alpha chains in rat thyroid cells even when cultured in the presence of bovine TSH (10). We, therefore, extended our analysis of MHC class II gene expression in the rat by preparing an homologous probe for the RT1.D alpha chain transcripts (14). This rat cDNA probe is considerably more sensitive (at least

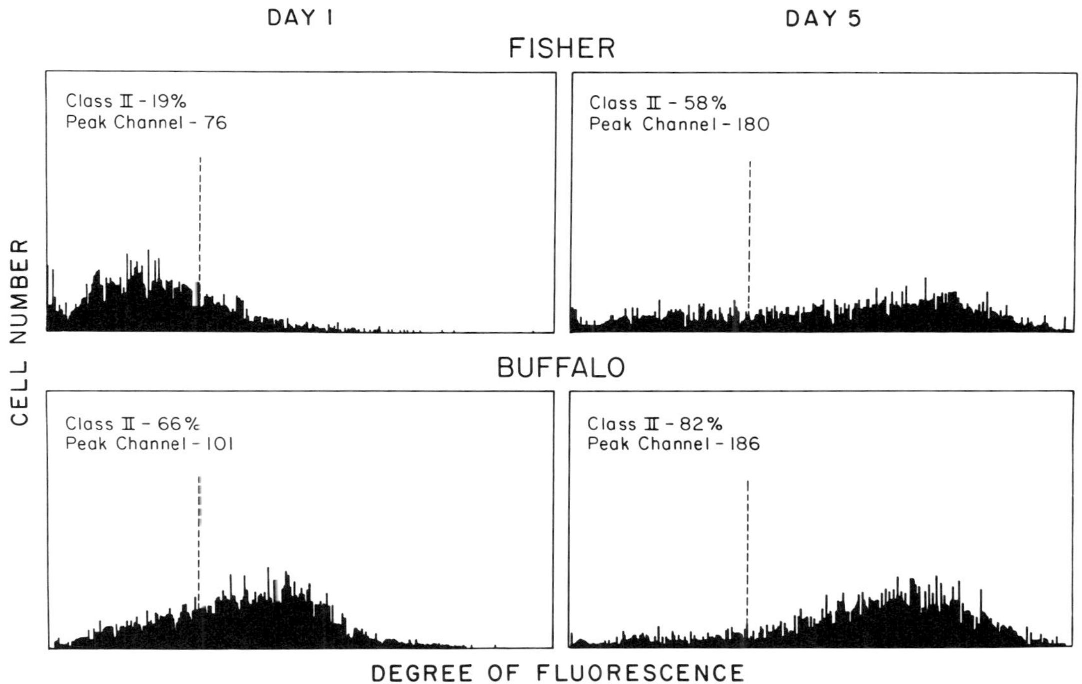

Figure 3. Comparison of flow cytometric analyses of rat thyroid cell MHC class II antigens after exposure to 100U/ml rat gamma interferon. Data from Fisher (upper) and Buffalo (lower) thyroid monolayer cells are shown.

100-fold) than the human probe. Despite this increased sensitivity, we have found no constitutive MHC class II transcription in the 1B-6 or WRT cell cultures during the proliferative (with TSH) and non-proliferative (without TSH) parts of the growth cycle. Hence, these data are consistent with our earlier observations on unstimulated human thyroid monolayers, where both basal and induced induction of class II transcripts were inhibited by antibody to gamma IF (15). In the human thyroid cell model, contaminating lymphocytes in primary thyroid cell cultures are the likely source of gamma IF responsible for low basal class II transcript levels. In the cloned rat thyroid cells, where no such lymphocyte contamination exists, no basal class II transcripts can be detected.

Some diversity of the MHC gene response to gamma IF has been found among cells although in general both mRNA and protein levels increase. Kinetic studies indicated that the rat thyroid class II alpha mRNA was detectable much earlier than antigen, as soon as 4 hours, and continues to rise under gamma IF stimulation. We found that the rat RT1.D beta2 gene and the RT1.D alpha gene were equally sensitive to gamma IF. However, antigen expression peaks by day 3 although the mRNA transcript levels continue to increase. Some of this incongruity may be due to our failure to adequately assess intensity of antigen expression on the thyroidcell surface and deserves further study.

6. T CELL INTERACTION WITH RAT THYROID CELLS

To determine whether MHC class II positive thyrocytes can be recognized by MHC restricted T cells, we utilized our clone of rat thyroid cells (1B-6) to express MHC class II antigens in response to recombinant rat gamma IF. $CD4^+$ and $CD8^+$ normal syngeneic Fisher rat spleen T cells were selected by flow cytometry and averaged >96% purity. We demonstrated that irradiated MHC class II positive 1B-6 thyrocytes, but not class II negative 1B-6 thyrocytes, stimulated $CD4^+$ T cells in a primary sensititzation reaction over 4 days. In contrast, $CD8^+$ T cells had no response in similar experiments. This stimulation of $CD4^+$ T cells was dose-dependent for 1B-6 thyrocytes and was abrogated by monoclonal anti-rat MHC class II antibody

(MRC OX-6). Autoreactive (Fisher) and alloreactive (Buffalo) T cell lines, and isolated CD4$^+$ T cells derived from these lines, which were developed against Fisher rat spleen cells, similarly recognized MHC class II antigens expressed on 1B-6 cells but had no detectable response to 1B-6 MHC class II negative thyrocytes or MHC class II positive human thyroid cells.

Hence, using our cloned rat thyrocytes (1B-6), we have been able to demonstrate that MHC class II positive thyroid cells can function as stimulators of T cells in syngeneic mixed cell reactions in a similar way to lymphocytes reacting within classical MLRs. The results support our previous human data and imply that MHC class II positive thyrocytes can serve as potent activators of T cells within the thyroid and have the potential to act as antigen-presenting cells. Once T cells are activated, they will secrete lymphokines, including gamma IF, which will perpetuate thyrocyte class II antigen expression. It is likely, of course, that activated T cells themselves initiate this cycle rather than the thyrocyte and our recent production of Fisher rat T cell clones which are thyroglobulin specific should help clarify this situation (16).

In contrast to our data, murine T cell unresponsiveness to MHC class II positive murine thyrocytes has been reported (17). Although these investigators used responder lymph node cells from mice immunized with Tg and tried to observe the specific antigen-presenting capacity of MHC class II positive thyrocytes in a syngeneic system, they failed to detect any stimulatory effects. Such data led them to deny a primary role for thyrocytes in the inductive phase of thyroiditis even though they were unable to demonstrate T cell activation by MHC class II positive thyroid monolayer cells. Our results are in disagreement with such data and support our previous observations in human thyroid/T cell co-cultures which have also been confirmed by other investigators (18).

7. VIRAL INITITATION OF MHC CLASS II ANTIGEN EXPRESSION

The initiating events in autoimmune thyroid disease are unknown. While it seems most likely that thyroid reactive T cells are important, the initiation of thyroid cell MHC class II antigen expression appears to be intimately linked to their propagation, perhaps by enhancing thyroid antigen presentation. In order to examine the possibility that a viral infection of thyroid cells may be involved in the primary event we have used both adenovirus and reovirus infection of our 1B-6 cells. Reovirus types 1 and 3 caused a dose-dependent induction of thyroid cell MHC class II antigen expression as determined by laser flow cytometry and FITC-labelled anti-RT1.B. As the number of viral particles/cell used for the infections increased up to 100, the number of antigen positive cells increased to 50% (19). Reovirus infection *in vivo* induces multiple autoimmune endocrine gland disease in rodents and our experiments demonstrated that reovirus may initiate rodent thyroid cell MHC class II gene expression *in vitro*. Type 1 reovirus infection also leads to production of autoantibodies that react with antigens in the pancreatic islets, the anterior pituitary, gastric mucosa and the thyroid (20). Similar, but less dramatic, data were generated with adenovirus infections. These experiments demonstrate that perhaps many viruses have the potential to initiate MHC class II antigen expression in cultured thyroid cells. Such expression may attract thyroid antigen-specific and non-specific T cells to the intrathyroidal environment and initiate thyroiditis in susceptible animals and humans with appropriate T cell and B cell clones.

REFERENCES

1. Davies, T.F. and Piccinini, L.A. (1987) Endocrinology and Metabolism Clinics of North America 16,247.
2. Hanafusa, T., Chiovato, L., Doniach, D., Pujol-Borrell, R., Russell, R.C.G. and Bottazzo, G.F. (1983) Lancet 2,1111.
3. Bottazzo, G.F., Pujol-Borrell, R. and Hanafusa, T. (1983) Lancet 2,1115.
4. Davies, T.F., Yang, C. and Platzer, M. (1987) Endocrinology 121,78.
5. Brandi, M.L., Rotella, C.M., Mavilia, C., Franceschelli, F., Tanini, A., Toccafondi, R. (1987) Molecular and Cellular Endocrinology 54,91.

6. Diamond, A.G., Hood, L.E., Howard, J. C., Windle, M., Winoto, A. (1989) Journal of Immunology 142,3268.
7. Huber, G.K., and Davies, T.F. (1989) (submitted for publication).
8. Cone, R.D., Platzer, M., Piccinini, L.A., Jaramillo, M., and Davies, T.F. (1988) Endocrinology 123:2067.
9. Martin, A., Platzer, M. and Davies, T.F. (1988) Molecular and Cellular Endocrinology 60:233.
10. Platzer, M., Neufeld, D.S., Piccinini, L.A., and Davies, T.F. (1987) Endocrinology 121:691.
11. Hirose, W., Lahat, N., Platzer, M., Schmitt, S. and Davies, T.F. (1988) Journal of Immunology 141,1098.
12. Graves, P., Neufeld, D.S., and Davies, T.F. (1989) Molecular and Cellular Endocrinology 3:758.
13. Lahat, N., Hirose, W., Davies, T.F. (1989) Endocrinology 124:1754.
14. Neufeld, D.S. and Davies, T.F. (1988) Molecular Endocrinology 2,507.
15. Piccinini, L.A., Mackenzie, W.A., Platzer, M. and Davies, T.F. (1987) Journal of Clinical Endocrinology and Metabolism 64,543.
16. Hirose, W. and Davies, T.F. (1988) Immunology 64,107.
17. Ebner, S.A., Stein, M.E., Minami, M., Dorf, M.E. and Stadecker, M.J. (1987) Journal of Immunology 104,154.
18. Matsunuga, M.K., Eguchi, K., Fakuda, T., Kurata, A., Tezuka, C., Shimomura, C., Otsubo, T., Ishikawa, N., Ito, K. and Nagataki, S. (1986) Journal of Clinical Endocrinology and Metabolism 62,723.
19. Neufeld, D.S., Platzer, M. and Davies, T.F. (1988) Endocrinology 124,543.
20. Onodera, T., Toniolo, A., Ray, U.R., Jenson, A.B., Knazek, R.A. and Notkins, A.L. (1981) Journal of Experimental Medicine 153,1457.

THE MOLECULAR BASIS OF MHC ASSOCIATION WITH DISEASE

Nadir R. Farid

Thyroid Research Laboratory
Health Sciences Centre
Memorial University of Newfoundland
St. John's, Newfoundland, AlB 3V6
Canada

The discovery that some endocrine disorders were associated with HLA alleles emphasized the genetic basis of these disease (1,2). Soon, diseases with an autoimmune basis were found to be primarily associated with MHC Class II alleles (1,2). It was, nevertheless, clear that not every person carrying a particular Class II allele would develop the disease. A substantial proportion of patients with a particular disease carry other Class II alleles and up to 30% normal control may also possess the Class II alleles in question. Explanations offered for the less than complete association between marker and disease include: disease heterogeneity, involvement of genes in linkage disequilibrium with the typable marker or "splits" of the marker alleles, with only subsets being related to the disease as well as the involvement of other factors, both genetic and environmental, in disease the emergence of disease phenotypes (3).

While better definition of disease subsets based on clinical and laboratory features have resulted in stronger association of a Class II allele with a disease subset, most diseases have remained relatively homogeneous. Advances in serology, cell-typing, identification of MHC II subsets by extended haplotypes, restriction fragment (RFLPs) polymorphism and nucleotide sequencing have allowed for stronger disease associations (2).

Genes other than MHC are involved in liability

to autoimmune endocrine disorders. These genes often interact with the MHC in influencing liability. Disease is then also only expressed in the "appropriate" environmental setting (4). The issue of polygenic nature of the endocrine autoimmune disorders will not be discussed here.

MHC CLASS II ANTIGENS

The MHC is by far the most polymorphic genetic system known. This polymorphism apparently arose by repeated gene duplication which generated multiple loci, and by repeated mutation and gene conversion, which produced at least 100 multiple alleles. There are, thus, more than a 100 (recognized) different allele products for Class I and Class II MHC molecules derived from six or more sets of closely linked loci. The number of possible combinations of these genes on a single chromosome are between 5,000 and 10,000. Given that each person has two haplotypes and that most people are heterozygous, it is clear that the number of possible genotypes runs into the millions. Population variation is, therefore, extra-ordinarily large. The MHC is also characterized by the non-random association (linkage disequilibrium) of alleles at different loci separated, in some instances, by substantial genetic distances (5).

Class II molecules (DR, DP and DQ in man, and I-A and I-E in mouse) are made up of two polypeptide chains, a 34,000 dalton A chain and a 28,000 dalton B chain (5,6). Recently, crystallographic studies have shown that two alpha helices of class I molecules form a cleft to serve as a peptide-binding site (7). A similar structure has been proposed for the class II molecules (8). The importance of MHC class II molecules is that they act as antigen-presenting molecules to Th cells (5,6) and they are involved in determining the T cell repertoire by a positive or negative selection process in the thymus (9-11). Class II antigens are expressed in a tissue-restricted manner, i.e., they are expressed constitutively in B cells, activated macrophages and thymic epithelial cells (6). Seemingly, whether a T cell is positively or negatively selected is determined by interaction respectively in thymic medulla or cortex and is related to different conformations of Class II molecules (12). Class II molecules can also be expressed in a number of cells which are normally surface antigen negative. The cells include pancreatic islet cells and thyroid epithelial cells (6). It is proposed that MHC molecules, especially the class II molecules, may present as autoantigens in certain circumstances, leading to autoimmune tissue damage (13).

In humans the class II genes are located within the HLA-D region which spans about 1100 kilobases of the short arm of chromosome 6. The HLA-D region contains three subregions, DP, DQ and Dr. The polymorphism in the D region was defined by mixed leukocyte reaction (Dw), primed lymphocyte typing (DP), and serologically by microcytotoxicity using alloantisera and monoclonal antibodies (DR and DQ). More recently, Class II polymorphism was refined by analysis of restriction fragment length polymorphisms (RFLP) and by direct gene sequencing. The DR region consists of 3 DR B genes and one DR A gene. The polymorphic DR B1 and non-polymorphic DR A gene products associate to form a heterodimeric glycoprotein on the cell surface which reacts with the alloantisera that define the HLA-DR1 through DRw14 specificities. DR BII is a pseudogene. The relatively nonpolymorphic DR BIII and DR A gene products encode DRw52 and DRw53 determinants (5,14).

The DQ locus consists of one A and one B gene; their products were detected serologically. The DQ antigens are associated with groups of DR antigen because of linkage disequilibrium between these loci. There are so far four DQ serological specificities (DQw1, DQw2, DQw3, and DQ blank). RFLP and DNA sequencing of DQA and B chains have, however, greatly extended the number of antigens coded for in this genetic region (14).

The DP (formerly SB) antigens were identified by primed lymphocyte typing or monoclonal antibodies. The DP locus consists of two A and two B genes, one set of which are pseudogenes. Currently, six DP antigens have been defined (DPwl-DPw6). No association have been found between DP antigens and DR or DQ antigens. Bugawan et al. (15) recently demonstrated that the degree of polymorphism of the DP region is more extensive. The DP B chain determines all the polymorphic epitopes recognized by primed T cells. DPA genes are less polymorphic than DPB genes.

Analysis of class II molecules at the DNA level provides more specific information about the structural basis of serological epitopes or those recognized by T cells. For example, there are at least seven distinct haplotypes which share the HLA-DR4 serologic specificity. Nucleotide sequencing of cDNA and genomic DNA of a number of DR and DQ genes have indicated limited differences in the hypervariable region between alleles of the same broad specificity (micropolymorphism) (14,16-20). Such microheterogeneity also exists within the DPw4 and DP blank specificities (15). This is important because different DR-associated diseases are related to different specific allelic variants of DR and DQ genes.

Recent studies indicate that much of Class I and Class II polymorphism had arisen before mammalian speciation (21,22). The relative stability of MHC polymorphism indicates that hypermutational mechanisms are not necessary to account for Class I and Class II gene diversity and presumably function.

Class II gene structure and autoimmunity

The conviction that MHC Class II genes are the basis of the immune response led some laboratories to sequence class II genes and mutants thereof in the mouse. It was found that Class II polymorphism was localized to three areas in the first domain of I-A and I-E and that deletion of certain residues was associated with the abrogation of the immune response to some antigens but not others (23). With this as background, a similar effort was made to sequence human DRA and B and DQ, A and B chain genes. These efforts were recently greatly aided by the application of the polymerase chain reaction (PCR) in amplifying domains of these genes harboring polymorphism (14, 16-20). Polymorphic residues were also found to aggregate in certain domains of the DRA, DQA and B genes (14). When cDNA sequences derived from lymphocytes of patients with given HLA- associated disorders were compared with those of their counterparts derived from controls, no structural differences were seen, indicating that disease is not associated with mutant Class II alleles (14). Disease liability may be based on shared residues or epitopes among susceptibility alleles.

We will examine two scenarios which have emerged from these investigations. First, a discovery that DR alleles (DR1 and DR4-Dw4, Dw14, Dw15), found to be associated with rheumatoid arthritis are almost identical in residues 67 to 74 of the BI chain of DR (14,24). The fact that residues are also identical in the DR BIII chain of DRw53 may suggest that an additional class II domain may be involved in R.A. liability (14,25). This subject will be expanded upon in the chapter by Dr. R. Winchester (24). The other scenario is that of the negative association of DQ alleles carrying Asp at position 57 of DQB with type I diabetes (16). Whether positive association of rheumatoid arthritis with DR BI and the negative association of DQ B with type 1 diabetes reflect the fact that these two loci direct different subsets of T cells (helper and suppressors, respectively) remains to be seen. In the meanwhile, it is proposed that the negative association of IDDM with DQB Asp 57 is by way of deletion of the T cell receptor chain which recognize that specificity (16). While how the absence of this residue predispose to diabetes has not been considered, it is conceivable that the presence of ser, Ala Val at BQ 57 may positing select for T cell receptors which recognize beta cell antigens. It is also possible that haplotype-specific alternative splicing of DQ genes recently described by Briata et al (26) as opposed or in addition to micropolymorphism might contribute to disease liability. Alternative splicing of class II genes is not restricted to DR molecules.

Recent structural observation cast new light on the potential role of the residue at DQB 57 in immune recognition and immune responsiveness. First, using site- specific mutagenesis Kwok et al (27) found that monoclonals which recognize DQw 3.2 (DQw 8) no longer do so if DQ B position 45 was mutated. Of course, the dependence of monoclonal antibody on presence of glycine at DQB 45 may only reflect the fact that monoclonal recognize a different epitope from that seen by T cells, crucial to disease pathogenesis. It would be of interest to compare the effect of mutations at position DQB 57 versus 46 in their ability to bind peptides known to be restricted by DQw 8. Second, perusal of class II B chain sequences in sub-human primates showed the same distribution of residues at position 57 as that described for DQ B. It has been suggested selection of the position 57 residues forms a part of a balanced polymorphism (Asp on the one hand; Val, Ala, Ser on the other)(28). This also implies a basic role for these two types of polymorphism in the folding of class II beta chain and class II function; its association with type I diabetes may be coincidental.

A finding concerning the negative association between DQB asp 57 and IDDM in particular has raised a number of interesting issues. The proposal that MHC-linked liability to IDDM is related to homozygozity at DQB Asp-negative allele does not conform with the greatly increased risk for HLA-DR3/DR4 heterozygotes compared to homozygote DR3 or DR4 nor with the observation that liability in DR4 (non-DR3) patients is close to dominant and that in DR3 (non-DR4) patients is close to recessive (29). A similar situation pertains to HLA-DR4, DQw8/DRw8, DQw4 heterozygotes who are at much higher risk for IDDM compared to those carrying only one of the two haplotypes (30). DQ alpha/beta chain transcomplementation was proposed as a potential mechanism for the generation of crucial restriction molecules (30). The fact that DQw2 on a DR7 haplotype is Asp negative but carried no risk for IDDM (31) lead the authors to invoke a contribution of DQ A chain in IDDM liability. Interestingly, DQ A polymorphism turns out to be important to IDDM liability in the Blacks (32). The observation that the influence of DQB Asp 57 negative on IDDM liability is not independent of that of DR4- Dw10 and vice versa (33) also suggest strongly that more of the haplotype than DQ B chain may be necessary for the liability to IDDM. Moreover, while the Asp

57 negative status in the DQ B equivalent chain is maintained in the NOD mouse (15,16), it is not so in the diabetes prone BB rat (34). This important finding may imply that in the rat (as in some human populations) other class II domains may be important to diabetes liability or that the immune regulated dysfunction paramount in the rat in the genesis of islet-cell damage.

ASSOCIATION OF MULTIPLE MHC CLASS II ALLELES WITH THE SAME ANTIGEN

Apparent association of several HLA-DR alleles with an autoimmune disease may be due to their linkage disequilibrium with a DQ allele or to the sharing of sequential residues on the B chain. The reported association of Hashimoto's thyroiditis with HLA-DR5, DR4 and DR3 cannot seemingly be explained by the two above mechanism. The fact that in some population HLA-DR5 was found to be increased in a 1979 study and HLA-DR4 was, instead, associated with the disease in new patient cohorts studied 5 years later incriminates differences in triggering environmental factors (see 35). If this is indeed the case, then remaining the influence of the DR allele associated with the disease, the influence of an allele incriminated in another Caucasian population should become apparent. HLA-DR3 is associated with Hashimoto's thyroiditis in Eastern Hungary; when the influence of DR3 is removed a significant increase in DR4. On the other hand, DR4 and DR5 act as alternate susceptibility factors i.e. when one is increased in a population of patients with thyroiditis the other is reduced. Interestingly, the highest risk with Hashimoto's thyroiditis (35) was noted with DRw53 (O.R. = 7.51, $P < 1 \times 10^{-6}$) in the study showing an association with DR4: As DR3 and DR5 are in linkage disequilibrium with DRw52, one can either conclude that DRw53 is not the relevant restricting element or that DRw52 and DRw53, may lead to Hashimoto's thyroiditis by independent mechanisms. Alternate explanations include shared residues on DRB I chains, DQA chains or DQB chains in linkage disequilibrium with DR3, 4 & 5. Table 1 shows that the first proposal is unlikely. It cannot be discounted that the association may be accounted for by polymorphism at the DP B chain. A very striking multiple allele association is that presented by malaria antigens, overlapping residues of which are recognized by the majority of DR alleles.

ENVIRONMENTAL INFLUENCES

The association of differentiated epithelial thyroid cancer with MHC Class II may be used to introduce the influence of the environment in disease liability. The evidence for our arguments, it has to be stressed, is circumstantial. Thyroid epithelial cancers are associated with HLA DR1 in iodide deficient areas and show no association whatsoever in iodide sufficient areas. An association with DR7 was found in iodide sufficient areas where other environmental factors were incriminated. While the "environmental" influence may be different to prove, it might be feasible to explore how iodide deficiency would cause a transformation of thyroid cells from a given MHC phenotype versus that of another (35).

This issue has not been closely scrutinized in the past except in the case of drug-induced autoimmune disorders (37,38). We feel that it may be relevant in understanding molecular basis of association of endocrine disorder with MHC alleles.

ARE MHC HAPLOTYPES RELEVANT TO DISEASE LIABILITY

Graves' disease is one of a few DR3 associated disorders in which there is a high prevalence of the haplotype A1, C_, B8, C4AQO, C4B3, DQ2 in Graves' disease (50% of DR3 positives in one study) as compared to controls. This observation is remarkable in that haplotype extends over 3,000 Kb and must have been preserved with little recombination over a considerable period of time. The association is specific for Graves' disease (39). When Hashimoto's thyroiditis is associated with DR3 no consistent extended haplotypes are observed (35). To what measure MHC class I alleles, complement alleles and tumor necrosis factors alpha and beta carried on DR3 haplotype contribute to disease liability and progression remains to be seen. In the meanwhile, a report indicating that TNF alpha production is greater in DR3 positive patients with SLE is of interest in this context (40). It is unlikely that they would account for Graves' hyperthyroidism being associated with thyroid stimulation.

In several other disorders, identification of extended haplotypes has aided in identifying class II subtypes more closely associated with the disease as compared to the broad specificity (41). The same argument as forwarded for Graves' disease for potential influence of haplotype components. In no other disorder, however, are extended haplotypes as frequent as in Graves' disease.

In conclusion, even in the most restricted association of MHC alleles with disease it is clear that there is interaction between DR B1 and DQ B as well as DQ A in contributing to disease liability. Whether this reflects positive susceptibility contributed by DR as opposed to deletion of T cell receptor chains in the thymus imposed by DQ is unclear.

TABLE 1

A.A. residue of DRB1 in antigens incriminated in Hashimoto's thyroiditis

	57	60	61	67	70	7L	74	77	78
DR3	D	Y	W	L	Q	K	R	M	Y
DR4.W4		"	"	L	Q	K	A	T	Y
DR5	"	"	"	F	D	R	A	T	Y
DR52	"	"	"	L	Q	K	O	M	Y
DR53	"	"	"	L	R	R	E	T	Y

REFERENCES

1. Svejgaard, A., Platz, P., and Ryder, L.R. (1983). Immunol. Rev. 70, 193.
2. Farid, N.R. (Editor) "Immunogenetics of Endocrine Disorders". Alan R. Liss Inc., New York, 1988.
3. Farid, N.R., Bear, J.C. (1983). In "Autoimmune Endocrine Disorders" (T.F. Davies, ed.) p. 59. John Wiley & Sons, New York.
4. Farid, N.R. (1987). Endocrine Metab. Clin. N. Amer. 16, 229-245.
5. Degos, L. (1988). In "Immunogenetics of Endocrine Disorders" (N.R. Farid, ed.) p. 1. Alan R. Liss Inc., New York.
6. Mach, B. (1988). In "Immunogenetics of Endocrine Disorders" (N.R. Farid, ed.) p.49. Alan R. Liss Inc., New York.
7. Bjorkman, P.J., Saper, M.A., Samraoui, B., Bennet, W.S., Strominger, J.L., Wiley, D.C. (1987). Nature 329, 512.
8. Brown, J.H., Jardetzky, T. Saper, M.A., Samraoui, B., Bjorkman, P.J., Wiley, D.C. (1988). Nature 332, 845.
9. Pullen, A.M., Marrack, P., Kappler, J.W. (1988). Nature 335, 796.
10. Kisielow, P., Teh, H.S. Bluthmann, H., van Boehmer, H. (1988). Nature 335, 730.
11. Sha, W.C., Nelson, C.A., Newberry, R.D., Kranz, D.M. Russell, J.H., Loh, D.Y. (1988). Nature 336, 73.
12. Murphy, D.B., Lo, D., Rath, S., Brinster, R.L., Flakell, R.A., Slatez, A. and Janeway, Jr. C.A. (1989). Nature 338, 765-768.
13. Pujol-Borrell, R., Todd, I., Londei, M., Foulis, A., Feldmann, M. Bottazzo, G.F. (1986). Mol. Biol. Bed. 3, 159.
14. Todd, J.A., Acha-Orbea, H., Bell, J.I., Chao, N,, Fronek, Z., Jacob, C.O., McDermott, M., Sinha, A.A., Timmerman, L., Steinman, L., McDevitt, H.O. (1988). Science 240 1003.
15. Bugwan, T.L., Horn, G.T., Long, C.L., Mickelson, E., Hansen, J.A., Ferrara, G.B., Angelini, G. and Erlich, H.A. (1988), J. Immunol. 141, 4024.

16. Todd, J.A., Bell, J.I., McDevitt, H.O. (1987) Nature. 329, 599.
17. Hardy, D.A., Bell, J.I., Long, E.O., Lindstem, T., McDevitt, H.O. (1986), 323, 453.
18. Bell, J.I., Denney, J.R., D., Foster, L., Belt, T., Todd, J.A., McDevitt, H.O. (1987) Proc. Nat. Acad. Sci. 84, 4591.
19. Lee, B.S.M., Rust, N.A., McMichael, A.J., McDevitt, H.O. (1987), PNAS, 84, 4591.
20. Gregerson, P.K., Moriuchiu, T., Karr, R.W., et al. (1986). 335, 265.
21. Figueroa, F., Gunther, E., Klein, J. (1988), 335, 268.
22. Lalor, D.A., Ward, F.E., Ennis, P.D., Jackson, A.P., Pardiam, P. (1988). 85, 6012.
23. Mengle-Gaw L. and McDevitt, H.O. (1985). Ann. Rev. Immunol. 3, 367.
24. Winchester, R. (1988) This volumne.
25. Scharf, S.J., Freidmann, A., Brautbar, C., Szafer, F., Steinman, L., Horn, G., Gyllensten, U. and Erlich, H.A. (1988) Proc. Nat. Acad. Sci. USA 85, 3504.
26. Briata, P., Radka, S., Sartoris, S. and Lee, J.S. (1989). Proc. Nat. Acad. Sci. USA 86, 1003.
27. Kwok, W.W., Lotshaw, C., Milner, E.C., Knotter-Jack, N. and Nepom, G.T. (1989). Proc. Nat. Acad. Sci. USA. 86, 1027.
28. Erlich, H.A., (1989). Nature, 337, 4151.
29. Thomson, G., Robinson, W.P., Kuhner, M.K., Joe, S., MacDonald, M.J., Gottschall, J., Barbosa, J., Rich, S.S., Bertrams, J., Baur, M.P., Partanen, J.I., TAit, B.I.D., Schober, E., Mayr, W.M., Ludvingsson, J., Lindblom, B., Farid, N.R. (1988). Am. J. Hum. Genet. 43, 799.
30. Ronningen, K.S., Markussen, G., Iwe, T., Thorsby, E. (1989). Human Immunol. 24, 165.
31. Klitz, W. (1988). Nature, 333, 402.
32. Todd, J.A. Mijovic, C.,Fletcher, J. Jenkins, D., Bradwell, A.R., Barnett, A.H. (1989) Nature 338, 587.
33. Sheehy, M.J., Rowe, J.R., Nepom. (1988). Abstract, Diabetes [suppl.] 37, 1,91A.
34. Holowachu, E.W., Greer, M.K. (1989) Diabetes 38, 267.
35. Farid, N.R. and Balazs, C. (1988). In

"Immunogenetics of Endocrine Disorders", (N.R. Farid, ed.) Allan R. Liss Inc., New York, p. 267.

36. Sinigaglia, F., Guttinger, M., Kilgus, J., Doran, D.M., Matile, H., Etlinger, H., Trzeciak, A., Gillessen, D., Pink, J.R.L. (1988). Nature 336 778.
37. Batchelor, J.R., Welsh, K.I., Tinoco, M., Dollery, C.T., Hughes, G.R.V., Bernstein, R., Ryan, P., Naish, P.F., Aber, G.M., Bing, R.F., Russell, G.I. (1980). Lancet i, 1107-1109.
38. Speirs, C, Fielder, A.H.L., Chapel, H., Davey, N.J. and Batchelor, J.R. (1989). Lancet i, 922.
39. Farid, N.R. and Stenszky, V. (1988), in "Immunogenetics of Endocrine Disorders" (N.R. Farid, ed.) Alan R. Liss, Inc., New York, p.223.
40. Jacobs, C.O., Fronek, Z. and McDevitt, H.O. (1980). Clinical Research 37, 412A.
41. Dawkins, R.L., Christiansen, F.T., Kay, P.H., Garlepp, M.J., McCluskey, J., Hollingsworth, P.H., Zilko, P.J. (1983). Immunol. Rev. 70, 5.

BASIC ROLE FOR ANTI-IDIOTYPE AUTOANTIBODIES IN THE PREVENTION OF EXPERIMENTAL AUTOIMMUNE THYROIDITIS

C. Bédin, C. Roubaty,* B. Texier, H. Tang, M.A. Franco,* J. Charreire

INSERM U. 283, Hôpital Cochin, 75674 Paris Cedex 14 France

1. INTRODUCTION

The goal of therapy in autoimmune diseases is to develop potent tools to exert specific control of the immune response to self antigen (S-Ag). Anti-idiotype autoantibodies (anti-id) may provide such specific immunomodulators since the relevance of the id network in autoimmunity is well documented. If autoimmune disease is the pathological expression of an immune response to S-Ags and if interactions between id and anti-id are crucial for the regulation of the immune responses to S-Ags, then it follows from the network theory (Jerne, 1974) that the regulation of the immune response to S-Ag could play a basic role in autoimmune reactivity.

On this basis, we investigated whether modulating an id network could interfere with the production of experimental autoimmune thyroiditis (EAT). To precisely answer this question, we had previously defined each parameter of an idiotypic network: the A-Ag, the B cells producing A-Ag specific Ab1 and Ab2, and a cytotoxic T cell hybridoma clone specific for this A-Ag.

In our model, the A-Ag is a small tryptic fragment (TF) of the porcine Tg (PTg) molecule which induces EAT when injected into susceptible strains of mice (Salamero et al., 1987a). We also produced monoclonal anti-Tg auto-Abs able to recognize this TF and to block the proliferative response of TF specific helper T cells (Salamero et al., 1987b). Lastly, we selected two anti-id A-Abs, one of which recognizes the

The Molecular Aspects of Autoimmunity

Ag binding site of one m anti-Tg A-Ab specific for the PTg TF (Charreire, 1989).

Because in EAT cytotoxic T cells play a major role in the thyroid gland damage (Creemers et al., 1983 ; Salamero and Charreire, 1985), we selected cytotoxic T cell hybridomas recognizing the TF of the Tg molecule normally expressed on murine TEC (Remy et al., in press).

With these T or B cells, both specific to the 5-10 Kd pathogenic TF from the Tg molecule inducing EAT, we studied the mechanisms of murine EAT protection using a T cell vaccination strategy.

2. T CELL VACCINATION

T cell vaccination was performed using a protocol similar to that previously described by Maron et al. (1983). Briefly, mice were inoculated 21 days before Tg challenge with one million mitomycin-attenuated T cell clone HTC2 (H-2^k) or with the fusion partner, BW 5147 (H-2^k), as a control. Then mice were immunized s.c. with 50 µg porcine Tg (PTg) emulsified in complete Freund's adjuvant (day 0) and boosted on day 14, with the same amounts of PTg in incomplete Freund's adjuvant. These experiments were conducted in H-2^k, EAT-susceptible CBA strain of mice (Vladutiu and Rose, 1971). Each experimental group included 5-8 mice 6-8 weeks old. The animals were killed 28 days after Tg challenge.

Histological studies show 76% reduction of lymphocytic infiltration in the thyroid glands of animals inoculated exclusively with HTC2 cells. Moreover, considering the incidence and the mean grade of EAT, it appears that in mice receiving HTC2 cells, the severity of the disease was markedly decreased: no animals presenting acute or severe EAT were observed. In contrast, such animals were predominant in the two control groups of mice (Table I).

3. ANTIBODY RESPONSES

Autoantibody (A-Ab) responses were analyzed on day 0, three weeks after HTC2 cell inoculation and on day 28, after Tg challenge when EAT is in the acute phase (Table II). An enzyme-linked immunoassay (ELISA) was used for their quantification. Briefly, murine sera diluted 1/250, 1/500 and 1/1000 were deposited for 2 hours at room temperature in 96-well polyvinyl microplates previously coated with 50 µg

PTg and saturated with 1% bovine serum albumin in phosphate buffered saline. Binding of alkaline phosphatase-conjugated goat anti-mouse (GAM) IgG was detected using p-nitrophenyl phosphate disodium as the substrate.

On day 28, high levels of A-Abs to Tg were found in each group of mice immunized with Tg, independent of the nature of the T cell hybridoma inoculated on day - 21. In contrast, on day 0 before Tg challenge, only mice receiving HTC2 cells developed an anti-Tg A-Ab response which represented approximately 65% of the post-immunization maximum immune response. We define this unexpected Tg-specific response as Ab3 A-Abs because these mice never came into contact with Tg in the past and the two control groups of mice, naive or BW-inoculated, did not mount any anti-Tg response.

Table I. Prevention of EAT by clonotype-specific T cell clone vaccination

Tg challenge	T cell clone inoculated	EAT: Incidence	EAT: Grade No. of mice	EAT: Infiltration index ± SEM (relative EAT %)
-	None	0/5	acute / 0 severe / 0 mild / 0 negative/ 5	0.40 ± 0.04 (-)
+	None	8/8	acute / 7 severe / 1 mild / 0 negative/ 0	4.20 ± 0.40 (100)
+	BW 5147	8/8	acute / 3 severe / 3 mild / 2 negative/ 0	3.10 ± 0.30 (76)
+	HTC2	3/8	acute / 0 severe / 0 mild / 3 negative/ 0	1.00 ± 0.23 (24)

Table II. Anti-Tg A-Abs in sera (diluted 1:1000) from CBA mice vaccinated with Tg specific T cell clone (mean ± SEM of 5-8 sera)

Cell injected[a]	After Tg challenge (D = 28)	Prior to Tg challenge (D = 0)
None	1126[b] ± 63	N.D.[c]
BW 5147	1132 ± 109	N.D.
HTC2	1142 ± 97	756 ± 47 (66.2)[d]

[a] 1 x 10^6 mitomycin inactivated cells were injected s.c. on day -21 before Tg challenge.
[b] Optical density at 405 nm.
[c] N.D. = not detectable.
[d] Percentage of D28 response.

To further establish that the anti-Tg A-Abs detected on day 0 were Ab3 in exclusively HTC2-inoculated mice, we analyzed the ability of these A-Abs to bind the two anti-id A-Abs (Ab2) directed against the anti-Tg A-Abs specific for the pathogenic epitope (Table III). An ELISA was performed as described above for anti-Tg A-Abs. Anti-id A-Abs were determined in sera diluted twice from 1:125 to 1:1000 on plates coated with 3 µg of F(ab')2 fragment from anti-id A-Abs. Then a peroxidase conjugated GAM IgG (anti-Fc) was added, before binding was detected using O-phenylendiamine as the substrate. As predicted by our previous results, only sera from mice inoculated with HTC2 cells and producing anti-Tg A-Abs were able to bind to m alpha or beta Ab2 A-Abs.

4. SPECIFICITIES OF ANTIIDIOTYPIC ANTIBODIES

The detection of anti-Tg A-Abs on day 0 before Tg challenge led us to look for anti-anti-Tg A-Abs in mouse sera both before and after nominal Ag challenge. We then attempted to define their fine specificities using their ability to bind F(ab')2 from polyclonal and from two m anti-Tg A-Abs. An ELISA was performed in technical conditions identical to those reported on Table III.

Table III. Anti- anti-idiotype A-Abs (day 0) in CBA mice sera (diluted 1:250) vaccinated with Tg specific T cell clone (mean ± SEM of 5-8 sera)

Cell injected	Nature of the F(ab')2 anti-id A-Abs coated	
	Ab2 alpha	Ab2 beta
None	0[a]	0
BW	0	0
HTC2	212 ± 28	256 ± 18

[a] Optical density at 492 nm.

Anti-id A-Abs directed against polyclonal or non pathogenic related m anti-Tg A-Abs were detected at similar levels in the three groups of mice studied prior to Tg challenge. These Abs have been described as natural Abs directed against public cross-reactive idiotypes (Zanetti *et al*., 1983; Male *et al*., 1985). The only striking difference we found concerns the response in mice inoculated with HTC2. Whereas control animals, naive or BW-injected, show background levels of anti-id A-Abs towards anti-Tg A-Abs specific for the pathogenic epitope of the PTg molecule, HTC2-injected animals exhibit an 200% increase in the level of these Abs (Table IV).

Study of the same responses on day 28 post-challenge still shows no significant differences in anti-id A-Abs responses towards polyclonal anti-Tg A-Abs or towards a non pathogenic epitope related m anti-Tg A-Ab. Moreover, it must be noted that their levels are not modified by the Tg immunization procedure. The only variations we detected were those of anti-id A-Abs to the anti-Tg A-Ab specific for the pathogenic epitope of the PTg molecule. Whereas these anti-id A-Abs were maximum in the two control groups of mice, they were greatly decreased in animals inoculated with HTC2 cells, reaching a level near that of the background detected in naive mouse sera (Table IV).

Table IV. Levels of anti-id A-Abs to various anti-Tg A-Abs in preimmune (D = 0) and immune (D = 28) sera[a] from mice vaccinated with Tg specific T cell clone (mean ± SEM of 5-8 determinations)

F(ab')2 from anti-Tg A-Abs coated	Cell injected	Before immunization (D = 0)	After immunization (D = 28)
Polyclonal anti-Tg A-Abs	None	1112 ± 102[b] (108.8[c])	1128 ± 127 (102.5)
	BW	1022 ± 86 (100.0)	1157 ± 110 (100.0)
	HTC2	988 ± 74 (96.6)	1032 ± 91 (89.1)
Pathogenic epitope related m anti-Tg A-Ab	None	431 ± 56 (105.3)	1456 ± 215 (123.2)
	BW	409 ± 43 (100.0)	1181 ± 106 (100.0)
	HTC2	826 ± 63 (191.6)	602 ± 54 (50.9)
Non-pathogenic epitope related m anti-Tg A-Ab	None	1227 ± 97 (118.6)	1297 ± 120 (91.0)
	BW	1034 ± 112 (100.0)	1181 ± 87 (100.0)
	HTC2	925 ± 105 (75.4)	909 ± 73 (76.9)

[a] Sera dilutions 1:250.
[b] Optical density at 492 nm.
[c] Percentage of A-Abs response in mice sera from animals injected with BW cells.

5. DISCUSSION

In the last few years, a role for anti-id has been sought in the prevention of several experimentally induced autoimmune diseases: autoimmune thyroiditis (Maron et al., 1983), encephalomyelitis (EAE) (Ben-Nun et al., 1981; Sun et al., 1988; Lider et al., 1988; Ellerman et al., 1988), collagen arthritis (Kakimoto et al., 1988; Arita et al., 1987), uveoretinitis (De Kozak, 1987), myasthenia gravis (Agius et al., 1986). Protection was effected using antigen-specific T cell lines or specific anti-id Abs.

We now describe, in a fully syngeneic system, the protective immunity against EAT induced exclusively by a Tg-specific cytotoxic T cell clone. This down regulation occurs through the generation of anti-id A-Abs (Ab2 beta) which recognize the paratope of a monoclonal anti-Tg specific to the pathogenic epitope of the Tg molecule. We further analyze the various steps of the antibody responses (Ab1, Ab2 and Ab3) in terms of poly-, mono- and auto-specificities defined by the pathogenic epitope of the Tg molecule or by the idiotope of the related antibodies recognized. The levels of these immunoreactants correlate with the incidence of EAT.

These experiments support Jerne's hypothesis of an EAT regulation pathway operating through the idiotypic network. The mechanism involves the generation of Ab2 A-Abs and their Ab3 A-Abs specific to the Tg epitope responsible for EAT. Probably, the Tg complementary structure of the T cell receptor borne by HTC2 cells generates A-Abs bearing the internal image of the nominal antigen, structurally similar to the anti-idiotypic Ab2 beta A-Abs. However, an alternative hypothesis is tenable. Cytotoxic T cells specific to syngeneic murine thyroid epithelial cells (TEC) can migrate specifically towards the thyroid gland, lyse TEC and consequently liberate syngeneic autologous Tg. In that pathway, anti-Tg A-Abs detected on day 0 prior to Tg challenge would be conventional anti-Tg A-Abs.

In our experiments, protection against EAT is mainly due to both the presence of pathogenic epitope specific to anti-Tg A-Abs and their Ab2 beta at the time of immunization by Tg. More precisely, these anti-Tg A-Abs block the pathogenic epitope(s) of the Tg molecule which cannot further stimulate specific T cells whereas anti-id A-Abs can also block the pathogenic epitope specific to B cells. Moreover, it can also be imagined that anti-id A-Abs, Ab2 beta, bind to specific helper T cell receptors and consequently inhibit their A-Ag recognition. It must be noted that the anti-Tg A-Ab response detected in HTC2 inoculated mice on day 0 prior to Tg challenge cannot be due to Tg borne by HTC2 cells because following hybridization these cells were propagated *in vitro* in the absence of nominal antigen.

In contrast to Zanetti et al. (1986) who found a decrease of A-Abs to Tg in mice immunized with isologous m anti-Tg A-Abs, we do not find a perturbation of anti-Tg A-Abs on day 28 post-immunization in mice inoculated with HTC2. This discrepancy could be due to both the fact that the m anti-Tg A-Ab that they used for their immunization had no evident

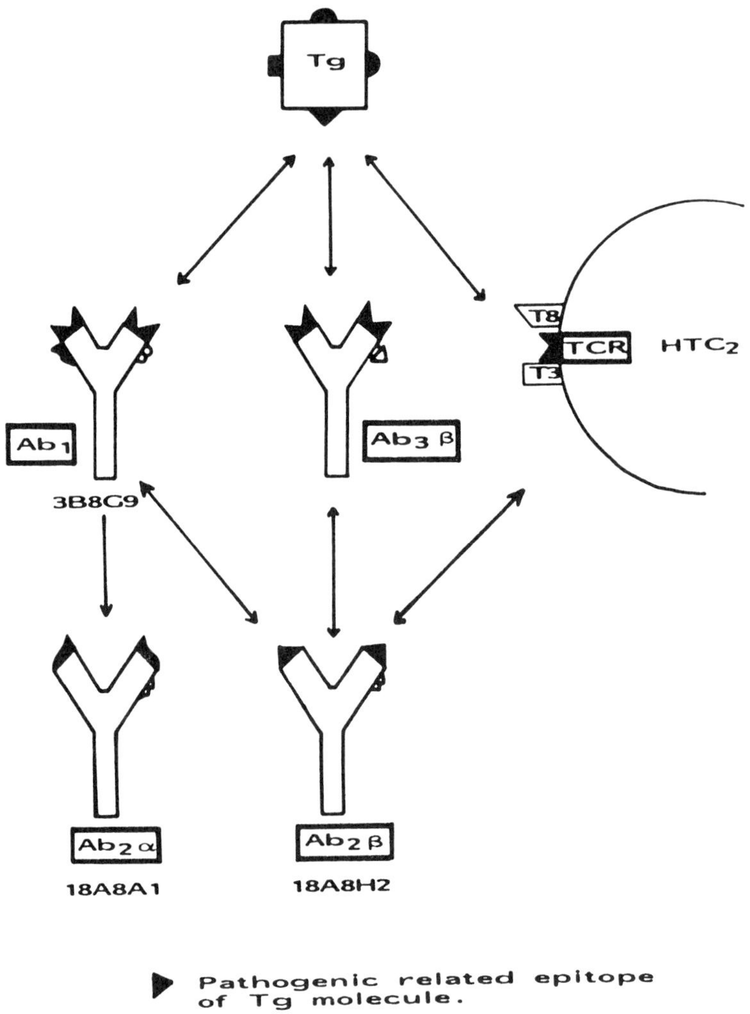

Fig. 1. Idiotypic network in EAT.

relationship with the pathogenic part of the Tg molecule and that they did not look for a correlation with the disease.

On the other hand, our results show that the main level of regulation of EAT is located at the anti-id A-Abs (beta A-Abs) as defined by Jerne et al. (1982). More precisely, Ab2 beta Abs are able to bind to the B cell producing Abl as well as to the T cell specific to Tg and represent the internal image of the nominal antigen; therefore it recognizes the paratope of the m anti-Tg A-Ab specific to the pathogenic epitope of the Tg molecule (Figure 1). This major role for Ab2 beta Ab is further evidenced by their correlation with the incidence of EAT. In the acute phase of EAT, mice exhibit maximum levels of Ab2 beta, whereas in naive or vaccinated mice, only background levels are detected.

Two principle observations result from this work: there is a link between the humoral and cellular Tg specific immune responses which could occur through idiotypic interactions and there is a correlation between anti-id A-Abs (beta Abs) and the incidence of EAT. Prior to this, no correlation between anti-Tg A-Abs (Abl) and the incidence or progression of EAT was observed (Polley et al., 1988; Okayasu, 1985). However, by virtue of the sensitivity of our experimental design, we are confident that such a correlation exists, allows new insight into the pathogenesis of EAT and suggests new pathways for modulating the disease.

ACKNOWLEDGMENTS

We wish to thank Ms. Eliette Lallemand and Mr. Jean-Louis Olivier for their technical assistance and Mrs. Jocelyne Decaix for typing of the manuscript and designing the figure.

REFERENCES

Agius, M., and Richman, D.P. (1986). J. Immunol. 137, 2195.

Arita, C., Kaibara, N., Jingushi, S., Takagishi, K., Hotokebuchi, T., and Arai, K. (1987). Clin. Immunol. Immunopathol. 43, 374.

Ben-Nun, A., Wekerle, H., and Cohen, I.R. (1981). Nature 292, 60.

Charreire, J. (1989). Adv. Immunol., in press.

De Kozak, Y., Mirshahi, M., Boucheix, C., and Faure, J.P. (1987). Eur. J. Immunol. 17, 541.
Ellerman, K.E., Powers, J.M., and Brostoff, S.W. (1988). Nature 331, 265.
Jerne, N.K. (1974). Ann. Immunol. Inst. Pasteur (Paris) 125C, 373.
Jerne, N.K., Roland, J., and Cazenave, P.A. (1982). EMBO J. 1, 243.
Kakimoto, K., Katsuki, M., Hirofuji, T., Iwata, H., and Koga, T. (1988). J. Immunol. 140, 78.
Lider, O., Reshef, T., Beraud, E., Ben-Nun, A., and Cohen, I.R. (1988). Science 239, 181.
Male, D., Pryce, G., and Roitt, I. (1985). Mol. Immunol. 22, 255.
Maron, R., Zerubavel, R., Friedman, A., and Cohen, I.R. (1983). J. Immunol. 131, 2316.
Okayasu, I. (1985). Clin. Immunol. Immunopathol. 36, 101.
Polley, C.R., Bacon, L.D., and Rose, N.R. (1981). J. Immunol. 127, 1465.
Remy, J.J., Texier, B., Chiocchia, G., and Charreire, J. (1989). J. Immunol. 142, in press.
Salamero, J., Remy, J.J., Michel-Béchet, M., and Charreire, J. (1987a). Eur. J. Immunol. 17, 843.
Salamero, J., Remy, J.J., and Charreire, J. (1987b). Clin. Immunol. Immunopathol. 43, 34.
Sun, D., Qin, Y., Chluba, J., Epplen, J.T., and Wekerle, H. (1988). Nature 332, 843.
Vladutiu, A.O., and Rose, N.R. (1971). Science 174, 1137.
Zanetti, M., Barton, R.W., and Bigazzi, P. (1983). Cell. Immunol. 75, 292.
Zanetti, M., Glotz, D., and Rogers, J. (1986). J. Immunol. 137, 3140.

FOOTNOTES

* C. Roubaty: Post-doctoral fellow of the Swiss National Foundation for Research.

* M.A. Franco: Fellowship of the National Institute for Health and Medical Research (INSERM).

This work was supported in part by a grant from the Fondation pour la Recherche Médicale, 54, rue de Varenne, 75007 Paris, France, and from the Association pour la Recherche sur le Cancer, Villejuif, France.

Index

A

Acetylcholine receptor, epibodies in immune response to, *see* Epibodies, acetylcholine receptor
AChR
  characteristics of epibodies from immune response to, 140–144
  V region similarities, 149–150
Alleles
  ethnic differences in structure of MHC class II alleles, 251, 253–254
  multiple MHC class II, with same antigen, 283–284
α–β heterodynamics complex, stable, evidence, 221–223
Amino acid sequences of immunoglobulin heavy and light chains, 147–149
Animal models, use of to study viruses
  congenital rubella syndrome, 232–233
  reovirus, 235–236
  retrovirus, 233–235
Antibodies, V genes encoding, structural characteristics, 16–24
Anti-BrMRBC antibodies, VH segment encoding, 98–99
Anti-BrMRBC hybridomas, VH nucleotide sequences, 95–95
Anti-BrMRBC VH repertoire, 101
Anti-DNA antibodies, human
  diversity gene usage, 68–70
  genetic diversity of VH and VL genes used, 61–64
  germline VH genes in IgM, 65
  preferential VH gene utilization, 64–65
  relatedness of VH subregions, 65–68
Anti-DNA idiotypic recurrence, 74–76
Anti-histone H1 autoantibodies
  detection, 162–163
  idiotypes, 167–171
  production, 161–162
  specificities, 163–167
Anti-idiotype autoantibodies in prevention of experimental autoimmune thyroiditis, 292–294, *see also* Experimental autoimmune thyroiditis
Anti-self-related genes, molecular configuration, 79–83
Anti-Sm antibodies, interspecies idiotypes
  discussion, 157–158
  SLE definition, 155–156
  SLE and interspecies Id expression, 156–157
Autoantibodies
  genetic origin, 107–108
  genetic restriction among, 119–120
  see also Murine lupus-associated humoral anti-self response
Autoantibodies, anti-histone, H1, *see* Anti-histone H1 autoantibodies
Autoantibodies, germline genes, preimmune repertoire, 83–85
Autoantibodies, human IgM, *see* Human IgM autoantibodies, structural characteristics
Autoantibodies, V gene families, 13–16
Autoantibody producing cells, VK family gene utilization, 78–79
Autoantibody-specific genetic elements, 116–119
Autoimmune murine models, genomic and expressed TCR repertoire, *see* T-cell antigen receptor repertoire
Autoimmune type I diabetes, *see* Diabetes, autoimmune type I
Autoreactive T cell clones, 184

B

B-cell compartments, establishment of different, 127
B-cell repertoires, V-region complementarities mediating selection, 125–126
BrMRBC hybridomas, VH nucleotide sequences, 94–95
  JH segment of anti-BrMRBC hybridomas, 95
BrMRBC VH-encoding DNA fragment, hybridization of genomic DNA with, 99–101

C

Cα and Cβ genes, 195–196
CDR1 and CDR2 abrogate Id expression, point mutations, 135
CDR2 and Id expression, mutations,125–126
Cis-acting regions, identification, 222–223
Class II antigens, MHC, 278–280
Class II gene structure and autoimmunity, MHC, 280–283
Class II genes, organization of, 251, 252
Class II molecule, structure of, 246–251
CMV, *see* Cytomegalovirus
Complementarity-determining region, *see* CDR
Congenital rubella syndrome (CRS)
  in animal models, 232–233
  in humans, 236
Conformational equivalence hypothesis, and mapping susceptibility to rheumatoid arthritis
  introduction to, 242–251
  association with classic HLA specificities, 243–246
  DR β chain gene, mapping, 254–256
  DR 1, relation, 256
  ethnic differences in structure of MHC class II alleles, 251, 253–254
  inferences, 256–259
  organization of class II genes, 251, 252
  structure of class II molecule, 246–251
CRS, *see* Congenital rubella syndrome
Cytomegalovirus (CMV), in humans, 236–237

D

Diabetes, autoimmune type I, viruses triggering
  animal models
    congenital rubella syndrome, 232–233
    reovirus, 235–236
    retrovirus, 233–235
  characterization of, 231–232
  conclusions, 237
  human system
    congenital rubella syndrome, 236
  cytomegalovirus, 236–237
  mumps, 237
DNA-binding specificity, structural basis for
  diversity gene usage in anti-DNA antibodies, 68–70
  relatedness of VH subregions of anti-DNA antibodies, 65–68
DNA-protein interactions, analysis, 223–224
DR β chain gene, mapping, 254–256

E

EAT, *see* Experimental autoimmune thyroiditis
Epibodies, in immune response to acetylcholine receptor
  characteristics, 140–144
    binding data, 142
  competitive binding assays with, 144
    origins and specificities, 141
    specificity, 143–144
  involvement of in immune response, 144–145
    function, 144
  recognition, molecular basis, 145–152
  role, 139–140
  summary and perspectives, 152–153
Ethnic groups, HLA-DR4 and susceptibility to RA in, 243–246, *see also* Rheumatoid arthritis
Experimental autoimmune thyroiditis (EAT), anti-idiotype autoantibodies in preventing
  antibody responses, 290–292
  discussion, 294–297
  goal of therapy, 289–290
  specificities, 292–294
  T cell vaccination, 290
Expressed TCR repertoire in autoimmune models, 199–212
  genomic impositions on TCR V β gene expression, 202
  multiprobe TCR RNAse protection assay, 199–202
  origin of *lpr* and *gld* cells, 208–212
  tolerance- or negative selection-related TCR V beta repertoire modifications, 203–208

F

Fisher rat thyroid cell lines, 268–269

G

Gene diversity and T-cell maturation, 190–194
Gene families, variable, *see* LY-1 and immunoglobulin variable gene families in hybridomas, expression
Genomic complexity of VK families, studies, 10

Genomic DNA with BrMRBC VH-encoding DNA fragment, 99–101
Genomic impositions on TCR V β gene expression, 202
Genomic TCR repertoire in autoimmune murine models
  genomic impositions on TCR V β gene expression, 202
    multiprobe TCR V beta RNAse protection assay, 199–202
    origin of *lpr* and *gld* cells, 208–212
    tolerance- or negative selection-related TCR V β repertoire modification, 203–208
Germline genes, autoantibodies, preimmune repertoire, 83–85
Germline TCR α and β genes, 194–199
  C α and C β genes, 195–196
  V α haplotype, 196–199
  V β haplotype, 196
Germ-line VH genes in IgM anti-DNA antibodies, 65
gld and *lpr* cells, origin, 208–212

H

Haplotype, relevancy to disease liability, 284–285
H chain, independent expression of Id62 on, 132–133
H1 autoantibodies, anti-histone, *see* Anti-histone H1 autoantibodies
HGG, *see* Human gamma globulin
Histone H1 molecule, representation of, 166–167, *see also* Anti-histone H1 autoantibodies
HIV-1 enhancer, 224–225
HLA specificities, disease association of rheumatoid arthritis with, 243–246, *see also* Rheumatoid Arthritis
HTLV-1, TNF alpha and tax protein, 226–227
Human anti-DNA antibody-associated 16/6 CRI, basis of, 51–52
Human autoantibodies, *see* Molecular characteristics of human anti-DNA antibodies; Molecular genetics of human autoantibodies
Human gamma globulin (HGG)
  induction of tolerance, 176–177
  tolerance in HGG-specific T cell clones, 183
  tolerance to *in vivo*, 177–181
Human IgM autoantibodies, structural characteristics
  characterization, 29–30
  conclusions, 37
  materials and methods, 30
  results and discussion
    serological idiotypy, 33–35
    somatic mutation, 35–36
    specificity, 32–33
    structural similarities, 30–32
    switching, 36–37
Human interleukin 2 receptor, structure of, *see* Interleukin 2 receptor, human
Humkv 325 gene, identification and characterization of, 42–45
Humkv 328 gene, identification and characterization of, 45–49
  immunochemical studies, 41–42
Hybridomas, LY-1 and immunoglobulin variable gene families in, *see* LY-1 and immunoglobulin variable gene families in hybridomas, expression

I

Id62 on H chain, independent expression, 132–133
Idiotope mapping by site-directed mutagenesis, 133–136
  mutations in CDR2 and Id expression, 125–126
  point mutations in CDR1 and CDR2 abrogate Id expression, 135
Idiotypes of anti-histone H1 autoantibodies, 167–171, *see also* Anti-histone H1 autoantibodies
Ig gene segments encoding autoantibodies
  autoantibody-specific genetic elements, 116–119
  genetic restriction among auto-antibodies, 119–120
Ig germline genes
  Ig heavy chain gene loci, 108–110
  Ig kappa light chain loci, 110–115
Ig variable region genes, diversification, *see* Lupus anti-DNA antibodies, idiotypic expression of
Igh-V families with VCP12, comparison of nucleic acid sequences from, 98
Immune response, to acetylcholine receptors, *see* Epibodies in immune response to acetylcholine receptor
  possible involvement of epibodies, 144–145

Immunoglobulin variable gene families and LY-1, *see* LY-1 and immunoglobulin variable gene families in hybridomas, expression
In vitro model systems for study of thyroid autoimmunity, *see* Thyroid autoimmunity, in vitro model systems for study
Interleukin 2 receptor, structure and biochemical basis
  regulation, 222–227
  structure, 220–223
  summary, 227

J

JK2 or JK4 joining segment, association of same VK9 gene with, 96–97

K

Kinetics of binding to IL-2R α and IL-2R β subunits, contrasting, 220–221
Kinetics of HGG-induced unresponsiveness and involvement of T-suppressor lymphocytes, 179

L

Lpr and *gld* cells, origin, 208–212
  tolerance- or negative selection-related TCR V β repertoire modifications, 203–208
Lupus Anti-DNA antibodies, idiotypic expression of
  anti-DNA idiotypic recurrence, 74–76
  autoantibodies, germline genes, preimmune repertoire, 83–85
  molecular configuration of anti-self-related genes, 79–83
  SLE history, 73–74
  VK family gene utilization in autoantibody producing cells, 78–79
  VK locus in human lupus, 76–78
LY-1 and immunoglobulin variable gene families in hybridomas, expression
  expression, 3–9
  history, 1–3
  V gene families in autoantibodies, expression, 13–16
  V gene utilization by murine B lymphocytes, 9–13
  V genes encoding antibodies, structural characteristics, 16–24
Lymph node T cells, proliferation, 178
Lymphocyte population dynamics, observation of characteristics, 125–126

M

Major histocompatibility (MHC) class I antigens, description, 265–267, *see also* MHC
MHC association with disease, molecular basis
  class II antigens, 278–280
  class II gene structure and autoimmunity, 280–283
  definitions, 277–278
  environmental influences, 284
  haplotype, relevancy to disease liability, 284–285
  multiple MHC class II alleles with same antigen, 283–284
MHC class II alleles, ethnic differences in structure, 251, 253–254
MHC class II molecules encoded by different alleles, mapping susceptibility to RA into conformationally equivalent region, *see* Rheumatoid arthritis, mapping susceptibility
Molecular basis of MHC association with disease, *see* MHC association with disease, molecular basis
Molecular characteristics of human anti-DNA antibodies
  structural basis for DNA-binding specificity, 65–68
    diversity gene usage in anti-DNA antibodies, 68–70
    relatedness of VH subregions of anti-DNA antibodies, 65–68
  studies of, 59–60
  summary, 70–71
  variable region genes encoding
    genetic diversity of VH and VL genes, 61–64
    germ-line VH genes in IgM anti-DNA antibodies, 65
    preferential VH gene utilization and anti-DNA antibodies, 64–65
Molecular genetics of human autoantibodies, discussion, 52–55
  human anti-DNA antibody-associated 16/6 CRI, basis of, 51–52
  humkv 325 gene, identification and characterization of, 42–45

humkv 328 gene, identification and characterization of, 45–49
immunochemical studies, 41–42
Vh gene for human rheumatoid factors, defining, 49–51
Molecular mechanisms of T cell unresponsiveness, 183–184
Multiple affinity forms, and IL-2 receptor, 220
Multiprobe TCR RNAse protection assay, 199–202
Mumps virus, in humans 237
Murine autoantibodies specific for bromelinized red blood cells
autoimmune phenomena, 92–93
discussion, 101–103
materials and methods, 93
results, 94–101
variable regions, nucleotide sequences, 91
Murine B lymphocytes, V gene utilization, 9–13
Murine lupus-associated humoral anti-self response, molecular analysis
conclusions, 120–121
Ig gene segments encoding autoantibodies
autoantibody-specific genetic elements, 116–119
genetic restriction among autoantibodies, 119–120
Ig germline genes
Ig heavy chain gene loci, 108–110
Ig kappa light chain loci, 110–115
origins, 107–108

N

Nucleic acid sequences from known Igh-V tamilies with VCP12, 98
Nucleotide and amino acid sequences
of autoantibodies light chain V regions, comparison of with corresponding germline genes or consensus sequences, 21, 23
of autoantibody heavy chain variable regions, comparison of with corresponding germline genes, 21, 22
Nucleotide sequencing, origin and specificity of autoantibodies subsequently analyzed by, 19, 20

P

Phorbol esters, sequence requirements for activations, 226–227
Polymerase chain reaction (PCR), application of in amplifying domains of genes, 280–281
Preimmune repertoire, germline genes, autoantibodies, preimmune repertoire, 83–85
Protein-protein interactions mediated by regions of homology, 150–152
Proteins specifically binding, characterizations, 225–226

R

RA, *see* Rheumatoid arthritis
Rat MHC gene region, 267
Rat thyroid cell lines, 267–268
Rat thyroid cell MHC class II antigens
Fisher rat thyroid cell lines, 268–269
short-term preparations of rat thyroid monolayer cells, 270
Wistar rat thyroid cell line, 270
Rat thyroid MHC class II (RT1.D) transcripts, 270–272
Rat thyroid monolayer cells, short-term preparations of rat thyroid monolayer cells, 270
Regulatory idiotope by antibody engineering, characterization
discussion, 136–137
idiotope mapping by site-directed mutagenesis, 133–136
independent expression of Id62 on H chain, 132–133
primary sequence data, 130–132
studies on, 129–130
Reovirus, in animal models, 235–236
Retrovirus, in animal models, 233–235
Rheumatoid arthritis, mapping susceptibility to
characterization of, 241
conformational equivalence hypothesis, introduction to, 242–251
association with classic HLA specificities, 243–246
DR β chain gene, mapping, 254–256
DR1, relation, 256
ethnic differences in structure of MHC class II alleles, 251, 253–254
inferences, 256–259
organization of class II genes, 251, 252
structure of class II molecule, 246–251

Rheumatoid factors, human Vh gene for, 49–51
Rheumatoid synovial fluid, immunochemical studies, 41–42
Rubella virus, *see* Congenital rubella syndrome (CRS)

S

Serological markers and gene segments
  present in human monoclonal IgM autoantibodies, 34–35
  present in human monoclonal RF, 33–34
Short-term preparations of rat thyroid monolayer cells, 270
Signal transduction through IL-2R beta subunit, 222
SLE, *see* Systemic lupus erythematosus
Somatic mutation, 35–36
Specificities of anti-histone H1 autoantibodies, 162–167, *see also* Anti-histone H1 autoantibodies
Systemic lupus erythematosus (SLE), 51–52, 59, *see also*, Lupus anti-DNA antibodies, idiotypic expression
  VK locus in, 76–78
Systemic lupus erythematosus (SLE) and interspecies idiotypes on anti-Sm antibodies
  definition of, 155–156
  interspecies Id expression, 156–157

T

T-cell antigen receptor repertoire in autoimmune models, genomic and expressed
  conclusions on, 212–213
  expressed repertoire, 199–212
    genomic impositions on TCR V β gene expression, 202
    multiprobe TCR V β RNAse protection assay, 199–202
    origin of *lpr* and *gld* cells, 208–212
    tolerance- or negative selection-related TCR V β repertoire modification, 203–208
  gene diversity and T-cell maturation, 190–194
  germline TCR α and β genes, 194–199
    C α and C β genes, 195–196
    V α haplotype, 196–199
    V β haplotype, 196
  studies on, 189–190
T cell interaction with rat thyroid cells, 272–273
T-cell tolerance, experimental models
  autoreactive T cell clones, 184
  conclusions on, 185
  induction of to HGG, 176–177
  molecular mechanisms of T cell unresponsiveness, 183–184
  role of thymus in HGG-induced tolerance, 181–183
  tolerance in HGG-specific T cell clones, 183
  tolerance to HGG, 177–181
T cell vaccination, prevention of EAT by, 290, 291, *see also* Experimental autoimmune thyroiditis
TCR, *see* T-cell antigen receptor repertoire
Thymus, role of in HGG-induced tolerance, 181–183
Thyroid autoimmunity, in vitro model systems for study of
  MHC class I antigens, description, 265–267
  rat MHC gene region, 267
  rat thyroid cell lines, 267–268
  rat thyroid cell MHC class II antigens
    Fisher rat thyroid cell lines, 268–269
    short-term preparations of rat thyroid monolayer cells, 270
    Wistar rat thyroid cell line, 270
  rat thyroid MHC class II (RT1.D) transcripts, 270–272
  T cell interaction with rat thyroid cells, 272–273
  viral initiation of MHC class II antigen expression, 273–274
Thyroid lesions with cloned T-cells, transfer to, 183
Thyroiditis, *see* Experimental autoimmune thyroiditis
TNF α and *tax* protein of HTLV-1, 226–227
Tolerance- or negative selection-related TCR V beta repertoire modifications, 203–208
Type I diabetes, *see* Diabetes, autoimmune type I, virus as triggering

V

Vaccination, T cell, 290
V α haplotype, 196–199
V β haplotype, 196
V gene families in autoantibodies
  encoding antibodies, structural characteristics, 16–24
  expression of, 13–16
  utilization by murine B lymphocytes, 9–13
V-gene repertoires in normal mice, establishment
  during establishment of different b-cell compartments, 127
  selection of B-cell repertoires, 125–127
  summary on, 127
VH families
  frequency of among monoclonal autoantibodies with various specificities, 13, 14
  frequency of among 164 monoclonal antibodies obtained from various strains, 16, 17
VH gene for human rheumatoid factors, defining, 49–51
VH gene utilization and anti-DNA antibodies, preferential, 64–65
VH nucleotide sequences of anti-BrMRBC hybridomas, 94–95
VH and VL genes, genetic diversity, 61–64
Viral initiation of MHC class II antigen expression, 273–274
Viruses, as triggering factor of autoimmune type 1 diabetes, *see* Diabetes, autoimmune type 1, viruses as triggering
VK domains, encoded by vk9 gene, 96–97
VK families
  frequency of among monoclonal autoantibodies with various specificities, 13, 15
  frequency of among 168 monoclonal antibodies obtained from various strains, 16, 17
VK family gene utilization in autoantibody producing cells, 78–79
VK locus in human lupus, 76–78
V region similarities with AChR, 149–150

W

Wistar rat thyroid cell line, 270